THE NEW WAY FORWARD TO BETTER HEALTH

BALANCED DAYS

BALANCED LIVES

Eight Guiding Truths for Lifelong
Weight Control and Nutritional Balance

A **HEALTH REFLECTION**™ BOOK

by Prepak Products Inc

CREDITS

BUCHANANDESIGN

Design / Art Direction
buchanandesign.com

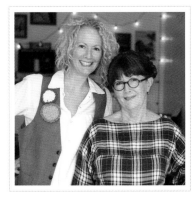

Bethany Jensen   **Tere Jensen**
Food Photography   *Food Stylist*

David Gouldthorp
Editing and Proofreading

Michael Ray
NutriMirror.com Software Development and Webmaster

Sheila Moore
Coordination of Contributor Graphics

Pam Ray
Coordination of Contributor Stories and Food Submissions

Susan Sanders
Sales

Judee Potter
Affirmations Research

Jim Ray
Dreamer

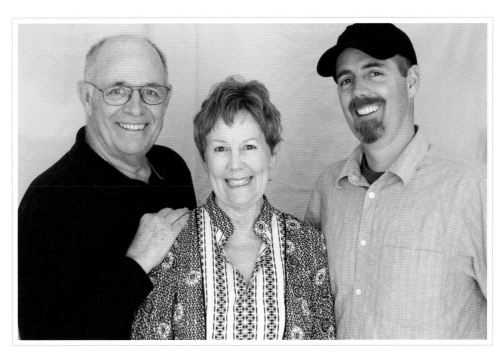

Jim Ray, Pam Ray, Michael Ray
Balanced Days, Balanced Lives *Creators and NutriMirror® Co-Founders*

PUBLISHED BY PrePak Products, Inc.
Oceanside, CA.

Library of Congress Control Number: 2009914237

ISBN: 978-1-936292-00-4

12 11 10 9 8 7 6 5 4 3 2 1
1st Edition, Fall 2010

Printed and bound in China

Acknowledgements

Judy Johnston has our deepest gratitude for allowing resources of her company, PrePak Products, Inc., to be used for the development of NutriMirror.com and this book. Her patient support and her faith in the soundness of our vision and mission gave us motivation to succeed and are most appreciated. She is also a co-founder of NutriMirror®.

Our thanks go to the PrePak Products Inc., family of employees who were some of the early testers of NutriMirror and who also did an admirable job in managing the logistics for publishing a work with the grand scope of *Balanced Days, Balanced Lives.* Thanks to Sheila Moore for coordinating the photographic and design elements of the book and for keeping all the office and support systems functioning smoothly; Susan Sanders for her able research, marketing, and sales help; and Carrie Gabel for so ably managing the accounting and record keeping functions. Thanks also go to Theresa Morales, Audon Ibanez, and DiAnna Lietzel.

David Gouldthorp generously contributed his time to proof and edit early drafts of *Balanced Days, Balanced Lives.* Thanks, David.

A special thanks goes to Therese Vannier for pitching in and being so helpful with copy development.

Monica Callan, RD, kept us straight on the nutritional science at the heart of the NutriMirror tool and this book. Thanks for your valuable consultation and friendship, Monica.

Thanks to our good friend Judee Potter for research of *Affirmations.*

Love and appreciation for early support and consistent cheerleading go to Tracy Reynolds and her husband Todd.

Hugs and thanks are sent to Tere and Bethany Jensen (a dynamic mother and daughter team) who took time out of their very busy schedules as owners of m•o•m (Encinitas, CA; www.42ndandorange.com) to cook, style, and photograph all the Green Day food submissions of contributors to *Balanced Days, Balanced Lives.* Tere expresses her gratitude to the friendly people at Seaside Market in Cardiff, CA. They believe in healthy living and helped make shopping there fun and easy.

We were impressed with the professionalism and talents of the Buchanan Design team that worked on the *Balanced Days, Balanced Lives* project. Especially, our gratitude goes to Bobby Buchanan and new father Ryan Skinner. (Ryan, the fact that you could help to change all those diapers and also happily meet every deadline is applauded.)

Our thanks and loving support go to the NutriMirror members who come to the Journal Room and are a part of our extended Internet family. As each of you know and have expressed, there is something very special happening there; we all feel it and embrace it.

And finally, we want to give a special hug and great respect to the forty-two members who have generously shared their stories and their Green Days in *Balanced Days, Balanced Lives.* We see you all as the pioneers of a new way forward that may, one day, lead to a reversal of the prevalent obesity and chronic disease trends in the nation.

Dedication

To our grandchildren Jake, Eden, and Savannah; and to Jilly and all the other children and grandchildren of the NutriMirror family. *Great happiness may be found through the loving and dedicated pursuit of worthy dreams.*

TABLE OF CONTENTS

INTRODUCTION

· ·

This book tells the stories of people just like you—people from all walks of life, from all around the country, who are taking action every day to live better, healthier lives.

While no two of us share the exact same set of challenges, we all face a brighter future since adopting the proven techniques that we'll share with you in these pages.

If you're looking to improve your own health—to regain your strength, increase your mobility, decrease your risk of disease or your dependence on medications, or simply to keep your weight in a healthy range—we think you'll love the results we've achieved—results that can be yours as well!

Welcome

There are things we all know: Regular exercise makes us stronger; A diet of wholesome, nutritious foods promotes a healthy body; We really shouldn't eat that entire bag of chips in one sitting.

In *Balanced Days, Balanced Lives,* we won't tell you any differently. We're not going to promise you any hidden magic that will instantly transform your life. We won't try to sell you a miracle.

What we will do is tell you our stories. We'll tell you who we are, what we're doing, and how we're changing and learning and growing—or shrinking!—every day. We'll share our successes and our failures, and we'll show you how you can apply what we've learned to your own life. We want you to benefit from what we've learned. We want you to win.

But who are we? We are adults just like you: mothers, fathers, brothers, sisters, sons, daughters, grandparents. We are young and old, we are healthy and active, we are recovering from illness or lifetimes of bad decisions.

More specifically, we are forty-two people—representative of thousands more—who have acted to take control of our own health through lifelong weight control and nutritional balance. We are real people overcoming the old habits, poor choices, and unfortunate circumstances that have held us back from our dreams for too long.

One thing we all have in common is membership in NutriMirror, a website (www.nutrimirror.com) that we use to monitor and analyze our daily food and exercise activities. But whether or not you decide to join us on the Internet, this book will serve as a valuable and inspirational resource for your own journey.

In these pages we'll share with you the basic yet fundamental changes that are leading us to remarkable transformations—not only in our weight loss and improved physical performance, but also in our rediscovery of newfound pleasures in the simple acts of day-to-day living. We'll share with you our *Eight Guiding Truths for Lifelong Weight Control and Nutritional Balance*. And you will see that a healthy weight does not have to mean deprivation, grueling workouts, and boring foods.

An Antidote to Decades of Falsehoods

By now we've all heard that the industrial world faces an epidemic of obesity and related problems, from high blood pressure to diabetes to heart disease. Our parents, our children, our friends and neighbors, everybody is affected. Whether it hits us personally, through someone we know and love, or indirectly through the rising costs of health care, we all suffer.

The solution is well known, and we hear it over and over again: *Don't eat more calories than we burn; balance our calories in versus our calories out.* But of course it's much more complicated than that when we're caught between the combined forces of powerful food and diet industries. One side tempts us endlessly with their latest double-fried chicken sandwich spectaculars, while the other generates an estimated $40 to $60 billion per year selling gimmicky, fingers-crossed promises of "easy" weight loss. These commercial diet interests exaggerate their claims, take our money, and six months later move on to the next big thing—always enticing us with dreams:

- The smoking hot body that could be ours in six easy payments.
- Pills, powders, meal replacements, serums, or miracle plants that put the responsibility for weight loss onto the product instead of our own efforts.
- Rapid weight loss, which is almost never maintainable because of severe calorie deprivation and/or boot camp style exercise regimens.
- Testimonials and amazing "before and after" photos which—when they're even authentic—imply that "after" is some permanent condition of the program, not just a fleeting moment in time.
- Eating plans and food delivery programs that offer sudden, 180-degree changes in lifestyle—but where does that leave us when our subscriptions end?

Unfortunately it's much easier to sell a miracle—or rather, a mirage—than to sell the difficult truth that the only guaranteed method for lifetime weight control does not come in a package.

But at NutriMirror and here in the pages of *Balanced Days, Balanced Lives,* we see ourselves as an antidote to the familiar falsehoods that the diet industry's commercial interests have promoted for decades—a New Way Forward, if you will. We don't expect to change the world that we all live in. But we hope to show you a way to change your own small place in it, for yourself and for those you love. For some it won't be easy, but the greatest rewards come from the greatest challenges.

Our methods and strategies have been gathered here in our *Eight Guiding Truths,* which you'll find later in these pages. It's no exaggeration to say that readers who live by these truths will achieve better health and will be successful at lifelong weight control.

Find Yourself in Our Personal Stories

In *Balanced Days, Balanced Lives* we'll show you what it's like to live by these principles. You'll learn of our setbacks and our triumphs, and you'll see the practical steps we take that keep us on the road to health.

Some of us have weight-related health issues while others are simply looking to feel better, to have more energy, or to avoid future problems. In these pages we open our life stories to you, sharing the circumstances that led us to seek self-improvement, and the choices we are making in pursuit of lasting health.

Our stories are but a small sample of the real life affirmations we hear daily from other NutriMirror members, who repeatedly tell us that something fresh and incredibly important is happening in their lives. We believe that these stories of transformation support a hopeful New Way Forward, one that will spur people in similar circumstances to take their own meaningful steps toward happiness through healthy, pleasurable living.

The Value of Self-Knowledge in Your Life

But what is healthy living? You've seen tables and charts and pyramids and you've heard about "calories in, calories out" and "five-a-day servings" and all those well-meaning but tough-to-implement diet tips and tricks. You walk into a grocery store and it seems that every label is shouting out "low fat," "non fat," "low carb," "no cholesterol," "no trans fat," "lite," or whatever else they can get away with.

Information and advice is everywhere and yet still we steadily add on the pounds, clog our arteries, raise our blood pressure, and take another step toward diabetes. How can so much knowledge help so little?

One thing we can all benefit from—and that we hope to share with you in the pages of *Balanced Days, Balanced Lives*—is a clear insight into the consequences of our own actions, past, present, and future. What we all need is a practical understanding of how our nutritional and physical activity choices stack up against our own personal needs as determined by sound, science-based standards. For example, how does this three-egg omelet affect my cholesterol? If I walk for half an hour each day, how much more can I eat? Are my food choices getting me enough iron?

These questions can be difficult without a calculator and reference tables. But if we make the effort to seek out the answers, we benefit enormously. This is the knowledge that prompts us to make better choices—the choices that can change our lives. This is also the knowledge that we've made easy to find through the tools freely available at NutriMirror, where the impacts of our decisions are reflected back to us as soon as—or even before—we make them.

The free NutriMirror system makes self-management of calorie and nutritional balance not only possible, but technically practical for daily, lifelong use.

Experience Forty-Two Balanced Days

Of course NutriMirror is just one tool that helps guide us to our goals. Whether we use that system or some other method of analysis, what ultimately matters are the practical steps we take. And so *Balanced Days, Balanced Lives* includes real life examples of people bringing their lives into calorie and nutritional balance.

In this book we will share our actual food and exercise choices with you—a total of forty-two unique, balanced days that we have lived. You'll see what we ate, how we exercised, and how it affected us—and how you could incorporate similar decisions into your own healthy lifestyle.

Balanced Days, Balanced Lives will show you that the pathway to health is not about magic pills or deprivation. With knowledge and work on your part, you will find that a healthy, balanced life is within your reach, and that the journey is filled with bounty and great pleasure.

Simple Truth and Free NutriMirror

Because we do not sell membership in NutriMirror—we give it away for free, all of it, unlimited and unconditionally—we have nothing to lose by being honest. So we'll tell you up front that, for some people, behavior change associated with successful weight control and nutritional balancing can be difficult to master. It is a never ending process. But it's not impossible, and once you get the hang of it ... wow! You'll be amazed by the joy it adds to your life.

We constantly remind members who want to give NutriMirror all the credit for their transformations that it is just a tool. Although it does exactly what it's supposed to do, every time, NutriMirror itself does not produce the result. Only each user can do that. So pat yourself on the back; all credit belongs to you.

As users of NutriMirror, there's one other thing we hear every day as we support and encourage one another, something that we all know is true and that we'd like to share with you now: *You can do it!*

The Eight Guiding Truths for Lifelong Weight Control and Nutritional Balance

1. Balancing calories and nutrition is a LIFELONG process; "After" does not exist.

2. The key to lifelong health is finding pleasure in the choices that bring us to balance.

3. A slow approach to weight loss and change is better than excessive calorie deprivation.

4. Eating snacks frequently, throughout the day, is a winning strategy!

5. Our nutritional needs are best met through wise food choices.

6. Physical activity is important for both health and effective weight control.

7. Perfection is a rocky road that leads to failure.

8. We cannot manage what we cannot measure.

BALANCED LIVES

The Eight Guiding Truths for Lifelong Weight Control and Nutritional Balance

The *Eight Guiding Truths* are essential to successful lifelong weight control and improved health. These truths are the antidote to the yo-yo world of diet churn and false promises, to decades of dietary guidance by a failing system.

1. Balancing calories and nutrition is a LIFELONG process; "After" does not exist.

Most commercial weight loss messages feature *Afters*—people living out their weight loss dreams. We feel their happiness; it is strong. We can't help but believe that their weight loss and their happiness are tied together and everlasting. We want to be an *After*. We want it bad and we want it now.

The merchants who want us to believe in *After* imply it is a permanent condition, a result of what they are selling. An entire lifetime in a Size One is inferred but, for understandable reasons, never explicitly guaranteed in the ads. Deep in our hearts and in our minds we may even know that this *After* messaging is a myth. Yet they keep hyping it and we keep buying it. Our desire is so strong that we are content to let truth pass us by.

Sadly, very few people—perhaps as few as five percent—who meet their dream weight to become an *After* are ever successful at maintaining that weight loss for the long term. Dietitians and other health professionals on the front lines of the obesity struggle know that our national problem is not weight loss. Most people who diet can lose weight successfully; the problem lies in developing *lifelong adherence* to behaviors that produce calorie balance and nutritional balance.

We see this disconnect between dream and reality everyday. Many people, perhaps even most of us, begin by thinking that when we meet our ultimate weight goal we are finished. We think the struggle, the roller coaster of emotions, and the deprivation, are finally over. "I have done the job I came here to do. I am an *After*. Today, I begin living the happier life I have imagined and longed for all this time."

And, of course, these feelings are reinforced by the reactions we receive from others. We are no longer invisible to the world. People begin to see us differently and are quick to praise. "You look fantastic. You should be so proud of what you've accomplished. Aren't you glad the struggle is over? No more eating foods that taste like cardboard. Now you can get back to living *normally*." But before too much time passes, we are no longer the *After* we had dreamed about. We become what we were, overweight and unhappy. During that entire period of weight loss struggle we learned little that was sustainable. And the results are as we see them: *We are a yo-yo nation, a nation in peril!*

When we are focused solely on losing weight, our journey is far different from when we seek new habits that can be sustained lifelong. *After*-seekers dream about life after the prize; the process itself is something to be despised, a thing to be tolerated only for a time. And the time of deprivation is always too long. Every weigh-in becomes a life and death matter. If we lose lots of weight we are euphoric; however if we stay even or lose less than expected, we become frustrated. And any weight gain brings on such unbearable stress that it can mark the end of the journey. It doesn't even matter that the weight gain may not have been real; it was just what the scale said at the moment. Eight hours later or earlier, that same scale might have brought cheers and smiles. "Life is too short for this," we rationalize. Many of us just quit the process and return to our old, unhealthy ways. We grab our remotes and get back to the comfortable, easy habits that make us fatter, sicker, and unhappier.

Alternatively, there are those of us who are guided by a more evolved truth: Successful weight control and nutritional balancing is a lifelong process. We see that instead of being part of the churn, success requires a lifelong commitment to learning about and being open to healthy foods and behaviors. As a result, our attitudes and actions during the weight loss phase are more relaxed, more productive, and more likely to yield better—and lasting—results.

When we take the long-term perspective, we are more likely to find pleasure in the process than those with only a drive to lose weight to become an *After*. And as explained in the following truth, finding pleasure in the process that brings us to balance is the behavioral key to lifetime health.

2. The key to lifelong health is finding pleasure in the choices that bring us to balance.

Contrary to what many "dieters" believe, our biggest challenge is not losing weight. Most of us who try to lose weight can, and do—over and over again. Instead, our most important mission is to consistently find pleasure in the choices that move us to *balance*. Only when we find pleasure in balancing our calories and meeting our nutritional needs does it become likely that we will maintain healthy habits for a *lifetime*.

To know if you, or anyone, will be successful in meeting or maintaining a *lifelong* standard, it may only be necessary to answer this simple question: *Do I consistently find pleasure in the choices that move me to balance?* If yes, the chances for long-term success are excellent; if *no*, there is still work to do.

Choose Your Pleasure

There are two kinds of pleasure to consider and choose. There are the easy pleasures that we not only like, but have made the staples of our diet—the choices that make us fat, sick, and unhappy. Then there are natural pleasures that satisfy our need for balance. We call these pleasures *natural* because our bodies are naturally inclined to find satisfaction in foods that sustain life, that make us healthy. But we've been driven by convenience, marketing, and the human impulses for ease and instant gratification to prefer the readily available "fake foods" loaded with fats, sodium, refined sugars, and nutritionally empty calories.

Most all of us have confronted this classic tension over what is *liked* and what is *healthy* at one time or another. And unfortunatley, the instant gratification choices usually win. We find the proof of that in more than 60% of the people we see today, in the prevalent national trend of rising obesity and chronic disease.

Resolving this *pleasure tension* is not easy for everyone. The vast majority of us repeatedly fail to maintain weight loss for any length of time. A key reason for failure is that we enter the challenge of weight loss seemingly bent on making it about deprivation of all our *likes*. We see the process as *all or nothing*; everything we were eating was bad for us, so the impulse is to make instant 180-degree change. All the foods we liked that got us in trouble are suddenly totally off limits. This all-or-nothing mindset is a pathway that repeatedly carries fellow weight-losing travelers back to where we began—overweight.

Balancing Pleasures Between the Foods You *Like* and the Foods You *Need*

Balance isn't just about controlling calories and nutrients; it is also about balancing pleasure. We must not deny ourselves the pleasure we take from food, because that is a guaranteed route to failure. Instead, we have to find a way to take pleasure in *all* of our dietary choices. That means moderating—but not necessarily eliminating—the convenient *likes* that have gotten us into trouble; and even more importantly, it means developing new *likes* for the neglected foods and activities that our bodies are *naturally inclined* to crave.

Yes, that means we do need to eat our fruits, vegetables, and whole grains. But we don't have to force down broccoli if we don't like broccoli! Instead, we need to find pleasure in the exploration of these healthy foods. We must take pleasure in the process of discovery, of preparation, of unexpected tastes and flavors that we miss when our senses are dulled by highly processed meals overladen with sodium and sugar.

We know that sounds like a lot of work, especially for those of us who are disasters in the kitchen, who can't tell a sauce pan from a steamer rack. But this is critically important: *If we can learn to love the process of healthy living, if we actually enjoy the way we live, we will succeed.*

Again, it's all about balance. We don't have to take hours out of every day planning and prepping our food. In moderation, we can keep our old *likes*, our convenient favorites, but we must not rely on them as a crutch at every meal. You'll learn in the Balanced Days section later in this book how easy—and how appealing—it can be. We'll show you real world examples of how we're incorporating wonderful, pleasurable new tastes into our own lifestyles. We're filling ourselves up with healthy, nutritious foods that we love to eat—and you can, too!

Finding pleasure in the choices that move us to balance—not simply losing weight—is our higher priority.

3. A slow approach to weight loss is better than excessive calorie deprivation.

It's only natural: when given the choice between "quick and easy" or "difficult and delayed," the quick and easy option wins every time. That's why we can't open a magazine or turn on the television without being bombarded by claims of "fast weight loss" or "amazing diet secrets."

The commercial diet industry earns billions of dollars every year pushing the idea that we can reach our goals quickly and with minimal effort—just eat this magic cookie, this trademarked meal replacement, this proprietary packaged food; take this wonder pill or serum; use this patented exercise device. In combination with a brief period of steep calorie deprivation, the body we dream about will be ours in short order.

And guess what? We *can* lose weight quickly. It's not that hard to do, and our initial successes are seductive. But there's a catch, and it's a catch that the miracle merchants are taking to the bank. We might look better after losing those first pounds, and we might feel better for a while, too, but rapid weight loss does nothing to address the problems that have caused us to gain weight in the first place. Those first pounds that come off so easily are often just water weight, while our bodies continue to carry the underlying fat stores that are the source of our troubles. And after two weeks or a month or two, after we've reached our goal and gone back to our regular lifestyle, the weight invariably comes back—often with a few extra pounds added for good measure. And when that happens, well, there's always another round of diet pills or potions ready to pick our pockets.

When we try to do it all at once, when we rush the process and starve ourselves for quick results as we are so often encouraged to do, the inconveniences and potential dangers can pile up. Among the possibilities: dehydration, headaches, irritability, fatigue, dizziness, hair loss, muscle loss, gallstones, malnutrition, and potential eating disorders. Where's the fun in that? It's no wonder so many of us give up before we reach our goals.

One of those points in particular—reduction in lean muscle mass—is important to note because it also results in a decrease in our metabolism. This occurs whether we lose weight quickly or slowly, but the ill effects are more likely to affect crash dieters because of what happens afterwards, when we return to our "normal" way of living. We start up again eating the same old foods, but because our bodies now burn fewer calories than they used to, those foods have an even greater impact than they once did. The bottom line is we now gain more weight more easily.

Slow Change Trains Our Bodies and Our Minds

And so there are two major reasons that we encourage slow, gradual weight loss:

1. To let our bodies naturally adjust to changes in diet and exercise.
2. To teach ourselves how to live these changes as a pleasurable lifestyle, rather than some temporary period of torment.

It's a common, wise recommendation that we hear repeatedly from knowledgeable professionals, including doctors and nutritionists. While some individuals who are extremely overweight or obese may benefit from losing weight more quickly in the beginning—and under the supervision of their physician—in general the thinking is that we should not try to lose weight at a rate greater than one to two pounds per week. Another way to look at it (as suggested by the National Institutes of Health) is to set an initial weight goal of no more than ten percent of our body weight over a six-month period. So, for example, a 250-pound person can set a goal of 25 pounds in six months—which works out to an average of just under one pound per week.

To add one more layer of math to the puzzle, there's an additional guideline that helps to reinforce this slow-change recommendation: women should try to keep their minimum calorie intake level at 1,200 per day, while men should try for at least 1,500. Below these levels, it can be quite difficult to get adequate nutrition—vitamins, minerals, fiber—from the foods you eat.

Here's an example of how this works in practice. Say you are a 5´5˝ woman, thirty years old and 150 pounds, with a sedentary lifestyle. Your estimated daily calories burned is 1,600. So if you eat the recommended 1,200 calories per day, that gives you a daily deficit of 400 calories. We'll spare you the calculations, but that works out to an estimated weight loss of 0.8 pounds per week—a healthy, sustainable rate. It's not super-fast, but it's steady, it's maintainable in the long term, and it allows you enough calories during the day—if you choose them wisely—to actually enjoy the foods you're eating.

And as we mentioned in Truth #2, that's critical if you want to maintain your new weight—and your health—for a lifetime.

4. Eating snacks frequently, throughout the day, is a winning strategy!

Any meal plan designed by a nutritionist will include small, frequent meals. The benefits of frequent eating are amply documented by scientific studies of metabolism, digestion, and dietary energy needs.

Although many contributors to *Balanced Days, Balanced Lives* may be in sync with the science of metabolism, most of us live the *frequent eating* truth simply because we have found it to be a winning strategy for pursuing better health through balancing. When readers look at the Green Days of the contributors later in these pages, they see that we usually enjoy many eating events throughout the day. Some of us speak to this frequent eating strategy in our My Green Day summaries; particularly it is seen in our snack selection comments.

Not only does frequent eating fuel our bodies in a way that keeps our metabolism working efficiently, it also controls those troublesome hunger spikes that come with missing meals or too much elapsed time between eating events. For example, by eating a healthy breakfast and always having nutrient-dense snacks at hand, it becomes much easier for us to say *no* to the workplace donuts, candies, and other troublesome goodies that provide lots of calories but little nutritional value. Instead of hunger impulsively steering us to convenient fast-food restaurants, we just reach into our pre-planned snack packs and pass by the temptation.

Also, when we snack frequently, we rarely sit down to any of our main meals in a ravenous state, which makes it much easier for us to control our portion sizes. At restaurants, where portion sizing has gone crazy, it is second nature now to many of us to ask for the go-container at the beginning of the meal, packing up half of what was served for another meal.

Another advantage that flows from controlling our portions and not eating out of hunger is that when there is less in front of us on a plate, the tendency may be to slow things down. We take smaller bites, chew our food more completely, and allow more time for digestion. By being more conscious of the foods we eat—mindful eating, we call it—we increase the sensual pleasures of the experience by giving greater attention to the smells, textures, and flavors within our meals. And by slowing things down we become more aware of the people in our company. We place a higher value on conversation when we are not primarily focused on the animal act of feeding.

Many of us in this book now begin each day by pre-planning and preparing nutrient-dense snacks to eat between our main meals. Pre-planning gives us measured nutrition and calorie roadmaps for the day that make the process of balancing much easier.

Here is the process many of us follow for managing our calories (*snack* calories in particular):

- First, we divide our daily calorie allotment roughly into four equal parts. For example, if we have 2,000 calories to eat for the day we divide by four and are left with an average of 500 calories to be allocated between our four daily eating events: *breakfast, lunch, dinner,* and *snacks*.

- Next, we select as many calorie friendly, nutritionally dense snacks (and low calorie treats) as possible for our *snack* group. For a representative sample of an actual day refer to page 283. There we see seven snacks totaling 438 calories that, by themselves, satisfy most of the daily nutritional requirements.

Enjoying frequent, nutrient-dense snacks not only adds pleasure to our day, but is also a key for lifelong success.

5. Our nutritional needs are best met through wise food choices.

We're all familiar with the standard Nutrition Facts label that we find on most packaged foods—the one that tells us how many calories and how much saturated fat are in a serving, and what percentage we're getting of our daily recommendations for such key vitamins and minerals as A, C, calcium, and iron. We might even be regular readers of these labels, taking care to avoid foods that are high in sodium or cholesterol, or choosing the ones that put more fiber into our diets. It's great information to have, and it's wonderful when we consistently use it to make wise, healthy choices.

Of course the Nutrition Facts label is just one small piece of the effort to keep us informed, and without additional guidance we can't really expect it to change our lives. For one thing, reading every label and figuring out our totals for the day requires a lot of math. And for another, the labels have been simplified for ease of use—our actual nutritional requirements could vary quite a bit from these generic guidelines.

And so the USDA and other government agencies have made additional tools available, the most prominent among these being the Food Pyramid. We're all familiar with this, although the guidelines are revised periodically and may not be what we remember from childhood. Here are highlights from the 2005 recommendations:

- **Grains**: Any food made from wheat, rice, oats, cornmeal, barley, or another cereal grain is a grain product. Bread, pasta, oatmeal, breakfast cereals, tortillas, and grits are examples of grain products. Grains are divided into two subgroups: whole grains and refined grains. RECOMMENDATIONS: *Eat at least three ounces of whole grain bread, rice, cereal, pasta, or crackers every day. At least half our daily grains should be whole.*

- **Vegetables**: Any vegetable or 100% vegetable juice counts as a member of the vegetable group. RECOMMENDATIONS: *Eat a wide variety of vegetables from each of the following categories: dark green vegetables (broccoli, spinach, etc.); orange vegetables (carrots, sweet potatoes, etc.); dry beans and peas (black beans, garbanzo beans, etc.); starchy vegetables (corn, potatoes, etc.); and "other" vegetables (artichokes, beats, cauliflower, etc.).*

- **Fruits**: Any fruit or 100% fruit juice counts as part of the fruit group. RECOMMENDATIONS: *Eat a wide variety of fruit. Remember that whole fruits supply fiber that is not available from juice..*

- **Oils**: Oils are fats that are liquid at room temperature, like the vegetable oils used in cooking. Oils come from many different plants and from fish. RECOMMENDATIONS: *Make most of your fat sources from fish, nuts, and vegetable oils. Limit solid fats like butter, stick margarine, shortening, and lard.*

- **Milk**: All fluid milk products and many foods made from milk are considered part of this food group. Foods made from milk that retain their calcium content are part of the group, while foods made from milk that have little to no calcium, such as cream cheese, cream, and butter, are not RECOMMENDATIONS: *Go low-fat or fat-free. If you don't or can't consume milk, choose lactose-free products or other calcium sources.*

- **Meat & Beans**: All foods made from meat, poultry, fish, dry beans or peas, eggs, nuts, and seeds are considered part of this group. Dry beans and peas are part of this group as well as the vegetable group. RECOMMENDATIONS: *Choose low-fat or lean meats and poultry. Bake, broil, or grill your selections. Vary your choices with more fish, beans, peas, nuts, and seeds.*

As with the Nutrition Facts label, the Food Pyramid provides general guidance that can most easily be applied to anyone's diet, rather than specific recommendations for each individual's needs. However, if we're able to incorporate all these recommendations into our daily choices, that's great.

The other thing to consider, of course, is our total calorie intake. This varies greatly depending on our individual circumstances and activity levels, and whether we're actively working to control our weight. Individual calorie needs might vary from 1,200 per day to as much as 3,000 per day or more.

The trick is to get all our nutritional needs into our diet while staying within our calorie needs—and keeping things like saturated fat, sodium, and cholesterol at reasonably low levels.

Depending on our calorie needs, the challenges we face can be quite different. Someone on a 1,200-calorie daily diet may find it hard to get enough calcium or iron within that limit; someone on a 3,000-calorie diet may have a hard time eating that many calories without going over on their sodium.

But the bottom line is, whatever our individual unique nutritional needs might be, we need to come as close as possible to meeting them through the real, whole foods we eat, rather than making high calorie, nutrient-deficient choices, and then making up our shortcomings through dietary supplements.

Supplements can be important tools in helping make up for deficiencies in our diet, but it's always best to get as much of our nutrition as possible from the foods we eat. For one thing, supplements can be expensive. For another, when our nutrition comes from whole foods rather than pills, then the vitamins, minerals, and antioxidants are often more "biologically available"—they are more easily taken in and used by our bodies than if they arrive in supplement form.

Taking it one step further, the process of choosing, selecting, and preparing our own whole foods provides a world of benefits over the cheap and easy diet of fast-food choices and quick supplements. When we actively work to choose a wide variety of foods that are rich in nutrients, we quickly discover that we are actually able to eat *more* than we otherwise would. Cravings for unhealthy foods disappear, along with hunger pangs. Energy levels rise along with overall satisfaction and the actual *enjoyment* of what we're eating.

6. Physical activity is important for both health and effective weight control.

When we read contributors' stories in *Balanced Days, Balanced Lives*, we learn that balancing calories is achievable at just about any level of physical activity. Some of us manage our weight goals through a commitment to regular, intense exercise. Others get there with sporadic, less strenuous physical activity by placing greater limits on the calories we eat. While most struggle at times with the motivation to remain physically active, we come to recognize that regular physical activity is a highly enjoyable part of a healthier lifestyle. The more active we are, the easier the process of balancing calories and nutrients becomes. And, of course, improved health and physical activity go hand-in-hand.

Every day in our NutriMirror community, we hear of the amazing benefits that come to our members who have decided to get off the couch to make even slight increases in physical activity. One such story is of a Chicago area woman who weighed close to four hundred pounds and had never met her next door neighbor because she didn't like going outside and was "unable to walk the distance to get next door." Today, she not only knows her neighbor well, she knows everyone all the way around a couple of her long neighborhood blocks. She reports amazing improvement in all facets of her life: health, self-esteem, and attitude. She was one who thought she "hated" exercise only to learn the opposite was true. We see similar stories day after day about the amazing emotional and physical benefits that exercise brings to people at all fitness levels and ages.

When we change our sedentary lifestyles and become more physically active, we promote health, psychological well-being, and a healthy body weight. The following recommendations for physical activity are taken from the *Dietary Guidelines for Americans*, published by the U.S. Department of Health and Human Services and the U.S. Department of Agriculture:

- To reduce the risk of chronic disease in adulthood, engage in at least thirty minutes of moderate-intensity physical activity most days of the week.
- For most people, greater health benefits can be obtained by engaging in physical activity of more vigorous intensity or longer duration.
- To help manage body weight and prevent gradual unhealthy body weight in adulthood, engage in approximately sixty minutes of moderate to vigorous intensity activity on most days of the week.

- To sustain weight loss in adulthood, participate in at least sixty to ninety minutes of daily moderate-intensity physical activity while not exceeding caloric intake requirements. Some people may need to consult with a healthcare provider before participating in this level of activity.
- Achieve physical fitness by including cardiovascular conditioning, stretching exercises for flexibility, and resistance exercises or calisthenics for muscle strength and endurance.

And here are key recommendations for specific adult population groups:

- **Pregnant women**. In the absence of medical or obstetric complications, incorporate thirty minutes or more of moderate-intensity physical activity on most, if not all, days of the week. Avoid activities with a high risk of falling or abdominal trauma.
- **Breastfeeding Women**. Be aware that neither acute nor regular exercise adversely affects the mother's ability to successfully breastfeed.
- **Older Adults**. Participate in regular physical activity to reduce functional declines associated with aging and to achieve the other benefits of physical activity identified for all adults.

Calorie Balancing For Weight Control Is A Lifelong Pursuit. Exercise Accordingly.

We see many beginners to the process who mistakenly revert to memories of a time when they were in training for athletics or the military and feel this is the only path to follow. Of course, because boot camp levels of exercise are not sustainable to a lifelong standard, this mindset typically results in failure. We need to remember that once our ideal weight has been realized, maintaining that healthy weight becomes a lifelong journey. Therefore, it is important that the type of physical activity we choose be sustainable for the long haul. Most of us would do well to note that good health and successful weight control do not require over-the-top efforts, nor do they include the words "boot camp."

To make physical activity sustainable, we must experience pleasure in the choices we make. Therefore, we look for activities that we enjoy enough to make part of a lifelong pattern of living. We start with small steps, slowly building up the time and intensity levels as we go. And we try to take advantage of common sense approaches to add physical activity whenever possible: we take the stairs instead of the escalator; park the car at far end of the parking lot; enjoy our pets and children more by increasing our physical activity with them; perform seated calisthenics while watching television; and we regularly perform simple stretching and strengthening exercises to improve our functional fitness levels.

7. Perfection is a rocky road that leads to failure.

Too many of us set unrealistic goals and subjectively apply standards of perfection to judge results of the actions we take. We expect that we must have the perfect body, quickly, make perfect food choices that always result in balance, and achieve perfect compliance with the exercise routines we set for ourselves.

Instead of setting a goal to slowly increase our physical activity based on our current capabilities, all too often we develop a mindset that leads us to do something unrealistic. We may resolve to immediately start a *boot camp* exercise regimen, completely ignoring that until yesterday, our lifestyle was totally sedentary. Typically the first couple of times we skip our self-imposed *boot camp*, we think, "I'm a failure; this is impossible; I can't do it." We retreat back to the couch, fall into a supine position, and quit exercising altogether.

Even though experts using science-based approaches to eating wisely may have told us we need only to "moderate" or "refine" our choices of calorie-rich, nutritionally empty foods, what we hear is "whatever you do, never again eat the foods you like so much that have gotten you into this mess." All too often we lock in mistaken mindsets that insist the journey must be about deprivation. We act as though we must be punished for those past transgressions that were centered on our easy and convenient choices for instant gratification. Then, when we inevitably eat ice cream and cake at a child's birthday party, or impulsively eat the food we now believe doesn't fit our new, "healthy" lifestyle goal, our perfectionist mindset tells us we are, once again, "complete and total failures."

When these same experts tell us to lose weight at a slow rate of about one pound a week—not more than ten percent of our body weight in six months—and not to eat fewer than 1,200 calories each day (1,500 for men), our desiring minds—and complicit weight loss merchants seeking our money—insist on a different strategy.

We severely restrict our calories to well below the minimum we require to function properly, insisting that we *instantly* lose the weight we've gained after years of self abuse.

Likewise, after we've been into the process of change for a period of time and look in the mirror and see flaws instead of the ideal of our dreams, or we step on a scale and don't see the results we expected, we judge ourselves harshly and often just throw in the towel.

Almost all of us feel the demands of busy lives. Additionally, many of us have unresolved emotional issues we deal with. We allow these to get in the way of healthy eating, physical activity, or just the times of quiet reflection we need to restore and care for ourselves. Compounding already difficult life issues are perfectionist mindsets that demand we need to "do it all and do it all perfectly." We have primed our feelings for failure. We bring unwarranted tensions into the difficult process of change and let them overwhelm and defeat us.

Contributors to *Balanced Days, Balanced Lives* are not immune from the pressures of living that can threaten the best of intentions. Some of us still struggle with the temptations for too much of the old foods and living patterns that are part of the human impulses for ease, convenience, and instant gratification. However, we know that despite any setbacks, when we apply the *Eight Guiding Truths* to our lives we will be successful. We find them to be antidotes to all the self-destructive, perfectionist thinking and behavior that would otherwise defeat our efforts.

And we have learned that what we do on any given day is not so important. We can have days where we impulsively eat more than we should. Instead of perfect days, we focus more on keeping our long-term balance trends in check.

Knowing we don't need to beat ourselves up over every poor choice has been a liberating discovery for many of us. It has made it so much easier for us to strategically incorporate "pleasure foods" from the past into our lifestyles, making the journey more sustainable for the long haul.

The path may not always be straight and we sometimes fall. But we own our behaviors and we control the bodies we have been given.

8. We cannot manage what we cannot measure.

Conditions of obesity and chronic disease are largely matters of behavior—the consequences of eating unwisely and moving too little. And since no one else can do our eating or moving for us, we must each accept our own personal responsibility for the behavior changes that can improve our health. However, many who are willing and able to make these changes still find that success remains elusive. The trouble is that when it comes to the choices involved in healthy living, we often don't instinctively know how much—or how little—we need: How big is a serving? Am I getting enough fiber? How many calories in a slice of pie? How far should I run, how fast, how often?

Fortunately, the information we need is available—thanks to many years of research by scientists dedicated to the study of human physiology, health, nutrition, and related fields. The details can be complicated and they aren't always easy to incorporate into our daily lives, but the information is there for anyone who seeks it out. Much of what we need to know can be grouped into two basic categories: calorie balance and nutritional balance.

- **Calorie Balance** This is the difference between the calories our bodies burn—due to exercise, daily activities, and our basic metabolic needs—and the calories we take in through the foods we eat. If we take in more calories than we burn, we gain weight; if we burn more calories than we take in, we lose weight.

- **Nutritional Balance** This refers to the vitamins, minerals, and macronutrients (carbs, protein, fat) that we need for a wide variety of both basic and complex bodily functions. Certain nutrients need constant replenishing; others can be dangerous at higher levels. Some are critical to daily living; others we can manage without for longer periods of time. But ideally, a proper diet will supply us with the nutrition we need without giving us too much of the things that can be unhealthy.

And that brings us to the core of this Eighth Truth: in order to successfully balance our calories and our nutritional needs, we must not only know what our calorie and nutritional needs are, but we must be able to successfully measure our progress toward meeting them.

Finding Our Targets

Finding general estimates of what we need is relatively easy, thanks to an abundance of science-based guidance from the federal government. At the most basic, the Food Pyramid is one place to start. We could do a lot worse than to follow the simple recommendations of eating appropriate servings of fruits, vegetables, and whole grains each day.

Of course, every person is different and our true nutritional needs vary based upon our age, sex, height, weight, activity level, and other factors. To find these more specific recommendations, we could refer to the Dietary Reference Intake (DRI) tables available from the USDA. Here's an example of the DRI table for Vitamin C:

DIETARY REFERENCE INTAKES FOR VITAMIN C
*Recommended Intakes for Individuals**

Age	Male	Female	Pregnant	Lactating
1-3 yrs.	15 mg	15 mg		
4-8	25 mg	25 mg		
9-13	45 mg	45 mg		
14-18	75 mg	65 mg	80 mg	115 mg
19-30	90 mg	75 mg	85 mg	120 mg
31-50	90 mg	75 mg	85 mg	120 mg
51-70	90 mg	75 mg		
70+	90 mg	75 mg		

Note that the Daily Value number for Vitamin C that we find on the Nutrition Facts labels of the foods we buy is based on 60 mg … so if we were to rely on that number alone, we could easily be shorting ourselves compared with the more specific DRI numbers.

These Recommended Dietary Allowances are set to meet the needs of almost all (97 to 98 percent) individuals in the groups listed.

As for our daily calorie needs, once again, every person is different. A number of formulas are available to calculate our resting metabolic rates, which must then be adjusted again based on our usual daily activity levels, then adjusted again to take into account digestive processes for the foods we eat, and adjusted once more when we exercise. The easiest method of figuring these numbers is to use any of the many online calculators available, such as at Mayoclinic.com or our own Nutrimirror.com.

Measuring Our Performance

Once we know what we need to do—the calorie and nutrition standards that we need to reach—we need to find a way to actually do it. And the closest thing to a true guarantee that anyone has come up with in the world of weight loss is that we should keep a food journal. Approval for this idea is near universal, with multiple studies showing that people who keep food journals are much more successful at losing weight and keeping it off than people who don't.

When we keep a food journal we know where our calories are coming from. We are better able to formulate plans to help us succeed. And we more easily motivate ourselves simply through the act of recording our actions.

A food journal can be as basic as writing our meals in a paper notebook, although that can get complicated if we manually calculate each day's exercise, or if we try to expand the analysis of our diet into areas beyond just calories. But even the simple act of writing our foods on paper gives us an advantage over our friends who fly blind into their diets, without any measured guidance to check their choices.

A Better Option

Computers and the Internet hold the promise to make so many things easier for us, and taking control of our food choices is no exception. A wealth of online tools and websites exist today that not only help us to keep track of our food and exercise, but take it far beyond what's possible when we're scratching out our own calculations on paper.

A good online food journal should do the math and measuring for us, instantly and easily, and would let us know exactly where we stand in relation to our own calorie and nutrition needs. When using a good online food journal, we can spend just a few minutes a day making note of our exercise and dietary choices, and the system should instantly show us the impact of these choices—personalized, measured feedback that makes it easier for us to manage a healthy lifestyle.

Acting in Our Own Best Interests

When our goal is to take control of our lifestyles and set ourselves on the road to health, the potential rewards are enormous. But always remember that we are ultimately the only ones responsible for our own choices. No one else can make them for us. If we are truly dedicated to this mission, then we had best make these choices wisely.

And so whichever route we choose—a paper journal or a computerized system— always remember that we will be better lifelong managers of our body weight and our health when we consciously control our measured calorie and nutritional needs. Without the ability to measure our performance against standards that define success, we cannot effectively manage the process of improvement.

If you cannot measure it, you cannot control it.
If you cannot control it, you cannot manage it.
If you cannot manage it, you cannot improve it.

The Health Reflection™ Nutrition Facts Report

The people you meet in the following Balanced Days section of this book all utilize the free NutriMirror food log. Each of us relies upon the information we get from our personalized Health Reflection™ Nutrition Facts Report, which helps provide the measured feedback we need to successfully control and manage the exercise and dietary choices we make every day.

After we log our daily food and exercise choices, this color-coded report instantly scores the impacts of our actions, telling us whether or not we have achieved calorie balance and nutritional balance. When our numbers are green, we've done well and have achieved balance. When we see the color red we know there is room for improvement.

Although the format may look like the familiar Nutrition Facts Label we see on packaged foods, it is different and far more detailed.

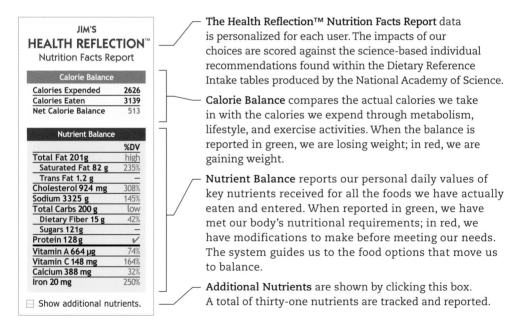

The Health Reflection™ Nutrition Facts Report data is personalized for each user. The impacts of our choices are scored against the science-based individual recommendations found within the Dietary Reference Intake tables produced by the National Academy of Science.

Calorie Balance compares the actual calories we take in with the calories we expend through metabolism, lifestyle, and exercise activities. When the balance is reported in green, we are losing weight; in red, we are gaining weight.

Nutrient Balance reports our personal daily values of key nutrients received for all the foods we have actually eaten and entered. When reported in green, we have met our body's nutritional requirements; in red, we have modifications to make before meeting our needs. The system guides us to the food options that move us to balance.

Additional Nutrients are shown by clicking this box. A total of thirty-one nutrients are tracked and reported.

NOTE: *While most Daily Value numbers (%DV) reported in the Health Reflection™ Nutrition Facts Label are based on Dietary Reference Intake standards specific to each user's needs, you'll note that total fat, carbohydrates, and protein show either a green check mark or a red "high" or "low." This indicates whether or not the percentage of calories from each of these sources falls within the following recommended ranges: 45–65% for carbohydrates; 20–35% for total fat; and 10–35% for protein.*

The recommendation for saturated fat is based on 10% of total calories; the recommendation for fiber is based on 14 g for every 1,000 calories eaten. Both of these recommendations follow the Dietary Guidelines for Americans 2005.

BALANCED DAYS

Whatever the life circumstances and health goals of the forty-two people you'll meet in the following pages, each has a common purpose and pursuit: balanced calories and balanced nutrition. Along with regular exercise, these are the two universal and key behavioral requisites for effective weight control and optimal health.

As contributors to *Balanced Days, Balanced Lives,* we have another thing in common. We all use the free NutriMirror.com website to help us track, monitor, and score the impacts of our food and exercise choices against our own unique, personal requirements for successful calorie and nutritional balance. After logging our choices at NutriMirror, the site gives us instant feedback in the form of personalized Health Reflection™ reports. Healthy, balanced choices are shown in the color green, while imbalances appear in red.

It is from these color-coded reports that a language naturally developed among users of the site, who began talking about "green days" and "living green"—shorthand for healthy, balanced choices.

As you'll see, *Live Green* has become a mantra by which many NutriMirror users now strive to live.

In our stories you may hear us speak glowingly about how we have been helped by the NutriMirror tool, but keep in mind that logging our food and exercise through the Internet is a personal choice. We recognize that not everyone will choose to do that, nor do they need to. But we do believe that everyone can benefit greatly by understanding our *Eight Guiding Truths* and by seeing the practical examples in the following Green Days.

At the very least, you will learn that weight control and good health are not achieved through deprivation. In fact, you will soon see that both bounty and great joy are possible—and essential—in balanced lives.

> **NOTICE**
> For the convience of readers, the nutritional facts for all recipes on the following pages are in the NutriMirror.com database.

"I'VE LEARNED TO LOVE THE FOODS THAT LOVE ME BACK"

username: Lmatava / *first name:* Lynn / *location:* Eastern Shore, MD

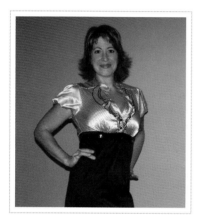

Lynn NOW: September '09 / age: 34
131 lbs. / BMI 22.3 / waist 28˝

"If Mom ran McDonald's, they'd serve sprouts on the burgers and prune juice instead of sodas," my sister and I would joke at our mother's expense. We came from a family that liked food and loved to eat. From my father's Southern roots, we learned to feast on slippery white flour dumplings, buttered lima beans, fried chicken, and sweet potato biscuits. It was all good, home-style cooking and even the vegetables were seasoned with precision and salty, cured hunks of pork fat.

My mother would send us girls to school with what seemed like the healthiest lunches in the cafeteria. We always had an apple, grapes, or carrot sticks, pretzels, a sandwich, and real fruit juice to drink. We never had the individually wrapped brownies, cupcakes, or fruit roll-ups that our friends had. Still, I managed to find plenty of places to sneak in the junk. By the time I was thirteen I was pronounced overweight. My pediatrician put me on a 1,200-calorie diet but gave little nutritional direction. I believe this is where the yo-yo dieting unofficially began.

By the time I was in high school, I began to play sports, took up running, and spent the next several years not even thinking twice about how much I weighed or what I put into my mouth. My physical activity counter-balanced the food I consumed and I remained at a healthy weight from the time I was sixteen until I turned twenty. As I progressed through college, I found plenty of non-active ways to spend my time. Beer-pong was the only athletic event that I participated in.

I met my future-husband, Joe, and when we got our own place we began entertaining often. I worked in an Italian-American restaurant and the food was so delicious that I often mimicked the 3,500-calorie dishes at home. I was consuming far more than my 5´4˝ frame needed. When I was twenty-seven years old, I weighed 213 pounds. I had officially hit my highest weight. I was altogether unhealthy and visibly unhappy. I also was

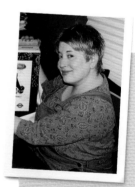

Lynn THEN: March '01
213 lbs. / BMI 36.4 / waist 44˝

suffering from hypoglycemia and my consumption habits did a number on both my physical and emotional well-being.

I was fortunate that my mother's love of unique foods and her try-anything-once attitude was still with me somewhere. My husband hunts and fishes. Early on, I had a sense that the meat he was bringing home was, in many ways, superior to what we'd been purchasing, but I did not know why. I also knew that I needed to lose a considerable amount of weight. I didn't know how.

I began yo-yo dieting. I tried cabbage soup and, apart from the side effect bar-tricks, had minimal success. The gelatin diet was a great one and I had all the sugar-free wiggly stuff I could stomach for three days. I tried the three-day diet, some paid programs, and even a medication with an embarrassing orange side effect.

Fad dieting and desperation had managed to help me shed about thirty pounds just in time to discover I was pregnant. The good news was that it was going to be impossible to consume anywhere near the amount of calories I had drunk in beer each day. When my beautiful baby girl was born, I was delighted to find out that I'd only gained about ten pounds during my pregnancy.

Having my first daughter was the official turning point in terms of my health. Wanting to change was not enough. I needed a catalyst. I had this beautiful little life in my arms and I did not want to be too unhealthy to care for her. I wanted to be able to run around and play with her. I needed to be a good example.

I made a lot of changes over the next year. I took up walking during my lunch and coffee breaks at work and usually went for another walk when I returned home. With a baby on my chest, and two large dogs on their leashes, by the time my daughter was eighteen months old I weighed 147 pounds. I kept it off for an entire month, then found out I was pregnant with our second daughter.

Because I ate so much during my first pregnancy, I really didn't pay attention to what I was eating during my second. When I gave birth, I learned that I had gained forty pounds. Even worse, I was unable to stick to any diet plans that would help me lose weight. I was desperate and would go days on end eating only a handful of almonds. I somehow convinced myself that this would sustain me.

I felt out of balance. Deep within myself, I knew I could change, but didn't know how. I had this deep love of natural foods and ancient grains like quinoa. I loved dark leafy vegetables like kale and collard greens. Not the salty, fatty greens of my youth but the garlic and olive oil sautéed ones. My husband's love of outdoor recreation provided my family with natural and low-fat protein sources. I realized it was all there in front of me. It all started to come together.

NutriMirror was the missing ingredient. I now have the tool that lets me measure the impacts of all my food choices. I am guided to a healthy nutritional balance. NutriMirror allows me to monitor the right amount of nutrients to fuel my body and mind. I am finally in control. Fresh, whole ingredients are the things that drive me now.

I weigh 131 pounds and know that, with maintenance ahead, I have only begun my journey. It has taken me a long time to learn that good health is not about deprivation or starvation. I love food and have a lot less guilt than before. I've learned to love the foods that love me back.

MY PHYSICAL ACTIVITY

Like most things in my life, exercise can quickly become monotonous and tiresome. If I eat too much of the same thing, I want to binge eat. If I do the same exercise again and again, I want to sleep in.

I joined a gym for several reasons, the most compelling being that they offer free daycare. With two young children, exercise quickly became something that I did only at six o'clock in the morning (no thank you) or avoided altogether. I enjoyed running but, again, it grew uninteresting really fast.

My gym possesses a host of equipment that I would not otherwise have access to. They also employ friendly and informative professionals who offer valuable tips and advice. Hiring a personal trainer really helped me learn about body mechanics and it further established the nutritional goals I've been working on at NutriMirror. Five to six days per week I do a ten-minute warm up on one of the many cardio/aerobic machines and then move on to a combination of free weights with core and balance exercises. This routine usually takes no more than an hour. In addition, I attend hour-long yoga classes three times per week and try to get in at least one good run. When I begin to lack motivation or feel the need for change, I attend a class or two, learn some new tricks and get my butt kicked by a drill instructor.

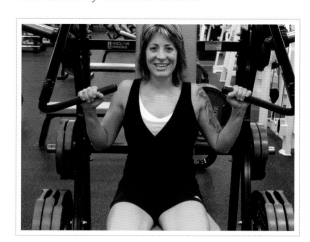

LYNN'S *GREEN* DAY 1

- Calories Expended: **2,550**
- Calories Eaten: **1,509**
- Net Calorie Balance: 1041

The NutriMirror tool has trained me in lifestyle balance. This particular day I happened to spend a lot of time at the gym. On average, I would say that my *calories expended* fall in the 1,500—1,700 calorie range. If I am hungry, I eat every calorie that I have earned. If I am not, I don't.

Eating is an unavoidable activity. You can't just say, "I overeat so I'll avoid food altogether." I like to think of it like the ebb and flow of the tide. I may not have eaten all of my calories today, but tomorrow I may just wish to eat a serving of real ice cream. I will eat it, too, and enjoy every guilt-free bite.

LYNN'S NUTRITION FACTS, GREEN DAY 1

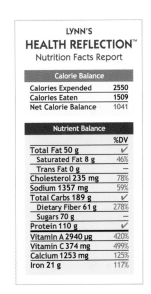

LYNN'S
HEALTH REFLECTION™
Nutrition Facts Report

Calorie Balance	
Calories Expended	2550
Calories Eaten	1509
Net Calorie Balance	1041

Nutrient Balance		
		%DV
Total Fat 50 g		✔
Saturated Fat 8 g		46%
Trans Fat 0 g		—
Cholesterol 235 mg		78%
Sodium 1357 mg		59%
Total Carbs 189 g		✔
Dietary Fiber 61 g		278%
Sugars 70 g		—
Protein 110 g		✔
Vitamin A 2940 µg		420%
Vitamin C 374 mg		499%
Calcium 1253 mg		125%
Iron 21 g		117%

MY BREAKFAST—196 calories

My first food log entry on NutriMirror was a real eye opener for me. I keyed in a vegetarian sausage breakfast sandwich that weighed in at 1,018 calories. Since I really enjoy eating the yolk, I make myself an over-easy egg and scoop out half of the yolk. The rich avocado, smeared on toast, more than makes up for the cheese I once loaded on. I enjoy this sandwich both for breakfast and lunch. Don't worry about the waste of the yolk; it is shared with two very appreciative pooches.

OPEN-FACED EGG SANDWICH (HALF YOLK) ON
EZEKIEL BREAD WITH AVOCADO
- 1 egg white, 17 calories
- 1/2 egg yolk, 27 calories
- 1.5 oz. avocado, 68 calories
- 12 oz. coffee, 4 calories
- 1 piece Ezekiel sprouted grain bread, 80 calories

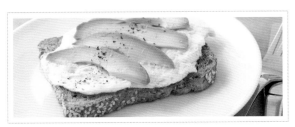

MY LUNCH–356 calories

In playing the "Get to Green (balance)" game, I quickly learned that spinach is a go-to food for pushing my logs into the green. I try to eat vegetarian at lunch each day and tofu is a protein source that I occasionally throw into the mix. Balsamic vinegar is one of those items I grab when dishes need some pizzazz because it is rich and full of flavor but low in calories and sodium. Kamut is one of the several ancient grains that you would find at our dinner table during the course of the week. The addition of lemon juice and zest turn this side dish into a great leftover lunch salad that is nutty and flavorful right out of the icebox.

SALAD WITH LEMON-Y KAMUT
- 1 serving Lemon-y Kamut (see recipe), 228 calories
- 1/2 tsp. garlic, 2 calories
- 1/2 cup firm tofu, 88 calories
- 1 tbsp. balsamic vinegar, 10 calories
- 1 1/2 oz. tomatoes, 14 calories
- 2 cups spinach, 14 calories

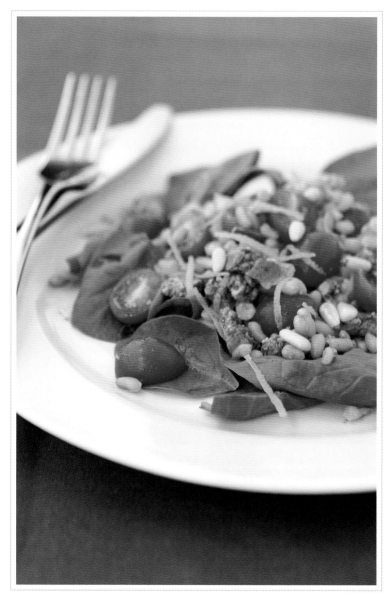

LEMON-Y KAMUT WITH PINE NUTS

Makes four and a half servings of three ounces each.

INGREDIENTS

1/3 tsp. kosher salt
1 cup Kamut grain, uncooked
1 tbsp. lemon juice
2 tbsp. extra virgin olive oil
1 tbsp. lemon zest
2 tbsp. parmesan cheese, freshly grated
1/3 tsp. grated nutmeg
1/2 tsp. black pepper
1/4 tsp. red pepper flakes
1 tbsp. pine nuts

PREPARATION

1. Add salt to three cups water and bring to a boil. Add Kamut grain and simmer, covered, for ninety minutes.

2. Drain Kamut grain and allow to cool.

3. In a large mixing bowl, whisk together lemon juice, olive oil, and lemon zest.

4. Add parmesan cheese, nutmeg, black pepper, and red pepper to the olive oil/lemon mixture.

5. Toast pine nuts in a skillet on medium-high heat, stirring constantly for about a minute or until slightly brown and fragrant.

6. Combine all Kamut, pine nuts, and previously mixed ingredients, and toss together.

7. Refrigerate for several hours. If made one day in advance, the flavors really have a chance to meld.

MY SNACKS—604 calories

It almost seems odd to me to be discussing my day in terms of three meals and a snack or two. Many days, rather than eating scheduled meals, I eat all day long—one mini meal or snack after another. Fresh fruit, Greek yogurt sweetened with agave nector, and chia seeds are in my snack repertoire almost every day.

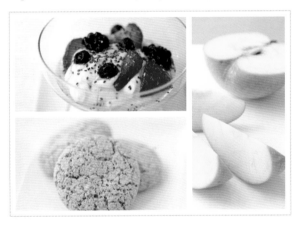

LOTS OF FOOD
- 1 apple, 55 calories
- 3/4 cup blackberries, 46 calories
- 1/3 cup strawberries, 19 calories
- 2 oz. sweet red peppers, 15 calories
- 2 oz. sweet yellow peppers, 15 calories
- 1/2 tsp. honey, 11 calories
- Protein supplement, 100 calories
- 3/4 tsp. raw agave nectar, 15 calories
- 1/4 cup blueberries, 23 calories
- 1 1/2 tbsp. chia seeds, 76 calories
- 18 amarettini cookies, 97 calories
- 1/3 cup Greek yogurt, reduced fat, 49 calories
- 2 tsp. chia bran, 83 calories

MY DINNER—353 calories

Venison is served in our home three nights per week. In days gone by, I may have topped it with béarnaise sauce or a Merlot-reduction butter. Today's preparation might involve a little olive oil with fresh pepper, thyme, and crushed garlic. Roasted root veggies is one of my all-time favorite cold weather comfort dishes. It is delicious and pretty enough for Thanksgiving dinner, yet humble, and perfect for a weeknight meal. Since the beets always come with greens attached, I sauté them, too. I am the only one in my house interested in eating them, which is okay, because I usually only have enough greens for one serving. If I am ever asked what I'd like for my last meal, this is it

VENISON WITH ROASTED ROOT VEGGIES AND
SAUTÉED BEET GREENS
- 3.5 oz. venison, 149 calories
- 1/4 tsp. black pepper, 1 calorie
- Dash salt, 0 calories
- 1 serving sautéed beet greens (see recipe), 53 calories
- 3/4 cup roasted root veggies (see recipe), 150 calories

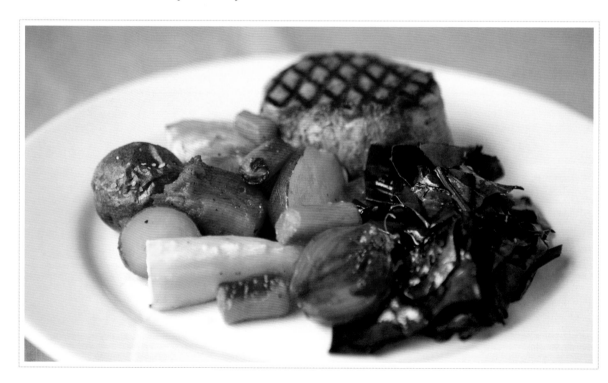

ROASTED ROOT VEGGIES

Makes approximately eighteen 3/4-cup servings.

INGREDIENTS

3 beets, fresh, peeled
3 large carrots, peeled
10 cloves garlic, fresh, roughly chopped
3 parsnip, peeled
5 small red potatoes, unpeeled
1 large rutabaga, peeled
2 large sweet potatoes, unpeeled
2 turnips, peeled
4 shallots, chopped
1 large celery root, peeled
1 large red onion
3/4 cup balsamic vinegar
1/4 cup olive oil, extra virgin
Salt and freshly cracked pepper, to taste
Optional: 1 bouquet garni (I used 1 sprig each fresh rosemary, parsley, oregano, and thyme)

PREPARATION

1. Peel all root vegetables except the sweet potatoes and red skin potatoes.
2. Chop all veggies into 1 1/2″ to 2″ chunks
3. In a large roasting pan, drizzle all roots with olive oil and toss liberally until well coated.
4. Add balsamic vinegar and toss until coated.
5. If desired, toss in bouquet garni of fresh herbs, salt and pepper.
6. Roast in 400°F oven for 1 hour and 15 minutes, stirring every 15 minutes. Watching carefully after one hour to prevent burning.
7. When veggies have carmelized, they are finished.
8. If desired, garnish with long, thin lengthwise strips of left-over beet greens.

TIP: I cut the veggies with gloves on so the beets do not stain my hands. This also makes tossing the roots in olive oil and vinegar much easier. You may also wish to cover cutting board with plastic wrap to keep from staining it with the beets.

SAUTÉED BEET GREENS

Makes one serving.

INGREDIENTS

4 oz. green leafy tops of beets
2 cloves garlic, smashed
1/3 tsp. extra virgin olive oil
Pot of boiling water

PREPARATION

1. Roll beet greens inside of each other so the stem runs from one end to the other.
2. Using a sharp knife, make 1/4″ slices in the greens so that once unrolled, they make long strips.
3. Blanch by cooking in a pot of water for 15–20 seconds.
4. Immediately dry on clean kitchen towel.
5. In a skillet on medium-high heat, add olive oil and garlic, and sauté for about thirty seconds before adding beet greens.
6. Cook, stirring occasionally for about two minutes.
7. Serve immediately.

LYNN'S NUTRITION FACTS, GREEN DAY 2

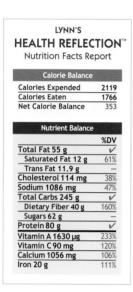

LYNN'S
HEALTH REFLECTION™
Nutrition Facts Report

Calorie Balance	
Calories Expended	2119
Calories Eaten	1766
Net Calorie Balance	353

Nutrient Balance	
	%DV
Total Fat 55 g	✔
Saturated Fat 12 g	61%
Trans Fat 11.9 g	—
Cholesterol 114 mg	38%
Sodium 1086 mg	47%
Total Carbs 245 g	✔
Dietary Fiber 40 g	160%
Sugars 62 g	—
Protein 80 g	✔
Vitamin A 1630 µg	233%
Vitamin C 90 mg	120%
Calcium 1056 mg	106%
Iron 20 g	111%

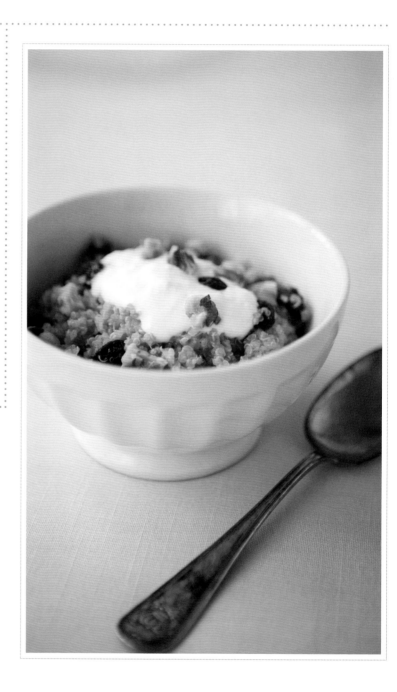

MY BREAKFAST
—384 Calories

HOT QUINOA BREAKFAST
- 1/2 cup milk, reduced fat, 68 calories
- 1 tsp. ground cinnamon, 6 calories
- 1/2 tsp. vanilla extract, 6 calories
- 1/2 oz. seedless raisins, 43 calories
- 1/4 oz. walnuts, 46 calories
- 1/2 tbsp. blackstrap molasses, 24 calories
- 1/4 oz. quinoa (uncooked weight), 159 calories
- 3 tbsp. Greek yogurt, nonfat, 22 calories
- 1/2 tsp. raw agave nectar, 10 calories

MY SNACKS–516 Calories

- 2 tbsp. parmesan cheese, shredded, 42 calories
- 6 cups popcorn, air-popped, 183 calories
- 1 apple, 59 calories
- 8 oz. Almond Breeze, non-dairy, 60 calories
- 2/3 cup ice cream, 172 calories

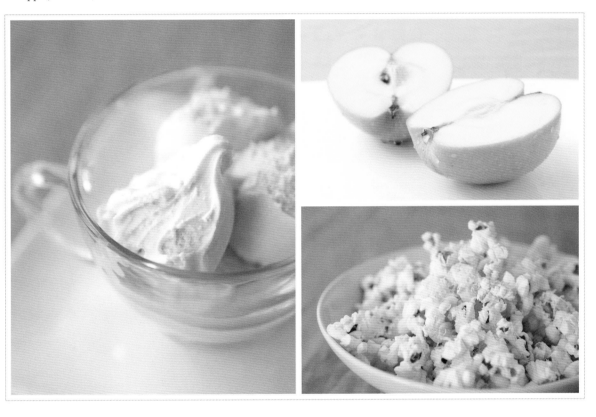

MY LUNCH–400 Calories

SANDWICH

- 1 1/2 tbsp. sunflower seed butter, 138 calories
- 2 pieces Ezekiel sprouted grain bread, 160 calories
- 1 tsp. chia bran, 42 calories
- 1 tbsp. SuperFood spread, 30 calories
- 3 oz. carrots, 30 calories

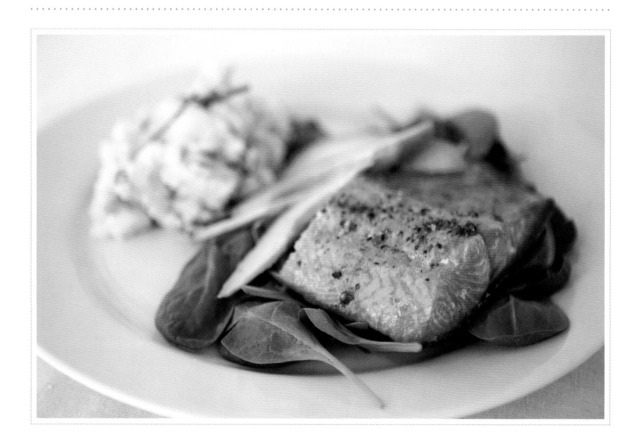

MY DINNER—466 Calories

WARM SALMON SALAD
- 4 oz. salmon, 130 calories
- 1/2 tsp. chili powder, 4 calories
- 1/2 tsp. cumin seed, 4 calories
- 1/2 tsp. paprika, 3 calories
- 1/4 tsp. black pepper, 1 calorie
- 1 1/2 oz. avocado, 68 calories

- 1/2 tsp. fresh garlic, 2 calories
- 1/2 tbsp. extra virgin olive oil, 60 calories
- 1/8 tbsp. cayenne pepper, 2 calories
- 1 1/2 cups spinach, 10 calories

SMASHED CREAMY POTATOES WITH CHIVES AND YOGURT
- 3 tsp. fresh chives, 1 calorie
- 6 oz. red potatoes, baked with skin, 151 calories
- 1/4 cup Greek yogurt, nonfat, 30 calories

I have a great breakfast recipe for any leftovers. You might even want to make extra to set aside for the morning. Trust me, it's worth it!

LYNN'S NUTRITION FACTS, GREEN DAY 3

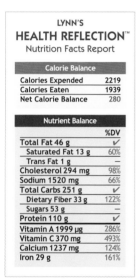

LYNN'S
HEALTH REFLECTION™
Nutrition Facts Report

Calorie Balance	
Calories Expended	2219
Calories Eaten	1939
Net Calorie Balance	280

Nutrient Balance	
	%DV
Total Fat 46 g	✔
Saturated Fat 13 g	60%
Trans Fat 1 g	—
Cholesterol 294 mg	98%
Sodium 1520 mg	66%
Total Carbs 251 g	✔
Dietary Fiber 33 g	122%
Sugars 53 g	—
Protein 110 g	✔
Vitamin A 1999 µg	286%
Vitamin C 370 mg	493%
Calcium 1237 mg	124%
Iron 29 g	161%

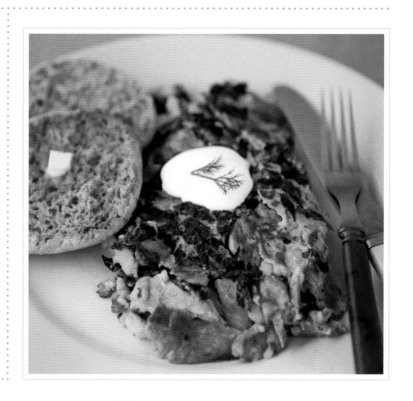

MY BREAKFAST—373 Calories

- 1/2 tsp. salted butter, 17 calories
- 1 egg white, 17 calories
- 1/4 tsp. black pepper, 1 calories
- 5 sprigs dill weed, 0 calories
- 1 cup fresh kale, 34 calories
- 4 oz. red potatoes, baked with skin, 101 calories
- 1 tbsp. fresh shallots, 7 calories
- 2 tbsp. Greek yogurt, nonfat, 15 calories
- 1 tsp. extra virgin olive oil, 40 calories
- 1/2 English muffin, spelt, 60 calories
- 2 1/2 oz. salmon, 81 calories

SALMON HASH

Cook kale in water until soft, then drain. Combine with some of the leftover salmon and smashed creamy potatoes that were set aside from the evening before. Add in 1 tbsp. shallots (or onions would work) and black pepper. Heat olive oil in a small round (omelet) pan. Press mixture into pan. Heat until browned. Using spatula, fold mixture in half like an omelet and slide onto plate. Top with a dollop of greek yogurt and dill.

MY SNACKS—678 Calories

GINGERSNAPS WITH MILK. PRE-DINNER APPETIZER OF
GRILLED CLAMS AND TWO GLASSES RED WINE.

- 1 1/2 cups milk, nonfat, 129 calories
- 1 1/2 cooked clams, 63 calories
- 1 apple, 55 calories
- 1/3 cup vanilla ice cream, light, 83 calories
- 6 oz. red wine, 152 calories
- 4 ginger snaps, 120 calories
- 3/4 oz. honey almond & flax whole grain crunch cereal,
  76 calories

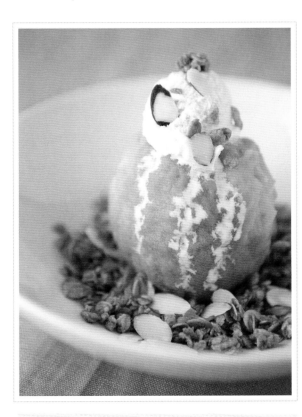

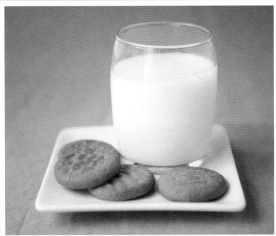

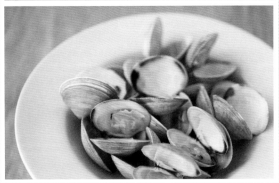

BAKED APPLE WITH ICE CREAM AND GRANOLA

Peel and core apple, sprinkle with turbinado
sugar and cinnamon mixture.

Wrap in foil and cook on grill (or in oven) until
soft. Top with 1/3 cup light vanilla ice cream and
sprinkle with Honey Almond & Flax, 9 Whole
Grain Crunch Cereal (Trader Joe's).

MY LUNCH—364 Calories

- 1/2 oz. queso añejo (Mexican cheese), 53 calories
- 1 oz. avocado, 45 calories
- 2 oz. sweet red peppers, 15 calories
- 2 tbsp. sweet white corn, cut from cob, cooked, 17 calories
- 2 oz. sweet yellow peppers, 15 calories
- 1/2 cup black beans, cooked without salt, 114 calories
- 1 tbsp. fire roasted vegetable salsa, 5 calories
- 1 tortilla (organic sprouted whole grain), 100 calories

BEAN WRAP

Smash precooked beans with salsa and stir in corn. Fill mixture into whole grain tortilla and top with crumbled cheese and avocado. Serve with raw red and yellow pepper "sticks."

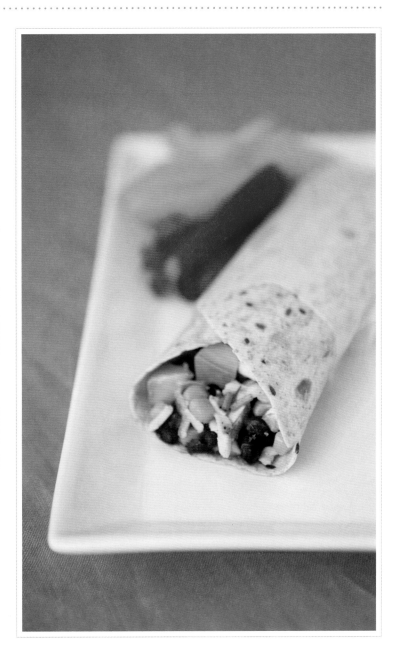

MY DINNER–524 Calories

• 1 serving shrimp and butternut squash with whole spelt noodles, 524 calories

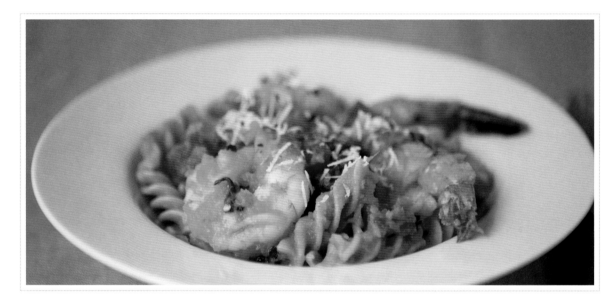

PASTA WITH SHRIMP AND BUTTERNUT SQUASH

INGREDIENTS

2 oz. whole spelt noodles
3 oz. raw shrimp
4 oz. butternut squash
1 tsp. fresh ginger root
1 clove garlic
1 tsp. extra virgin olive oil
1/2 cup fresh spinach
3 tbsp. grated fresh parmesan
1/8 tsp. ground nutmeg
1/4 cup tomato sauce
1/4 tsp. red pepper

PREPARATION

1. Boil pasta. When it is almost cooked, throw in shrimp for two minutes. Drain and set aside.

2. While pasta is cooking, sauté butternut squash, ginger, and garlic in olive oil, adding water as necessary to keep from sticking. When it begins to soften, add spinach and cook until creamy. Stir in 2 tbsp. parmesan and the grated nutmeg.

3. Return to pasta and shrimp to heat. Add tomato sauce. Add squash and spinach mixture. Serve topped with crushed red pepper and the remaining tablespoon parmesan cheese.

LYNN'S NUTRITION FACTS, GREEN DAY 4

LYNN'S
HEALTH REFLECTION™
Nutrition Facts Report

Calorie Balance	
Calories Expended	2443
Calories Eaten	1904
Net Calorie Balance	539

Nutrient Balance	
	%DV
Total Fat 46 g	✔
Saturated Fat 15 g	71%
Trans Fat 0 g	—
Cholesterol 86 mg	29%
Sodium 1370 mg	60%
Total Carbs 297 g	✔
Dietary Fiber 49 g	213%
Sugars 90 g	—
Protein 100 g	✔
Vitamin A 3483 µg	498%
Vitamin C 123 mg	164%
Calcium 1277 mg	128%
Iron 28 g	156%

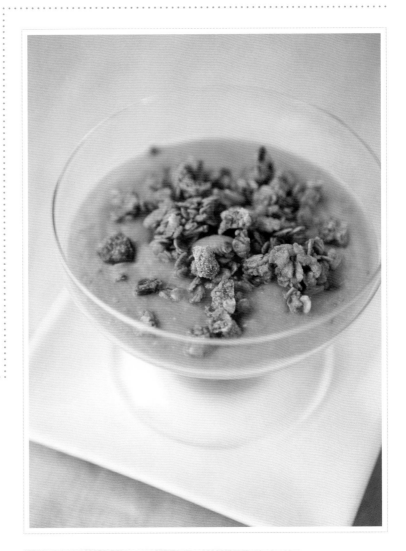

MY BREAKFAST
—335 Calories

- 1/2 tsp. ground cinnamon, 3 calories
- 1 tbsp. maple syrup, 52 calories
- 1/2 cup Greek yogurt, nonfat, 60 calories
- 1/2 oz. fruit & nut granola, 57 calories
- 1 tbsp. chia seeds, 51 calories
- 1 tbsp. white chia seeds, 30 calories
- 2 tbsp. chopped dates, 55 calories
- 1/3 cup canned pumpkin, 26 calories

PUMPKIN "MOUSSE"

Combine 1/2 cup yogurt, 1/3 cup canned pumpkin, 1/2 tsp. ground cinnamon, 1 tbsp. maple syrup, and 1 tbsp. chia seeds. Stir until smooth. Top with granola and dates.

MY LUNCH—581 Calories

- Lentils with chickpeas (see recipe), 318 calories
- Quinoa (see recipe), 263 calories

LENTILS WITH CHICKPEAS

INGREDIENTS
1/4 cup chopped onions
1 tsp. fresh garlic
1/2 tsp. extra virgin olive oil
1/4 cup uncooked lentils
1 tsp. turmeric
1 tsp. cumin
1 tsp. curry powder
1 tsp. fresh grated ginger
1/2 cup canned tomatoes
1/4 cup canned chickpeas

PREPARATION
Boil lentils with turmeric, cumin, curry powder, grated ginger, and canned tomatoes. Sauté onions and garlic in olive oil, then add the onion mixture to the lentils. Continue cooking until the lentils are soft and most liquid has been absorbed, adding water as necessary. Stir in chickpeas in the last five minutes to heat and soften slightly.

QUINOA

INGREDIENTS
1 oz. carrot
2 tbsp. chopped onion
1/2 tsp. extra virgin olive oil
1/4 cup quinoa
1/2 cup chicken stock
1 oz. watercress

PREPARATION
Sauté carrot and onion in olive oil. Add quinoa and cook until toasted. Add 1/2 cup chicken stock, then continue adding water as needed and cook until germ around the grain is beginning to peel off (about 10 minutes).

Serve alongside lentils and chickpeas, topping lentils with chopped, fresh watercress.

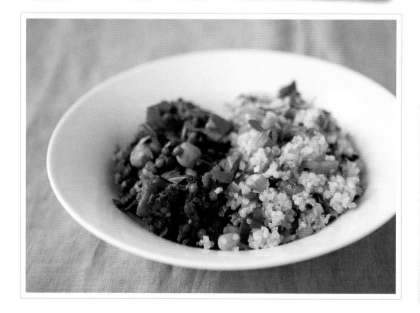

MY SNACKS—535 Calories

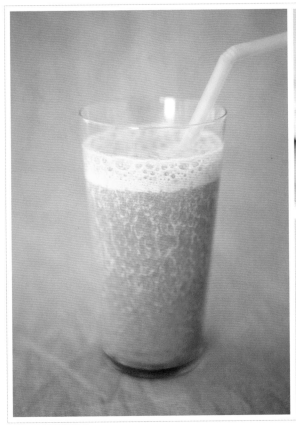

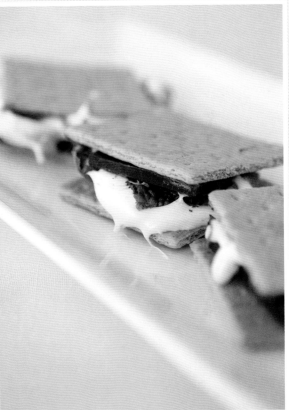

- 1 cup milk, nonfat, 86 calories
- 1/2 tsp. fresh ginger root, 1 calorie
- 1 tbsp. blackstrap molasses, 47 calories
- Designer whey protein supplement, 100 calories

- 4 oat bran graham crackers, 80 calories
- 1/2 bar dark chocolate with hazelnut toffee, 110 calories
- 2 marshmallows, 46 calories
- 5 oz. orange, 65 calories

PROTEIN SHAKE

Great after a strenuous workout. Tastes like liquid gingerbread.

Blend milk, molasses, ginger, and protein supplement. Sprinkle with cinnamon.

MY DINNER—453 Calories

- 5 leaves fresh basil, 1 calorie
- 1/3 cup tomato sauce, no salt added, 30 calories
- 2 servings homemade pizza dough, 302 calories
- 1 1/2 oz. fresh mozzarella cheese, 120 calories

GRILLED PIZZA

Dough is grilled on one side, flipped over, then topped with sauce, fresh basil, and fresh mozzarella cheese.

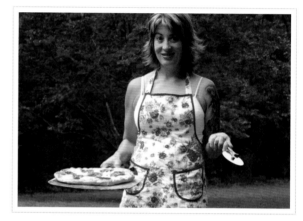

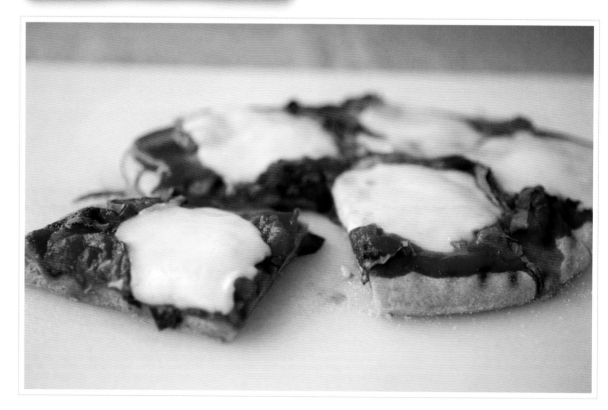

LYNN'S NUTRITION FACTS, GREEN DAY 5

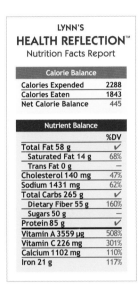

LYNN'S
HEALTH REFLECTION™
Nutrition Facts Report

Calorie Balance	
Calories Expended	2288
Calories Eaten	1843
Net Calorie Balance	445

Nutrient Balance	
	%DV
Total Fat 58 g	✔
Saturated Fat 14 g	68%
Trans Fat 0 g	—
Cholesterol 140 mg	47%
Sodium 1431 mg	62%
Total Carbs 265 g	✔
Dietary Fiber 55 g	160%
Sugars 50 g	—
Protein 85 g	✔
Vitamin A 3559 µg	508%
Vitamin C 226 mg	301%
Calcium 1102 mg	110%
Iron 21 g	117%

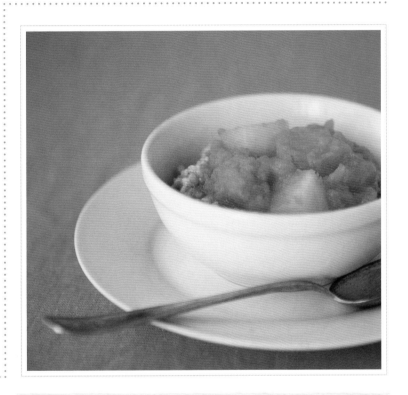

MY BREAKFAST
—374 Calories

- 2 tbsp. Greek yogurt, nonfat, 15 calories
- 1/3 raw agave nectar, 6 calories
- 1 cup steel cut oats, 200 calories
- 1 serving apples & butternut squash (see recipe), 153 calories

APPLES & BUTTERNUT SQUASH

INGREDIENTS
1 tbsp. butter, salted
1 tsp. ground cinnamon
8 oz. apples, without skin, fresh cubed
24 oz. butternut squash, fresh cubed
2 tbsp. maple syrup
3 tbsp. turbinado raw cane sugar

PREPARATION
Cook all ingredients (I use a dutch oven) atop the stove until apples are soft and squash has the look & texture of caramel. Serve over steel cut oats.

Note: Apples, squash, and oats may be cooked the night before.

MY LUNCH–364 Calories

- 2 1/2 cup baby spinach and spring mix, 10 calories
- 1 cup baby arugula, 15 calories
- 1 cup whole wheat couscous salad, 339 calories

WHOLE WHEAT COUSCOUS SALAD
Makes eight 1-cup servings.

INGREDIENTS

1/3 cup parmesan cheese, fresh grated
1/4 lemon, peeled
Zest from 1/8 of lemon
2 oz. pomegranates
1 tbsp. fresh garlic

1/4 cup red wine
1 oz. pine nuts, toasted atop
stove for 2–3 minutes
3 tbsp. extra virgin olive oil
1 cup peas

4 tsp. sunflower seed butter
2 cups whole wheat couscous
1 cup wild rice

PREPARATION

Cook couscous & wild rice according to packages, then combine. While hot, stir in sunflower seed butter. Make a dressing out of olive oil, red wine, lemon juice, lemon peel, and garlic. Toss into grains. Add Parmesan, lemon zest, pomegranate seeds, toasted pine nuts, and frozen peas. Allow to chill before serving atop a bed of greens.

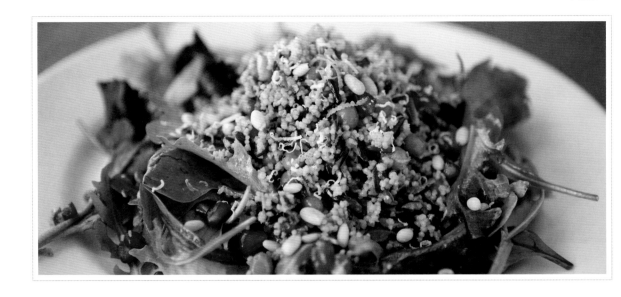

MY SNACKS
—605 Calories

- 1/8 cup pepitas, 80 calories
- 1/4 cup organic refried beans with green chilies, 66 calories
- 1/2 oz. queso asadero, 50 calories

MANGO CRAB SALSA
The following measurements are for a single serving. Multiply for more. Combine and chill before serving.
- 1/4 tsp. black pepper, 1 calorie
- 1/4 tsp. pepper sauce, 0 calories
- 1 oz. kiwi, 17 calories
- 1/2 tsp. lemon peel, 0 calories
- 1/4 tsp. lime juice, 2 calories
- 2 oz. mango, 38 calories
- 1/4 tbsp. fresh cilantro
- 1 oz. cucumber, peeled, 3 calories
- 2 oz. ripe tomatoes, 10 calories
- 1 oz. sweet red peppers, 7 calories
- 1/4 jalapeño, 2 calories
- 1 tbsp. red onion, 4 calories
- 3.5 oz. blue crab, cooked, 101 calories

May be served with chips (optional).

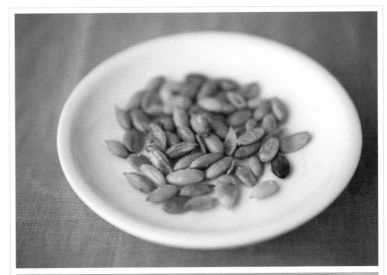

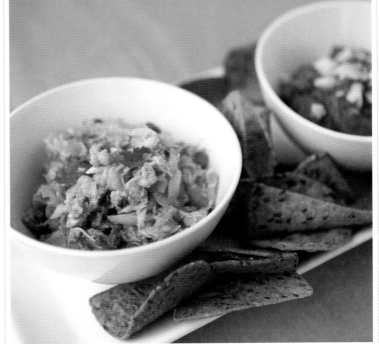

MY DINNER—500 Calories

- 1 cup collards, 49 calories
- 2 tsp. fresh garlic, 8 calories
- 3/4 cup chilaquiles de frijole, 443 calories

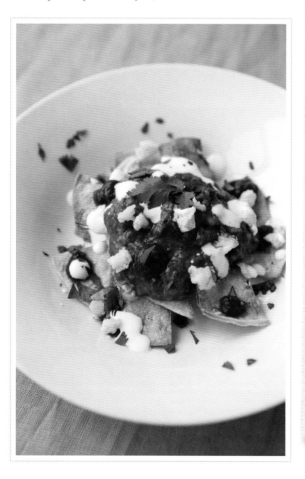

CHILAQUILES DE FRIJOLE

Makes six servings.

INGREDIENTS
Black beans (2 cans or 1 1/4 cup dried)
3 cups chicken broth
1 white onion, chopped
4 cloves garlic, chopped
1 chipotle chile (canned in adobo), chopped
2 tsp. adobe (from chipotle can)
1 epazote stem, with leaves
20 extra thin yellow corn tortillas, cut into strips
Corn oil for frying (or 2 tbsp. olive oil if baking)
Creme fresh (or 1/4 cup sour cream with 3 tbsp. milk)
4 oz. avocado
1/3 cup queso añejo

PREPARATION
1. Cook beans, chicken broth, onion, garlic, chipotle chile, adobe, and epazote together until beans are tender. Purée. Add broth as needed to make it the consistency of light cream soup.
2. Fry tortillas in corn oil until crispy (or bake in olive oil).
3. Pour puréed mixture over the tortilla strips. Add additional chipotle and epazote if desired. Top with creme fresh. Pour into casserole or large serving dish and garnish with avocado and queso añejo.

THE LOVE OF HEALTHY EATING: AN EVOLUTION

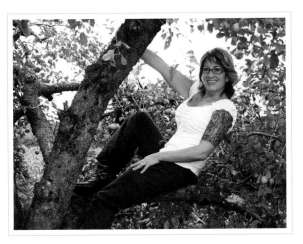

It occurs to me in previewing the stories and Green Days in this book that there are as many paths to balanced eating and living as there are people. No two people here eat to a fixed, one-size-fits-all diet plan.

What we do have in common is variety. We are eating the balanced selection from the three main sources of calories—proteins, carbohydrates, and fats—we need to meet our bodies' nutritional needs.

Another thing we have in common is that we are eating fewer of the nutrient-deficient foods that may have marked our previous diets. Processed foods laden with sodium and long lists of additives are rarer. You won't see a lot of those fast-foods that are heavy in not only sodium but saturated and trans fats. We don't often throw away our calories on nutritionally deficient carbohydrates heavy in refined sugars. Although we have our treats, most of us plan them into our diets to be eaten only when we know we've met our nutritional requirements.

The absolute key to lifelong success is that we learn to love the foods that love us back; only when we have learned to love the foods that bring us to balance can we expect to be successful for a lifetime. Learning to find that love is an evolutionary process. It comes to us slowly, one day at a time. Although each of us in this book may be at different places in this most essential quest, there is ample demonstration that great pleasure and bounty are possible in the choices that are bringing us to balance and improved health.

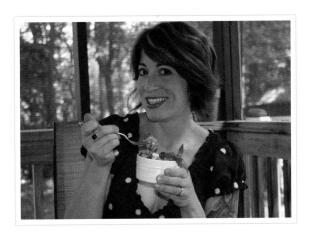

Lynn Matava's Serving Up A Smile column runs weekly at NutriMirror.com. Her Country Tart blog can be found at countrytart.blogspot.com. Currently she is writing a Health Reflection™ book dedicated to loving the foods that love you back.

HEALTHY LIVING: A POSITIVE ADDICTION

username: Alane67 / *first name:* Alane / *location:* Bloomington, MN

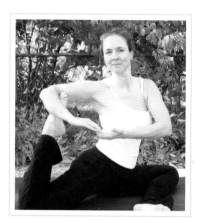

Alane NOW: October '09 / age: 42
160 lbs. / BMI 22.9 / waist 31˝

Food is not my problem. I am my problem. I will spare you the story of familial behaviors that set up my life pattern. Let's just say this, my name is Alane and I am an addict (support group chimes in with "Hi Alane"). I have used drugs, food, sex, work, relationships, alcohol, diets, exercise, cigarettes, and temper tantrums to try to make myself feel better. I have found that no "thing" can do that. At forty-one years old I realized that taking personal responsibility for my choices is the only way I can be empowered. That's what recovery from anything is all about.

On October 24, 2008, I stepped on the scale just like I did every morning. What I saw was the result of years of thinking I knew best. I weighed 179.4 pounds and I freaked out. Immediately I said out loud, "that's it … this is getting ridiculous." I walked out of the bathroom with a towel wrapped around me and sat down at the computer. I logged on to the Internet, entered "diet and exercise logs" in a search engine and found NutriMirror. I looked over the site, read a little about it, and decided to start logging my food and exercise, beginning right then!

Allow me to digress. I have never been seriously overweight. I was a healthy, active kid participating in all kinds of sports until I was in high school. Insert family problems here, and in an effort to control what felt to be out of control I found drugs. In my late teens and early 20s I weighed anywhere between 125 and 140 pounds. I received a lot of social reinforcement for being that thin. Never mind that I practically passed out when I

stood up. Enter some thoughtful personal assessments here, and in 1995 I admitted I was an addict. I began to learn how to take care of myself, eating better and exercising. I gained weight and felt good. I started teaching yoga classes and running. In June of 2001 I completed my first marathon. I weighed roughly 160 pounds—nearly the heaviest I'd ever been in my life. Over the next four years I graduated from college, completed four more marathons, lost ten pounds and managed to keep my weight around 150 the entire time. At the end of May 2005,

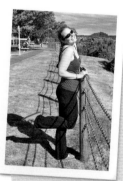

Alane THEN: October '08
179.4 lbs. / BMI 25.7 / waist 35˝

two weeks before I was to run my sixth marathon, my doctor informed me I was in adrenal fatigue. He told me I'd better stop running before I started causing some real physical damage. I cried all the way home. I am a highly educated woman. I am a certified yoga instructor with a bachelor's degree in human biology and a doctorate in chiropractic. I know the human body and how it works. I stopped running and began to do what my doctor told me to do in order to heal. What I didn't do was stop eating like a runner. I gained five pounds in the first year. Not all at once: it was up three, down two; up five, down one. I got used to 155 pounds. Slowly I got used to 160, 165, and 170 where I hung out at for the longest time. I hit 175 and wasn't happy but I believed there must be something wrong with my metabolism. Maybe I was just unlucky, or maybe there was some other excuse.

After all, I eat well, I am smart, I've taken multiple nutrition classes, and I know biochemistry. I teach yoga, I lift weights, and I walk every day. I didn't want

to admit that my choices and my stubbornness were perhaps getting in the way.

The day I saw 179.4 on the scale, I knew I didn't want to get used to 180. I got used to 175, and knew 200 was just around the corner. 179.4 pounds doesn't sound awful on someone who is five feet ten inches tall and I can carry a good amount of weight and not look too bad. What is bad is that in just under five years I had put on nearly 30 pounds. I was not comfortable with that extra weight.

My education has exposed me to diet and exercise logs, which I tried on paper and know is the best way to assess diet in order to make reasonable changes. I used notebooks to keep track of what I ate including carbs, fats, protein, and fiber. That lasted about a week. It's very time-consuming and cumbersome to carry a spiral bound notebook with you everywhere. On top of that I had to look up nutritional values, calculate percentages, etc.

When I typed "diet and exercise log" into the search engine, I knew what I wanted. I am glad I

found exactly what I needed.

It hasn't been easy. Over the months I realized that I struggle with letting go of control of what I think is best. I have lost nearly twenty of the thirty pounds I want to lose. That isn't the best part of this process. I am conscious about my choices. I accept responsibility for what I put into my mouth. I know I am not a victim of slow metabolism or some other genetic issue. Food or drugs or cigarettes don't jump into my mouth. I put them there. Since October of 2008, I have logged what I eat and what I do for exercise. When I see my numbers and percentages in color on my NutriMirror home page it makes it easy for me to see what I need to do to get to where I want to be. Together with an open mind and a great place to connect with other people that are also learning and growing, I know I will become healthy and stay healthy.

MY PHYSICAL ACTIVITY

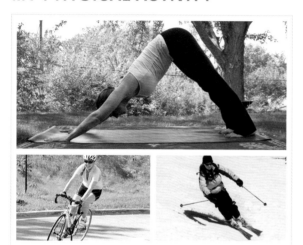

I love to exercise … I love to sweat. I know that sounds a bit odd but it feels cleansing to my body. In addition to lifting weights, I walk and jog in the morning. I teach yoga and go rock climbing twice a week. I don't really think of all this as exercise, it's just who I am. Last year my boyfriend bought me an awesome road bike. We try to hit the road at least once a week. Since Minnesota roads don't lend themselves to biking in the winter, I ski … have since I was six. All this activity helps keep me fit now and will into my old age.

ALANE'S *GREEN* DAY

- Calories Expended: **2,878**
- Calories Eaten: **2,651**
- Net Calorie Balance: **227**

Keeping track of my food intake really helps put things into perspective. Since I am so active it was a little confusing to me as to why my weight slowly kept creeping up. I wanted to blame it on getting older, declining metabolism or heck … just bad luck.

Now I see exactly what is happening, no denying it. I decided to make different choices. No deprivation here … just modifications and room to have some old favorites every once in a while.

MY GREEN DAY NUTRITIONAL FACTS

ALANE'S
HEALTH REFLECTION™
Nutrition Facts Report

Calorie Balance	
Calories Expended	2878
Calories Eaten	2651
Net Calorie Balance	227

Nutrient Balance	
	%DV
Total Fat 58 g	✔
Saturated Fat 8 g	27%
Trans Fat 0 g	—
Cholesterol 68 mg	23%
Sodium 1625 mg	71%
Total Carbs 405 g	✔
Dietary Fiber 39 g	106%
Sugars 146 g	—
Protein 132 g	✔
Vitamin A 3949 µg	564%
Vitamin C 196 mg	141%
Calcium 1755 mg	176%
Iron 28 g	156%

MY BREAKFAST
−626 calories

In order to have the necessary energy for a morning workout I usually start with a liquid concoction of protein and carbs. The mix I use has evolved over time to include greens that provide a variety of nutrients. After workout usually includes a grain cereal or granola along with rice milk or kefir and a piece of fruit.

MY WORKOUT BREAKFAST
- Soy protein powder, 110 calories
- Revitalizing Green Foods Protein Energy Shake, 110 calories
- 4 tsp. whole husk psyllium, 33 calories
- 4 oz. apple juice, 60 calories
- 3/4 cup multigrain oat bran cereal, 110 calories
- 6 oz. rice milk, 98 calories
- Banana, 105 calories

MY SNACKS−416 calories

A cup of yogurt before climbing gives me a little boost of energy without making me feel heavy. And again since I am not into deprivation, an afternoon iced mocha hits the spot. I used to drink a blended concoction that weighed in at roughly 400 calories. Easy enough to change to a skim milk iced mocha, 190 calories and zero fat.

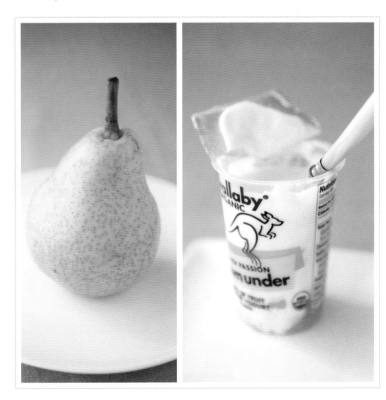

YOGURT, ICED MOCHA, AND PEAR
- Pear, 96 calories
- Iced mocha, nonfat, 190 calories
- 6 oz. peach yogurt, nonfat, 130 calories

MY LUNCH–953 calories

Since I am not into deprivation I indulge occasionally on take-out. This lunch was from a local Chinese food chain. It includes chicken in a sauce with white rice. A big lunch helps me prepare for a big evening of indoor rock climbing.

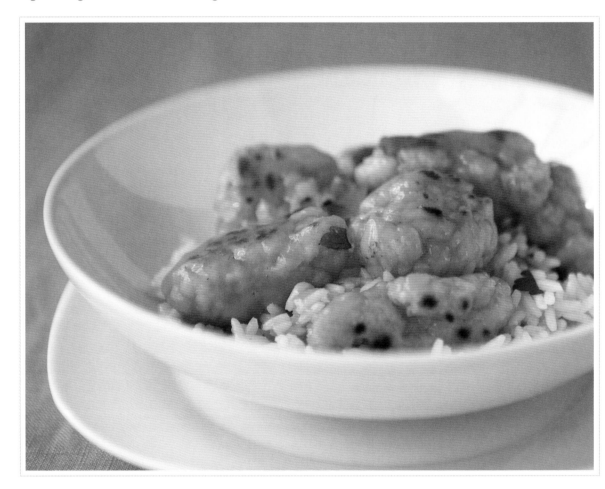

CHICKEN & RICE
- 8 oz. medium-grain white rice, 295 calories
- 10 oz. orange chicken, 658 calories

MY DINNER–656 calories

I've always enjoyed a good salad. My mixed field greens salad rounds out a great day with plenty of vitamins and minerals. The sweetness of the carrots and apple keeps me from wanting to eat sugary snacks into the night. I found the recipe for the flax oil dressing a while ago. The benefit of the omega 3s is too long to list here.

THAI PITA PIZZA AND SALAD
- Apple, 55 calories
- Carrot, 30 calories
- 1 tbsp. roasted pumpkin seeds, 74 calories
- 1/2 oz. feta cheese, 35 calories
- 2 oz. baby lettuce, 10 calories
- 1/4 serving flax oil dressing, 84 calories
- 1 serving Thai chicken pita, 368 calories

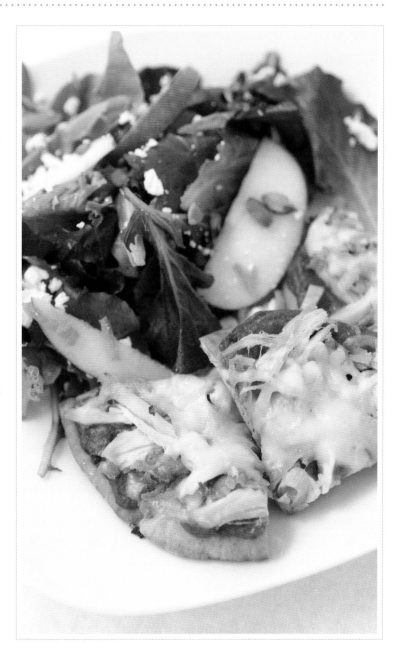

"A HEALTHY LIFESTYLE, IT'S LIKE MONEY IN THE BANK."

username: hungrymongo / *first name:* Brent / *location:* Flower Mound, TX

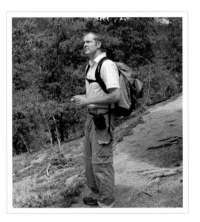

Brent NOW: September '09 / age: 38
178 lbs. / BMI 22.8 / waist 34˝

My wife and I entered our sixth year of marriage with a sense of complacency. We ate out several times a week, selecting food from the menu based on what looked good. I would ask the waiter for another beer without thinking. We went home at night and plopped down on the couch. My wife watched TV and I worked on the computer. Exercise consisted of walking the dogs a few times a week.

Without saying it, we both knew we had packed on a few pounds. From time to time we would verbalize a desire to do something about it. We needed to start working out again, but there was always the next day. With no tangible plan and no real sense of personal commitment, the days ticked away and our waistlines slowly crept outward.

In January 2009, my wife went in for a health exam. The results came back. She faced the possibility of blood pressure medication for the first time in her life. A week later I went in for my annual health exam. The results showed that I was in the worse shape of my life. At 220 pounds, my weight had hit a new high, and my blood pressure was also twenty points above normal. That night as I started my evening routine in front of the computer, I laid out my annual physical results for the last three years side by side and began to do the math. I remember thinking, "at this rate, I'll weigh a thousand pounds when I'm fifty."

That night, we agreed that complacency was no longer an option. We jumped into a commitment to new behaviors. We started walking on our lunch breaks at work. We bought some videos and started working out several times a week. We scaled back what we ate and tried to cook at home more often.

After several weeks, we started seeing results. We were down a few pounds and we had successfully built some exercise into our evening routines. Happy with our progress, we pushed onward, but we still had no goals. We knew we were moving more and eating less, and it seemed to be working.

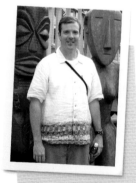

Brent THEN: February '09
220 lbs. / BMI 28.2 / waist 41˝

After about a month, I was discussing weight loss results with a coworker. She mentioned that she kept a food and exercise journal through a website called NutriMirror. She explained journaling as a much more structured approach to managing food intake and exercise regimen. I watched her navigate the NutriMirror website. I nodded as if I followed her every move on the site even though I didn't really get it.

I returned to my office and dismissed the idea of a food and exercise journal. It sounded like a lot of work. I wondered how accurate it could really be. I eventually forgot about the whole thing.

Then a few days later I was reconciling our bank statement when it hit me. The journaling concept might actually make sense. I wouldn't feel comfortable banking, spending money, or paying bills without keeping track of what I had spent. My wife and I manage our finances like most people do, keeping track of our expenses and making decisions based on what's available to us. Perhaps a similar disciplined approach applied to the choices we made for meals or exercise. The next day I approached my coworker and asked for the "name of that website again."

We gave NutriMirror a try. The process was immediately eye opening. Holy cow! I couldn't believe my favorite breakfast burrito really had that many calories. Geez! I thought for sure I was getting more of a workout by walking twenty minutes at lunch than that. As my wife and I began logging our food intake and daily exercise, we realized we were all over the place. Some days we were way under on our intake, other days we were way over.

Food and exercise journaling is a real learning process. This isn't just about counting calories, and it isn't about deprivation. We began to realize that journaling did not simply mean mindless data entry; it meant making informed choices throughout the day. We began to sculpt our routines and choices based on what was available to us.

Along the way we began to eat consciously. We became mindful of the interplay between carbohydrates, proteins, and fats. We are now aware of the sodium content in foods and the importance of vitamins and fiber and the benefits of exercise. We are disciplined in the daily management of food and exercise.

Over the following weeks and months, we gradually replaced bad habits with good ones. Journaling is now second nature. Exercising is an expectation, not something we needed to fit into our evening. Our patience and discipline have been paying off. The weight has fallen and taken the blood pressure down with it.

This doesn't mean that we turned our lives completely upside down. We find ways to maintain old habits by tailoring them to fit within a healthy framework. For example, when we eat out, we put more thought into menu choices. We still enjoy TV and computer time, just not at the expense of an evening workout.

We monitor our intake and we're enjoying the heck out of life as a result.

A few days ago I strapped a forty-pound backpack on my shoulders to hike in the mountains, and smiled to myself as I realized that last year that's how much I would have weighed without the pack. I have never enjoyed a hike more.

We realize that the most important concept in this process is that *it is a process*. We may have reached our target weight, blood pressure, and so on, but now we must choose what to do from here. We have built healthy habits; now we must maintain them for good.

Complacency creeps in if you're not watching for it. We have already found ourselves fighting thoughts such as, "it's only one more night off," and "that extra slice of pizza won't hurt me." Those thoughts might be individually true, but collectively they add up. We continue to manage those thoughts just as we would our bank account. We're making sure we don't end up overdrawn.

MY PHYSICAL ACTIVITY

My wife and I both work, and like so many people we are constantly pulled in many directions. Our exercise philosophy: keep it short and simple, so that it's harder to use the excuse that "we don't have time."

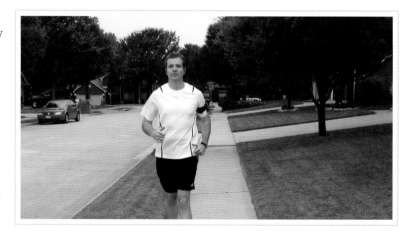

We exercise four or five nights a week, for about twenty to thirty minutes. We don't belong to a gym and we don't own any expensive workout equipment.

We have selected activities we both enjoy doing, so that it's easier for us to hold each other accountable for sticking to them. We alternate between circuit training videos at home and one of our two favorite outdoor activities—bicycling or running around the neighborhood.

We love this approach. It's quick, inexpensive, and easy to maintain. We feel energized afterward and enjoy the rest of our evening as a result. We're getting a good blend of weight training and cardiovascular activity, and we have fun in the process!

BRENT'S *GREEN* DAY

- Calories Expended: **2,287**
- Calories Eaten: **2,034**
- Net Calorie Balance: **253**

Although my wife loves to cook, our work schedule makes that difficult on most weekdays. Over the past few years we found ourselves going out to eat often—at lunch with coworkers and in the evenings together. This pattern of constant eating out was a big contributor to packing on the pounds!

Along with food journaling, we have changed our approach to weekday meals. We recognize that finding time to cook is difficult, but we can still minimize the impact on our waistlines (and wallets) from eating out often. Now we take lunch kits to work containing several items that can be mixed and matched into meals and snacks. When we do eat out in the evenings, we split entrées—saving on both cost and calories.

MY GREEN DAY NUTRITIONAL FACTS

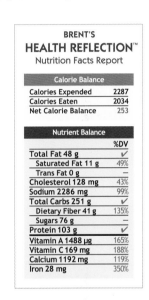

BRENT'S
HEALTH REFLECTION™
Nutrition Facts Report

Calorie Balance	
Calories Expended	2287
Calories Eaten	2034
Net Calorie Balance	253

Nutrient Balance	
	%DV
Total Fat 48 g	✔
Saturated Fat 11 g	49%
Trans Fat 0 g	
Cholesterol 128 mg	43%
Sodium 2286 mg	99%
Total Carbs 251 g	✔
Dietary Fiber 41 g	135%
Sugars 76 g	—
Protein 103 g	✔
Vitamin A 1488 µg	165%
Vitamin C 169 mg	188%
Calcium 1192 mg	119%
Iron 28 mg	350%

MY BREAKFAST—303 calories

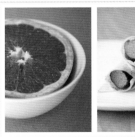 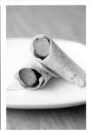

This breakfast only takes a couple of minutes to make. A bowl of healthy cereal, then a quick tortilla sausage wrap heated up in the microwave. By keeping breakfast quick and easy, I avoid the temptation to skip breakfast (something that I used to do often). I added a half grapefruit on this morning, a source of vitamins that is also low in calories and sodium.

CEREAL, MILK, AND COFFEE WITH TORTILLA AND SAUSAGE

- 1 cup milk, nonfat, 86 calories
- 1 cup multigrain Cheerios, 108 calories
- Grapefruit, 32 calories
- 64 oz. coffee, 19 calories
- 1/3 whole wheat tortilla, 25 calories
- 3/5 oz. smoked sausage, 33 calories
- Men's health vitamin, 0 calories

MY LUNCH–379 calories

This lunch is also intended to be quick and easy to put together, either the night before or in the morning. Thought has been put into the choices of meat, cheese, bread, and condiments—these are low sodium, low fat, without artificial preservatives or high-fructose corn syrup.

SANDWICH WITH YOGURT AND FRUIT
- 1 ground beef patty, extra lean, 140 calories
- 1 slice whole wheat Sandwich Thin, 100 calories
- 1/2 tbsp. mayonnaise, 16 calories
- 4 oz. strawberry yogurt, 70 calories
- Peaches in light syrup, 53 calories

MY SNACKS–552 calories

Snacks are my "secret weapon" during the day. I take several items that don't require much preparation, such as fruit, cheese, and a PBJ sandwich. Snacking on these throughout the day prevents me from stuffing myself at lunch or making bad decisions at the vending machine. I refer to eating my snacks as "grazing," and I don't let myself get overly hungry by the time I leave work—which helps prevent bad decisions in the evening.

SANDWICH, FRUIT, AND CHEESE
- Apple, 72 calories
- Banana, 105 calories
- String cheese, 50 calories
- 1 slice whole grain & flax bread, 100 calories
- 2 tbsp. peanut butter, 200 calories
- 1/2 tbsp. strawberry jelly, 25 calories

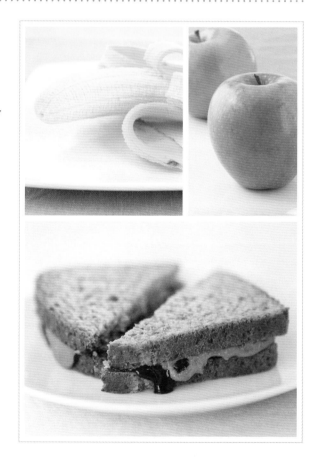

MY DINNER–800 calories

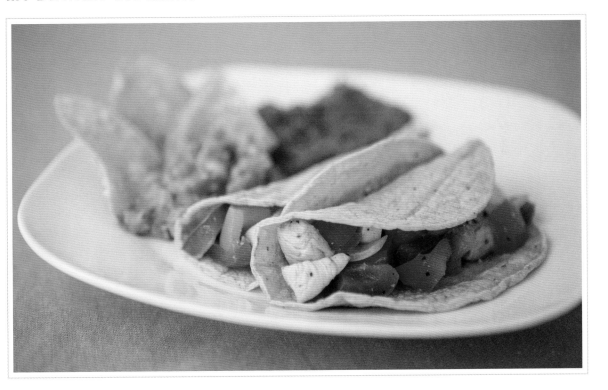

For this dinner, my wife and I elected to go to a Mexican restaurant (our favorite). I ordered two beers with dinner, because the point of this whole process is not to deprive myself of the things I enjoy, but to enjoy them in moderation. However, in keeping with the spirit of making good choices, my wife and I decided to split an entrée of fajitas. Like many restaurant entrées, the portion size is big enough that two people can split it and still enjoy a good meal. This way we save money, don't overeat, and leave without a takeout container. I avoid the temptation of tortilla chips on the table, which would put me over on sodium!

SHARE A MEAL (TACOS, CHIPS, AND BEER)
- 24 oz. beer, 278 calories
- 3 oz. refried beans, 132 calories
- 1/2 oz. tortilla chips, 69 calories
- 3/4 serving guacamole, 128 calories
- 2 corn tortillas, 104 calories
- 3 oz. grilled chicken breast, 89 calories

"ONCE AGAIN THE STORY WAS THE SAME. THE WEIGHT CAME BACK ON AND SO MUCH MORE."

username: czoerun / *first name:* Carla / *location:* Escondido, CA

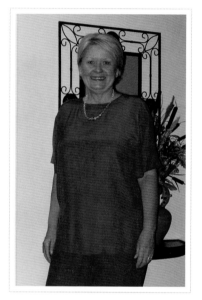

Carla NOW: October '09 / age: 56
159 lbs. / BMI 26.5 / waist 30.5˝

Weight loss, weight gain. This best describes most of my adult life. I did not have weight issues as a child, teen, or young adult. I always maintained a healthy weight of 120 to 125 for my 5´5˝ frame.

I began gaining weight in my thirties. My first real diet was in 1988. I was thirty-five years old and decided I wanted to lose weight for a friend's wedding. I found a diet in a popular women's magazine. The weight came off quickly: twenty-seven pounds in about five weeks. I was happy and excited. I was thin again and it felt great. But the weight loss did not last because I quickly went back to my old way of eating. It took less than six months to put all the weight back on. I felt like such a failure. I could not figure out why the diet did not work. That was the beginning of years of diets, weight gain, weight loss, and much frustration.

In 1989, I planned a trip to Hawaii—another good reason to lose weight. I decided to try the popular Jenny Craig weight loss program. It was designed to be easy. Just buy the food, follow the program, and lose the weight. Since I had put on even more weight, I needed to lose at least thirty-five pounds this time. The weight came off in about two months. I had my trip to Hawaii. I was thin again and done with that diet. In less than six months I put all the weight back on and more.

In 1992, I planned a cruise to Alaska. I had another good reason to lose weight. Since I had purchased the lifetime membership from Jenny Craig, I decided to try it again. After all, I lost weight when I was purchasing the diet food before. This time I needed to lose forty-five pounds. After several months with the program I lost the weight. I took the cruise and I felt great. I was home again. I was once more done with that diet. Once again the story was the same. The weight came back on and so much more.

Over the next seventeen years I tried diet after diet. I always grew tired of following special

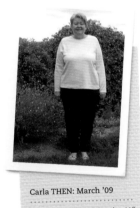

Carla THEN: March '09
215 lbs. / BMI 35.8 / waist 41˝

menus and recipes that simply did not fit my lifestyle. And I would always give up with the end result of gaining more and more weight.

In 2008, my doctor discovered a growth on my thyroid. I felt relieved to possibly have a reason for being fat. I had surgery to remove the growth and one side of my thyroid. I felt good after surgery and thought that I would finally lose weight, but I was wrong. By the end of 2008, I had gained fifteen more pounds to top me out at a whopping 215. I was devastated. I was placed on prescription thyroid medication, but still no weight loss. I came to a belief that I was just going to be an obese person and that was all there was to it. I donated my scale and my full-length mirror to a local thrift store. I did not want to look at my body anymore.

In March of 2009, I was really suffering with pain in my knees and legs. I also lacked energy from being so heavy. My cholesterol and blood pressure were elevated. My father had died of coronary disease when he was only sixty-one years old. I was fifty-five and headed

in the same direction. I did not want to diet again. I wrote down each thing I ate. To help get my cholesterol in check, I revamped my old recipes so that they became to healthier.

I began an online search for food logs and food calorie charts. I came across the NutriMirror website and started with the food log I could print out. I kept a manual log of my food intake for three days. I didn't know my next step. I still had to find and calculate the calories and did not know how to figure out how much cholesterol was in my food.

I went back to NutriMirror and read more. I learned that I could enter in my three days of food into the online food log and immediately see the calculations. I could not believe how badly I had done. My fat and calories were high as well as my sodium and cholesterol levels. This was amazing information to me. Not my figures, but that I could actually SEE the information that I wanted to know. After a week of using the site and seeing how easy it was to track my calories,

I went out and bought a new scale and a full length mirror.

I've learned that by using the tools on NutriMirror, I can have the foods I love to eat. I need to watch my portion sizes and the amount of fat and sodium I use. I can choose what I want each and every day. I enjoy cooking the majority of my meals and with the recipe tool I can now create my favorite recipes in a healthy way.

I have lost some weight, averaging about one pound a week during the weight loss phase. I see changes in my body shape and feel stronger every day. I am enjoying exercise now and I look forward to each day.

I do not have a weight goal in sight. I have taken that downhill fast lane too many times in my life and do not want to do that again. Using the NutriMirror tool has changed my outlook. Now, this is a lifetime journey about eating healthy. I have the tools that were missing in all those other failed attempts. I am finally eating healthier and feeling better than I ever thought possible.

MY PHYSICAL ACTIVITY

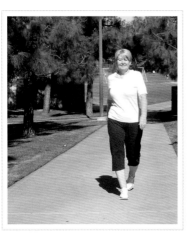

I have never been a person who works out at a gym. It is just not something that appeals to me. What I do enjoy is walking. It doesn't require any special equipment, just a pair of comfortable shoes; and I don't need to drive anywhere. My neighborhood is where I get my exercise. I regularly walk three to four days a week at a light pace of 2.5 mph for twenty to thirty minutes. There are a couple of nice hills in the neighborhood and I try to include these in my walk a couple of days a week.

When you walk you don't just lose weight in your legs, you get trimmer all over. My walks have helped me to lose fifty-six pounds. I also get "paid" back for my efforts with some additional calories to add to my day's allowance. That's nice when you want a snack while watching TV at night.

CARLA'S *GREEN* DAY

- Calories Expended: **1,925**
- Calories Eaten: **1,430**
- Net Calorie Balance: **495**

I have always loved cooking. I have a large collection of recipes and enjoy creating recipes of my own. Using the NutriMirror recipe tool has allowed me to modify my recipes to create healthier versions. Changing from butter to olive oil and the use of both sometimes; white rice to whole grains; using less salt or none at all—these are some of the changes I have made.

Both my lunch and dinner are recipes I have modified using the NutriMirror recipe tool. Having this tool available has enabled me to continue doing what I love to do: providing interesting, tasty, and now healthy meals for myself, family, and friends.

MY GREEN DAY NUTRITIONAL FACTS

CARLA'S
HEALTH REFLECTION™
Nutrition Facts Report

Calorie Balance	
Calories Expended	1925
Calories Eaten	1430
Net Calorie Balance	495

Nutrient Balance	
	%DV
Total Fat 40 g	✔
Saturated Fat 5 g	31%
Trans Fat 0 g	—
Cholesterol 101 mg	34%
Sodium 941 mg	41%
Total Carbs 205 g	✔
Dietary Fiber 27 g	160%
Sugars 80 g	—
Protein 75 g	✔
Vitamin A 4368 µg	624%
Vitamin C 194 mg	259%
Calcium 1344 mg	112%
Iron 13 g	163%

MY BREAKFAST—337 calories

I have never been much for eating breakfast. Most days in the past I would skip breakfast altogether, running out the door with just a cup of coffee in hand. By mid-morning I was starving and looking for anything that was around the office to eat! Usually a huge bagel topped with lots of cream cheese or some empty-calorie, high-fat donut or Danish.

Now, I look forward to taking just ten minutes to eat a small bowl of cereal with skim milk and some fresh fruit. I still run out the door with coffee in hand; but I feel much better knowing I have started my day out with a wholesome, whole grain, high fiber breakfast that supplies my body with 42% of my daily fiber. Not a bad way to start the day.

CEREAL, FRUIT, AND COFFEE
- 1 cup milk, nonfat, 86 calories
- Banana, 90 calories
- 8 oz. coffee, 14 calories
- 1 cup flax plus multibran cereal, 147 calories

MY SNACKS—262 calories

My choices for snacks are always plain yogurt with some fresh fruit. I generally have this in the morning and again in the evening, adding the granola bar too. This treat reminds me of cheesecake dessert, the granola bar being the yummy crust and the fruit and yogurt the "cheesecake."

I supplied my body with 70% of its calcium needs for this day using food alone; by adding a 500 mg tablet of calcium I am now at my daily requirement. Now that is remarkable.

FRUIT, YOGURT, GRANOLA BAR, AND VITAMINS
- 1/2 apple, 27 calories
- 1/2 cup plain yogurt, nonfat, 55 calories
- Oats-n-Honey granola bar, 180 calories
- Calcium + D supplement, 0 calories

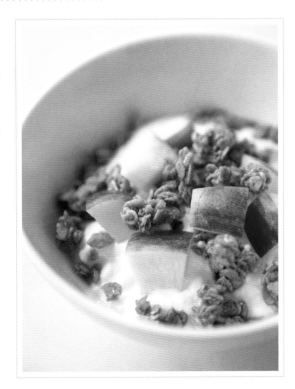

MY LUNCH–320 calories

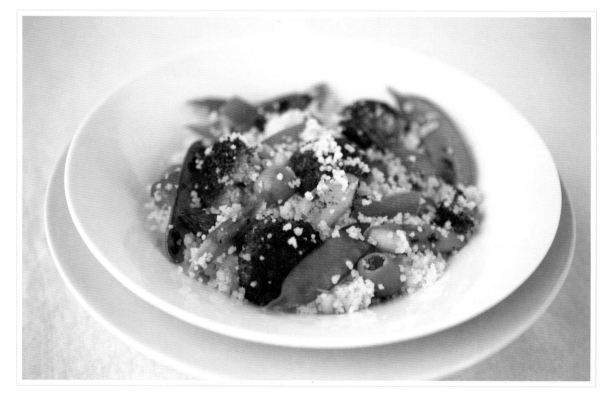

This is a quick, light, and healthy lunch of whole wheat couscous and some nice veggies. I toss the couscous with lemon juice and heart-healthy olive oil. I prepare several cups of couscous so that it is ready to go when I want to make up a quick, healthy lunch in a short amount of time.

Using a whole wheat couscous instead of white rice or white pasta adds more fiber and with the added vegetables supplies my body with lots of the vitamin A I need for the day.

COUSCOUS AND VEGGIES
- 1 tsp. lemon juice, 1 calorie
- 4 small olives, 15 calories
- 1 small spring onion, 2 calories
- 1 small red tomato, 16 calories
- 1 cup cooked couscous, 176 calories
- 2 tsp. extra virgin olive oil, 80 calories
- 3 oz. broccoli, 30 calories

MY DINNER–511 calories

I enjoy having a filling salad for dinner on warm summer evenings. This salad is simple to create with mixed greens with some roast chicken breast, pecans, tangerines, and sweet dried cranberries. I dress the greens with a Sweet Honey Mustard Tangerine and Thyme Vinaigrette.

In the past I would have used a large amount of olive oil to make the dressing for this salad—heart healthy yes, but not in the amounts I was using. By making some small changes in the way I prepare my salad dressing, I have reduced the calories in it by more than half.

This salad alone supplied my body with 100% of vitamin C for the day with only 30% of my calories coming from fat, very low in saturated fat too. Making these small changes has helped me to lower my cholesterol without medication.

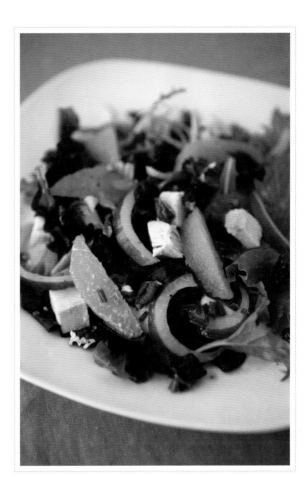

SALAD WITH CHICKEN
* 1/2 tsp. thyme, 0 calories
* 1/2 tsp. lemon juice, 1 calorie
* 2 tbsp. tangerine juice, 13 calories
* 1 tsp. honey mustard, 10 calories
* 1 tsp. extra virgin olive oil, 40 calories
* 1 tsp. honey, 21 calories
* 1/2 tsp. fresh chives, 0 calories
* 1/4 sweet onion, 26 calories
* 1/2 oz. pecans, 99 calories
* 4 oz. mixed baby greens, 20 calories
* 1 orange, 69 calories
* 1 tbsp. craisins, 25 calories
* 4 oz. roasted chicken breast, 187 calories

"I WAS GRASPING AT THE WALLS OF A SLIPPERY WELL."

username: carrieredhead / *first name:* Carrie / *location:* Modesto, CA

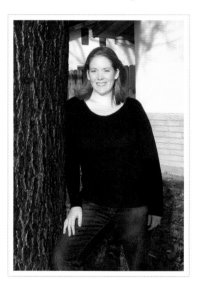

Carrie NOW: August '09 / age: 30
177.6 lbs. / BMI 28.5 / waist 33.5˝

This is taken from an entry I wrote on my NutriMirror journal: *"I was eight. My mother was in bed crying hysterically and had just literally lost her mind. My grandparents were there and the house was in upheaval, a flurry of activity in decision-making about what was to come next. I knew things were about to change in a big way, but no adult took the time to soothe my brother or I to explain what was going on. I just knew my mom had checked out and my life*

would never be the same. I got the chair from the kitchen and decided to take this opportunity to eat some ice cream. It was Neapolitan. I got a spoon and took a bite. It was heaven. It made everything better. This is where it started for me."

This set the stage for many years of my life. I used to eat my way through pain, anxiety, and every other emotion. I celebrated or intensified life with the high I got from food. This continued until the day I heard about bulimia from a girl in dance class. I could have all the food I wanted and then remove it from my stomach with a few uncomfortable moments in the bathroom. I went home and tried it out on a dry cheese sandwich. It did not work so well. I was desperate to lose the weight, because I would be performing on stage at the end of the year and I'd always been the fat girl. I wanted to be a star in all ways and I very much believed, at that age, being thin would make the moment so much better.

After my attempt at bulimia failed, I decided to invest my energy into not eating anything at all. I believed that if I could just do this and get thin then everything would be better. I tried it and it stuck. It became easier after a while. I cut down portions, eating just one bite. I gorged myself on zero calorie foods. When the end of the year rolled around I was thin and I wasn't feeling very good. I looked really good and everyone was complimenting me, but they didn't know how obsessed I had become with food or how sad and lonely

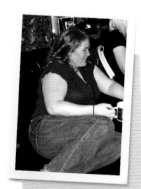

Carrie THEN: April '09
223.4 lbs. / BMI 36.3 / waist 41˝

I was inside. The year ended and the pressure was off, so I started eating again and gained all my weight back.

I spent the majority of 2003 to 2006 depressed and adjusting to being a mom. With my first pregnancy came more weight than I had ever carried on my frame. I was ashamed and lived in a cave most days with my young son. I never went out and my life was centered on a drive-thru window. I made sure I fed my son well and kept processed foods out of his body. When it came to me, I failed horribly.

I knew I didn't want to end up dying an ugly death. I didn't want to have a massive heart attack in my forties or be bed-ridden with cancer, as most of the people close to me have. My actions affect the people closest to me and it occurred to me how very selfish I was being. I attempted to numb myself with food and insulate my fear of life in fat. I could choose to have a positive impact or a negative one. The good nutrition I was teaching my son would be completely null and void if I didn't practice it myself.

I got on track and lost 15 pounds. I exercised and then got pregnant again. Being, once again, in an unhealthy pregnancy drove home my need to change. I promised myself during the second c-section, I would get healthy for my children, my husband and my loved ones.

While I was overweight, I went on a body makeover and diet-reading rampage. I tried Weight Watchers more times than I could count. I was grasping at the walls of a slippery well. I wanted to be thin, but nothing seemed to work. I wanted to starve myself and binge. I wanted weight loss to come easy and quick. When it became too difficult, I would quit.

I started NutriMirror in April of 2009. I actually signed up on March 29th and then didn't log in, putting it on the back burner. When my attempt to keep a written food journal failed, I logged in and haven't looked back. The diet book I was reading at the time, The Beck Diet Solution, was left in the

dust. Once I started honestly logging my food choices and looking at my pattern of behavior there was no turning away. The information I am getting is helping me help myself. The site doesn't log for me. No one tells me what I have to eat. I have my days when I have a beer or two or three, but I tell the truth. I log it and move on. I have become more focused on nutrition and the quality of food that goes into my mouth. For the first time I am enjoying what I eat on all levels. I don't dread the next meal. On the flipside, I know the next meal can redeem my last poor decision. It is all there in front of me and I see my choices; the good ones and the bad ones.

Most of my dieting life has been a combination of emotional eating and trying to fit into someone else's mold of what I should look like. The song "How to Save a Life" by The Fray was playing in the background of the operating room during my second c-section. There's more than one way of bringing someone back from the brink of death. It is time I save my own life, time to apply a defibrillator to the core of how I perceive food and choices concerning health. NutriMirror helps me make good choices every day. I wake up, I log on. I'm accountable and I know I've made another step towards living a healthy life.

MY PHYSICAL ACTIVITY

This is the way I have always approached exercise: "No pain, no gain," "All or nothing," "I have to do it right the first time." This time, after I started out too quickly I realized I needed to make myself a deal: start out small and build from there. I dialed the intensity down, loaded my iPod with cool tunes, took my workouts outside, and I tried to be more active in my home and while out running errands. More recently, I've added a gym membership and have found a renewed love of the elliptical machine. I still walk occasionally and have tried both yoga and biking outdoors. The rules now are: listen to your body, measure your physical success by where you have come from instead of what someone else is doing, and have FUN! Now both exercise and eating have become pleasurable events I look forward to.

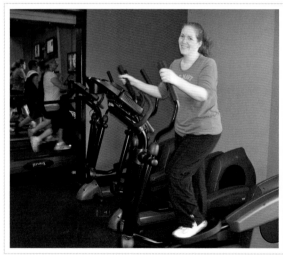 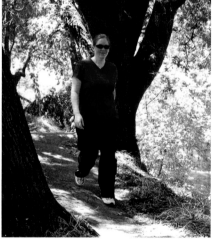

CARRIE'S *GREEN* DAY

- Calories Expended: **2,297**
- Calories Eaten: **1,744**
- Net Calorie Balance: 553

A lover of food is always what I thought I was. But really, my palate was so drenched in poor choices, there was never a chance for my mind or tongue to develop a sense of real food, real taste. I'm uncovering texture and flavors I never thought possible. I take a chance almost every week with something new I learn at NutriMirror: chia seeds, ancient grains like kamut, amaranth and quinoa, or blackstrap molasses. Learning that food is an experience, just like anything else in life, helps me to not take it for granted or waste my experiences on non-quality products. I'm beginning to understand the natural meaning of sweet, sour, salty, and bitter as God intended. For this Green Day I focused on making choices which prove to me that pleasure and my body's needs for health can be mutually satisfied while losing weight and achieving nutritional balance.

MY GREEN DAY NUTRITIONAL FACTS

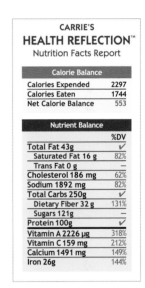

CARRIE'S
HEALTH REFLECTION™
Nutrition Facts Report

Calorie Balance	
Calories Expended	2297
Calories Eaten	1744
Net Calorie Balance	553

Nutrient Balance	
	%DV
Total Fat 43g	✔
Saturated Fat 16 g	82%
Trans Fat 0 g	—
Cholesterol 186 mg	62%
Sodium 1892 mg	82%
Total Carbs 250g	✔
Dietary Fiber 32 g	131%
Sugars 121g	—
Protein 100g	✔
Vitamin A 2226 µg	318%
Vitamin C 159 mg	212%
Calcium 1491 mg	149%
Iron 26g	144%

MY BREAKFAST–374 calories

This day was a light breakfast day. I've never been a huge fan of breakfast, so it needs to be quick, accessible, and sometimes sweet, like this day. I find I cycle through breakfast menus and during this period I was on a cereal kick. I try to keep it balanced with protein too, so I added kefir, which provided me with a dose of good bacteria too! Sweet and Simple.

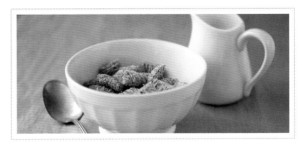

CEREAL WITH MILK AND KEFIR
- 1 cup Cinnamon Harvest Organic Promise cereal, 190 calories
- 4 oz. milk, low fat, 61 calories
- 6 1/2 oz. strawberry kefir, low fat, 123 calories

MY LUNCH–289 calories

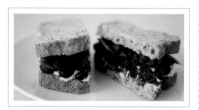

Being busy with the children means having to grab something quick and nutritious on occasion. One of my old stand-bys is the mighty sandwich. This one is much different from the sandwiches of yesteryear. Gone are the heavy mayo and multiple slices of cheese, with a copious side salad. Here I still get the salty flavor I crave, but also the fiber and iron from the beans and spinach. Throw in a cup of joe and I'm on my way!

SANDWICH, COFFEE WITH MILK
- 1/2 cup black beans, 110 calories
- 2 pieces flax seed bread, 100 calories
- 2 oz. spinach, 13 calories
- 1 serving garlic & herb cheese wedge, light, 35 calories
- 6 oz. coffee, decaf, 0 calories
- 2 oz. milk, low fat, 31 calories

MY SNACKS–726 calories

Ah, my beloved snacks! I never knew what a snacker I was until I started logging. Sometimes my snacks rival meals in bulk. This day was especially pleasurable. The cheese and pumpkin seeds really helped while on the go, the cinnamon, walnuts, and applesauce tasted like pie filling. I had a strawberry chocolate shake post-workout. Then, I added some frozen papaya, and ended the day with a hot cup of chamomile tea. I think this was the point, after entering all these delicious snacks, when the wisdom of my good Green Day choices hit me. I went to bed fulfilled and energized. Before using this simple Internet tool to get control over my food intake, I would likely have gone to bed starving and raided the pantry in the middle of the night. Never underestimate the snack!

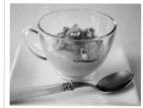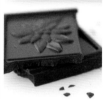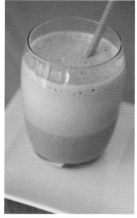

BELOVED SNACKS
- 1/8 tsp. cinnamon, 1 calorie
- 1/4 oz. walnuts, 40 calories
- 1/2 cup applesauce, unsweetened, 50 calories
- 1 oz. Swiss cheese, 110 calories
- 3/4 oz. pumpkin seeds, 114 calories
- 1 tbsp. chocolate syrup, 50 calories
- 1 3/4 oz. strawberries, frozen, 18 calories
- 1 cup milk, low fat, 130 calories
- 1/2 oz. dark chocolate, 82 calories
- 1 1/2 cup papaya chunks, frozen, 65 calories
- 6 oz. chamomile tea, 2 calories
- 1 tbsp. honey, 64 calories

MY DINNER–355 calories

This is where something new comes in, a time to experiment. I was trying out Quinoa after reading a suggestion in another member's journal. I found that not only is this grain high in nutritional value, but it cooks up quickly and is a good addition to my meal-in-a-bowl requirement (again, kids, fast-paced life, busy). The shrimp added protein and the peas added color and a bit of fiber to boot! I realize frequently that I can use old favorites (like Pomodoro Meat Sauce) for extra flavor and still come out on top with a healthy meal, loaded with flavor.

DINNER IN A BOWL (Shrimp & Quinoa)
- 1 tsp. red pepper flakes, 6 calories
- 1/4 cup quinoa (uncooked measure), 159 calories
- 3 oz. peas, 70 calories
- 3 oz. shrimp, 80 calories
- 1/4 cup pomodoro meat sauce, 40 calories

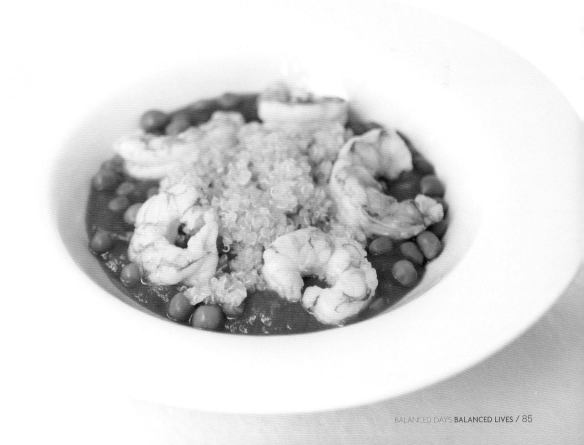

"I NO LONGER FEAR FOR MY LIFE."

username: CarrievanDev / *first name:* Carrie / *location:* Naperville, IL

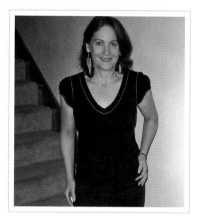

Carrie NOW: October '09 / age: 50
139.6 lbs. / BMI 23.3 / waist 29˝

My slow transition from healthy athlete to sad, obese, and carrying the weight of the world is now part of history. I'm back!

As an athlete, I had always been health conscious and aware of my weight fluctuations. I monitored my diet closely. I am a competitive swimmer and was on a local swim team, still competing into my forties. My fitness training included a couple of miles a day of swimming, lots of yoga, strength training, and various aerobic activities.

Then, in the late 1990s, my mother exhibited symptoms of Progressive Supranuclear Palsy (PSP) and needed around-the-clock care. My lifestyle and exercise routine changed. Providing her with homecare and taking her to doctor appointments no longer allowed time for swimming. I was also taking care of my four children. My husband was laid off from his job, so I began looking for work. We were barely able to afford our mortgage and health insurance.

When my father passed away in December 2003 my mother moved in with us. While working as a waitress I took care of her and my family full time. I was exhausted and depressed. I gained weight and developed health issues which added to my frustration and despair.

Mother's disease had progressed by the spring of 2007. I changed bedrooms to be closer to her, and slept lightly in case she needed anything. She endured many surgeries yet she outlived my brother who died from a heart attack. He had a poor diet and suffered from numerous health problems. Obesity played a contributing role in his early death at the age of forty-five.

My own weight ballooned to 202 pounds. And nothing I did seemed to help me lose any of it. I was scared and thought that I would die early, like my brother had done. Time passed slowly. My mother's health was dwindling. The stress in my life grew. I was tired of being fat. I was depressed. Life had been difficult and I was motivated to

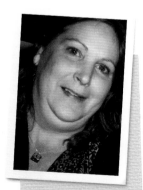

Carrie THEN: April '09

202.4 lbs. / BMI 33.7 / waist 45.5˝

do something but didn't know what. I decided to search the Internet for a food log website. The website needed to be quick and easy to use or I would stop doing it. I had logged food once before by hand. It was difficult and time consuming and I gave up. I knew I could do it if only I could find a good website.

After researching websites, NutriMirror stood out. It was free, seemed fairly easy to use and navigate, showed more nutrition information, and had none of the bothersome advertising of the others. Wow! I could immediately see I was finally going to have some control over this one area of my life—my physical health—even during those most difficult of times.

Using the site provided me with hope. It brought me joy to log and analyze my food choices every day. Soon I begin to see results. Shortly after beginning NutriMirror, my mother lost her battle and passed away. Saddened, hurt, and lost, I found purpose again in the focus on improving my own personal health. I wanted to lose more weight. I wanted to exercise and to start swimming again.

I found joy during a time of sadness and mourning as I continued to see improvement in my results. Being accountable for my health gave me satisfaction. I monitored my calorie intake exactly, lost weight, and made absolutely sure that I met my nutritional needs.

I became totally aware of portion control. I noticed right away how those heaping spoonfuls added calories to my diet. Measuring my portion sizes became a way of life. No heaping or cheating was allowed—subconsciously or otherwise.

I had never used salt much so I did not understand the sodium issues. On the very first day of logging, however, the sodium jumped out of the computer and practically slapped me in the face. Sodium is the first thing I read on nutrition labels now. As soon as I adjusted my sodium intake I noticed all my nutritional values improved. I had more energy, less swelling, more weight loss, and increased flexibility.

NutriMirror has been a hands-on nutrition class. I learned quickly through the instant, measured feedback which foods were good for me and which ones to avoid or limit. Even before taking my first bite, I was able to evaluate my food choices for the day and their nutritional impacts. It has been like doing a daily lab experiment where you are actually part of the experiment. There is no faster way to learn about nutrition.

After just two months I was able to derive most all of my nutritional needs just from the foods I ate, without supplements.

I no longer fear for my life. I have lost sixty-two pounds. I have gone from a size twenty to a size eight. I am no longer obese. I have more energy and my legs are not swollen. My stomach feels great and is getting flatter. My thinking is clearer. And, my hope for optimum health is restored because I know I can do this for life!

I am in the water again and hoping to be swimming

competitively soon. I feel much better about myself. I even let my daughter photograph me doing the butterfly stroke in the pool! I am also practicing yoga again and am more flexible than ever before. My mind is clear and focused. I love my eating and exercise habits. I love my life.

For those of you reading this who may have challenging life circumstances which rob your time, your energy, your sleep, and your peace of mind, you do not have to wait to make things better. I am the living proof that people in less-than-ideal conditions are still able to manage their bodies, achieve health, and a measure of happiness. You can do this!

MY PHYSICAL ACTIVITY

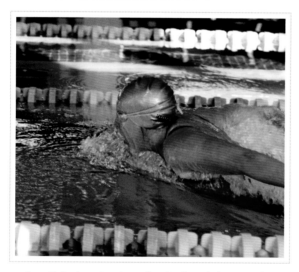

I love physical activities and exercise. My journey here at NutriMirror started with very little exercise and I still lost weight by logging my food. During the thirteenth week of food logging I returned to the pool to swim laps. I love to swim. I may return to Masters Swimming and competitions in the future. In the very short time back in the pool swimming, I have managed to increase my yardage up to two miles per training session. With balanced nutrition I feel healthy, strong and more flexible in the water. I add stretching and weights to my training as needed. Yoga is a must, I love yoga. It improves my swimming performance, flexibility, overall health, and well-being. I enjoy physical activity so when the opportunity arises I will participate in many other activities as well—walking, biking, dancing, skating, skiing, tennis, volleyball, etc.

CARRIE'S *GREEN* DAY

- Calories Expended: **2,148**
- Calories Eaten: **1,205**
- Net Calorie Balance: **943**

NutriMirror has made the challenge simple—just eat to get an all Green Day. The feedback I get is personal and accurate. I have the power to make food choices that affect my health. From the start, green days for me required managing portion sizes and being accountable for my nutrients (especially with getting sodium in check). Less sodium has also favorably impacted my fat scores and my calorie control. I am eating more veggies and fruits. As a result, I'm experiencing great benefits. I have become a more serous food label checker, especially where sodium is concerned—it's in everything. Achieving green days has become a new way to live life to me.

MY GREEN DAY NUTRITIONAL FACTS

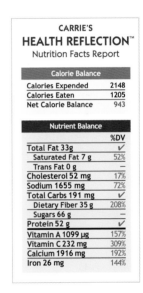

CARRIE'S
HEALTH REFLECTION™
Nutrition Facts Report

Calorie Balance	
Calories Expended	2148
Calories Eaten	1205
Net Calorie Balance	943

Nutrient Balance	
	%DV
Total Fat 33g	✔
Saturated Fat 7 g	52%
Trans Fat 0 g	–
Cholesterol 52 mg	17%
Sodium 1655 mg	72%
Total Carbs 191 mg	✔
Dietary Fiber 35 g	208%
Sugars 66 g	–
Protein 52 g	✔
Vitamin A 1099 µg	157%
Vitamin C 232 mg	309%
Calcium 1916 mg	192%
Iron 26 mg	144%

MY BREAKFAST–237 calories

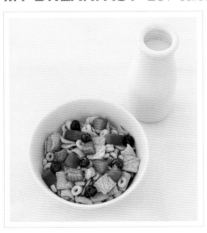

I begin almost every day with my "Red, White, and Blue Breakfast." It includes multigrain Cheerios with fresh blueberries and strawberries, usually with extra fruit. I add a bit of Benefiber and protein powder as well. For an extra boost of nutrition I will add goji berries.

MY RED, WHITE, AND BLUE BREAKFAST
- 1/2 cup multigrain Cheerios, 55 calories
- 12 blueberries, 10 calories
- 2 strawberries, 11 calories
- 6 oz. coffee, 2 calories
- 1/4 tsp. sugar, 4 calories
- 1 tsp. protein powder, 13 calories
- 1 tsp. Benefiber supplement, 7 calories
- 1/2 cup milk, skim, 40 calories
- 1/2 cup Cinnamon Crunch cereal, 95 calories

MY LUNCH–222 calories

For lunch I tried a "Mini Gyro" sandwich made with Morningstar sausage patties, whole wheat mini pita bread, cucumber, tomato, onion and a delicious cilantro & chive yogurt dip. I added red peppers and dill weed because I can. Yummy! On the side is pineapple, carrots and spinach. The spinach I toss in the microwave with a splash of water. Compare the 222 calories and good taste in this meal to a fast-food Gyro sandwich with fries…I dare you!

MINI GYRO SANDWICH WITH FRUIT AND VEGGIES

Mini Gyro Sandwich: 170 Calories
- 2 pieces mini pita bread, 52 calories
- Sausage patty, 79 calories
- 1 tbsp. cilantro & chive yogurt dip, 25 calories
- 1/2 oz. cucumber, 2 calories
- 1/4 oz. onions, 3 calories
- 1/2 oz. sweet red pepper, 3 calories
- 1 wedge red ripe tomato, 6 calories
- 1/8 tsp. dill weed, dried, 0 calories

Sides:
- 2.1 oz. pineapple, 29 calories
- 1.4 oz. carrots, 16 calories
- 1 cup spinach, 7 calories

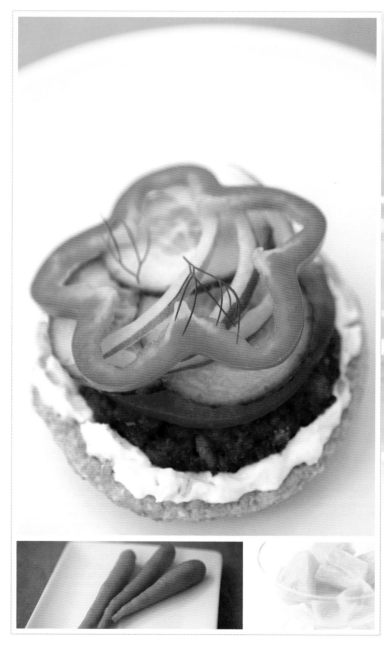

MY SNACKS–434 calories

With just 1,205 calories on this Green Day I still managed to eat some sweet treats and yummy snacks. Besides vanilla yogurt and crackers with avocado, I did enjoy one half of a Skinny Cow ice cream sandwich, carrot cake, and two chocolate orange sticks. I love snacks. There are so many delicious and nutritious snacks to choose from: fruits, veggies, nuts, yogurt, crackers, avocado, salsa, guacamole, hummus, PBJ, frozen treats, and chocolate. It's a genuine treat to have a Dark Chocolate Mocha Crunch Square from Trader Joe's knowing that all my nutritional needs have been met for the day!

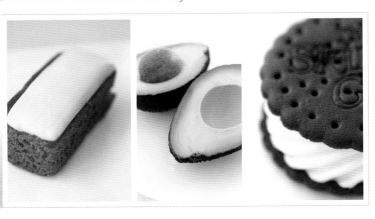

SNACKS
- 1.1 oz. avocado, 51 calories
- 2 chocolate orange candies, 75 calories
- 2 servings green tea, 0 calories
- 4 oz. vanilla yogurt, light, 70 calories
- 1/4 cup milk, nonfat, 20 calories
- Calcium + D supplement, 0 calories
- 8 All-Bran crackers, 58 calories
- 1/2 Skinny Cow ice cream sandwich, low fat, no sugar, 70 calories
- 1 serving carrot cake w/cream cheese icing, 90 calories

MY DINNER–312 calories

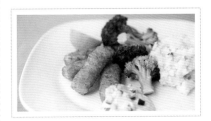

For only 312 calories this dinner is delicious. Before, I would have eaten a meal very similar to this but serving sizes were never measured. Who knows how many calories I used to consume? Obviously, it was too many. Now I know what my limits are and I stick to them.

FISH, POTATOES, BROCCOLI, AND SEASONING/TARTAR SAUCE
- 4 fish sticks, lightly breaded, reduced fat, 147 calories
- 1 cup broccoli, 54 calories
- 1/4 cup mashed potatoes, 55 calories
- 1/4 cup milk, nonfat, 20 calories

Homemade tartar sauce (1 serving)
- Pinch dill weed, 0 calories
- Pinch paprika, 1 calorie
- 1/4 tsp. parsley, 0 calories
- 1/3 tsp. lemon juice, 0 calories
- 1 tsp. mayonnaise, 30 calories
- 1/4 oz. cucumber, 1 calorie
- 1/4 tbsp. sweet pickle relish, 4 calories

"EVERY DAY I WAS TIRED AND THERE WAS LITTLE JOY IN MY DAILY GRIND."

username: ononnow / *first name:* Crystal / *location:* Upstate, NY

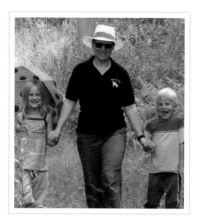

Crystal NOW: September '09 / age: 41
178 lbs. / BMI 28.6 / waist 32″

When I was younger, I was very strong and reasonably fit. I enjoyed running ten or fifteen miles on a regular basis. I was into biking, diving, hiking, and horseback riding. I didn't worry much about what I ate, and I enjoyed good health.

Due to a busy lifestyle, food during my pregnancies was very much grab-and-go. I had pizza frequently, as well as Taco Bell. I was good about getting my fruits and veggies in, but since I was eating for two, I also felt completely justified in eating as much junk food as I desired. At about five months into my first pregnancy, I was out for a run when my round ligament tore. That's the handy dandy ligament that holds the uterus in place. It tore pretty suddenly, and it hurt. This effectively put an end to my running for years to come. I now see that moment as the start of another phase in my life—the phase of ill health and health worries that only now am I finally conquering.

After I stopped running, I packed on the pregnancy pounds. I was miserable during the last two months of my two pregnancies. It seemed the only thing I could do was eat. I weighed 245 pounds before my son was born. I remember feeling as though death were right around the corner.

The next few years passed in a blur of finishing our home, working, caring for two young children, and moving to New York. I went on occasional diets and failed. I struggled with many illnesses.

I tried starvation, daytime fasts, no food after 6:00 p.m., Atkins, vegan, and a variety of "canned" meal recommendations from women's magazines. I joined Curves and I tried Weight Watchers. I joined some nutritional club down the road where I bought high protein shakes and bars. I kept a food diary and was regularly lectured on my failures. I failed repeatedly. Like everyone else, I'd go strong for a while, then give up and ravenously consume everything I had missed for the past week. Then I would hate myself for my gluttony.

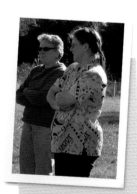

Crystal THEN: March '09
198 lbs. / BMI 31.8 / waist 36″

Everyone has his or her own reasons for failed diets. For me, I think it was pretty simple. Most of these diets assume I am an average woman with a daily requirement of 2,000 calories. On that basis, I'm usually allocated a daily intake of somewhere between 1,000 to 1,500 calories depending upon the speed the dietitians think I should lose weight. I am NOT an average woman with a daily requirement of 2,000. My calorie requirements range from 2,300 to 2,800, depending on exercise. Since we are always told to exercise while we diet, I did, with gusto. So I would go into diets all fired up, but with 1,000 + daily calorie deficits, I was bound for failure.

Starting about a year ago, I had more and more frequent and severe illnesses. Weighing was too upsetting, so I quit worrying about the scale.

When my breathing became progressively worse in January of 2009, I blamed it on anemia and a cold. It lingered like all the other illnesses. Finally, I collapsed trying to carry my son up the stairs. I was so afraid I was heading for an early grave.

Every day I was tired, and there was little joy in my daily grind. I was just trying to survive. I have lived a pretty long and very interesting life, so dying didn't seem so dreadful to me. But I couldn't stand the thought of my kids losing their mother. They need to have their mother alive and as healthy as possible.

I started going to doctors for diagnoses. Multiple tests were conducted. By March of 2009, we knew I was anemic with walking pneumonia and asthma, and I was early hypertensive even though my heart function appeared to be within normal limits. I had three courses of antibiotics, and I still wasn't better. I was scared. I stepped on the scale and weighed 198 pounds. I remembered the most successful program I ever did involved a food diary, so I looked online for one. NutriMirror was free. The price was right!

Before I started logging, I thought that all of my nutritional needs were being met, and that I had a healthy, balanced diet. After all, I ate plenty of fruits and vegetables, and exercised a fair amount. I ate meat sparingly. I only ate whole grain breads and cereals. I rarely indulged in fast foods and assumed I was eating right. I was in for a shocker. I learned that not only was I consuming far more calories than could possibly be burned off in even the most active of days. I also learned that I was getting too much fat and sodium, not enough iron, and frequently not enough calcium or vitamin A.

With the measured feedback I get from NutriMirror I've changed all of that. I track everything and have lost twenty pounds. My blood pressure is normal and the anemia is almost resolved. My pneumonia and asthma are gone and I have dropped two pant sizes. I can breathe, I am sleeping better, and I feel great. I can carry my son to bed at night, and I can run. I needed to eat better, smarter. However, without the necessary nutritional feedback that I needed I was unprepared to do it alone.

I am just another cyclical dieter. I am an overweight woman who has been struggling to lose weight and find balance for years. I know I will never be in that pit again, because as long as I log my choices daily, I will be able to avoid the pitfalls long before they become a reality. I plan to live a long healthy life and enjoy my kids and their kids.

MY PHYSICAL ACTIVITY

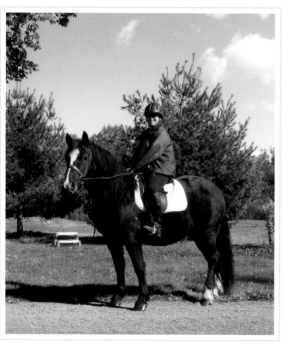

I am lucky to be one of those irritating people who literally LOVES to exercise. Running, horseback riding, biking, hiking, climbing, diving, swimming, skiing, snowshoeing, windsurfing—you name it, I do it. I have always loved almost all forms of outdoor sports, which is probably why I wasn't morbidly obese. The trouble with being just obese, however, is that it deters from one's ability to move. And that was a real drag for me.

Currently, I hike on our trails for thirty to sixty minutes on most days, I run cross country once a week, and I am training a young horse under saddle regularly. In addition, I do a large amount of heavy work around our small farm, bucking hay and cleaning the barn, etc., and I am an active mother who runs around with two kids, keeps house, and works outside the home as a veterinarian.

CRYSTAL'S *GREEN* DAY

- Calories Expended: **2,600**
- Calories Eaten: **2,173**
- Net Calorie Balance: **427**

I discovered after beginning Nutrimirror that I was consistently deficient in calcium and iron, and also that my sodium and fat levels were inordinantly high. Even meals that I used to think were healthy turned out to be very high in fat and sodium due to dressings, cheese, noodles and such.

I have steadily improved my food choices, choosing one goal every few weeks to "fix." At this point, I eat the breakfast, lunch and snacks in my Green Day on a regular basis. I try to vary my dinners quite a bit. The dinner here is unusual for me, as I eat red meat no more than once a week, but it was yummy so I decided to share it. And the meat was hormone and antibiotic free and humanely raised, thank you very much!

MY GREEN DAY NUTRITIONAL FACTS

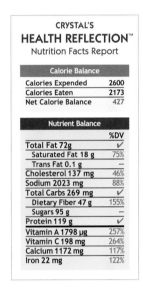

CRYSTAL'S
HEALTH REFLECTION™
Nutrition Facts Report

Calorie Balance	
Calories Expended	2600
Calories Eaten	2173
Net Calorie Balance	427

Nutrient Balance	
	%DV
Total Fat 72g	✔
Saturated Fat 18 g	75%
Trans Fat 0.1 g	—
Cholesterol 137 mg	46%
Sodium 2023 mg	88%
Total Carbs 269 mg	✔
Dietary Fiber 47 g	155%
Sugars 95 g	—
Protein 119 g	✔
Vitamin A 1798 µg	257%
Vitamin C 198 mg	264%
Calcium 1172 mg	117%
Iron 22 mg	122%

MY BREAKFAST–470 calories

This is by far my most common breakfast these days. As you can see, my "goop" is low fat, high fiber, and filled with nutrients. It is easy to make. I drink my coffee (okay, this isn't healthy, but I need it) first, and over the next one to two hours I take a bite here and there of breakfast. It has real staying power, and lasts me past lunch if there are too many emergencies for me to get to eat on time. I feel virtuous eating it in front of my colleagues, but I actually take huge enjoyment in every bite.

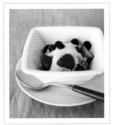

MY GOOP AND COFFEE
- 1 serving oatmeal, 150 calories
- 1 serving peach yogurt, nonfat, 140 calories
- 1 1/4 cups berry medley (strawberries, blackberries, blueberries, raspberries), 88 calories
- 26 oz. coffee, 14 calories
- 1 tbsp. light cream, 29 calories
- 1 tbsp. sugar, 49 calories

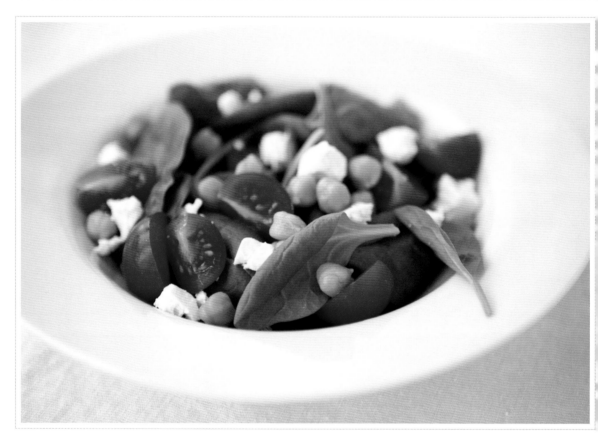

MY LUNCH–277 calories

I eat this meal at least three times a week. I bring the ingredients in separate containers and throw them together at work. I have found that I don't need dressing on this quick and healthy salad, but occasionally I'll squirt on a little lemon juice, chop in an olive or two, or sprinkle with some sesame seeds. It is so versatile, and although not as filling as breakfast, it takes a long time to eat and tastes great.

MY GO-TO SALAD
- 2 cups spinach, fresh, 15 calories
- 2 small red ripe tomatoes, 32 calories
- 1/2 cup chickpeas (garbanzo beans), 134 calories
- 1/3 cup feta cheese, reduced fat, 96 calories

MY SNACKS–737 calories

This is another menu I have created and eat regularly. I bring everything to work with me, washed, cut, and ready to go. Whenever I am hungry, I have something tasty to munch on. And the littles cubes of dark chocolate are scattered throughout the day and give me a quick pick-me-up. It's hard to feel deprived when one eats chocolate on a regular basis.

LOTS OF FLAVORS
- 14 Triscuit crackers, whole grain, reduced fat, 240 calories
- 2 tbsp. artichoke-spinach hummus, 70 calories
- Dark, bittersweet chocolate, 192 calories
- Carrot, 30 calories
- 2 stalks celery, 11 calories
- 1 tbsp. pumpkin/squash seeds, roasted, unsalted, 74 calories
- 2 oz. cheddar cheese, reduced fat, 120 calories

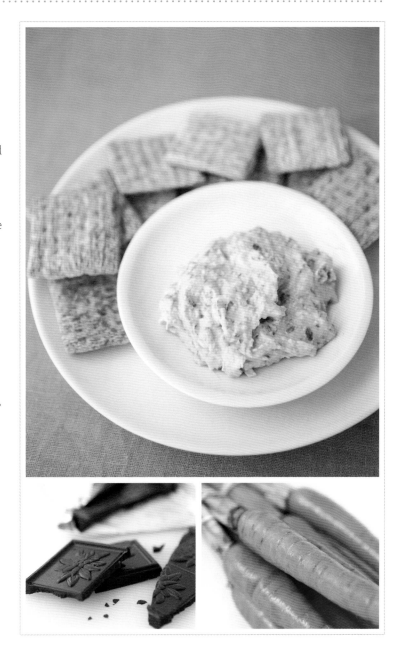

MY DINNER–689 calories

Dinner is the one meal that I vary widely. On my days off, I will experiment with new recipes. I used to go just for taste, but now I try hard to focus on nutritional value as well as taste. I usually have a dessert after dinner, and this is frequently a Skinny Cow product. This particular meal was great—fresh baby zucchini sprinkled with low fat Italian dressing, some steamed broccoli, a lovely roasted potato with smart butter, and a little medium-rare steak. The juice from the steak gave added flavor to the veggies. A perfect meal at the end of a long day.

STEAK, VEGGIES, AND DESSERT
- 1 tbsp. Italian dressing, reduced fat, 11 calories
- 1 tbsp. buttery spread (Smart Balance), 85 calories
- 2 spears broccoli, 38 calories
- 1 small zucchini, 19 calories
- 1 baked potato, medium, 161 calories
- 4 oz. New York strip steak, 235 calories
- Ice cream sandwich, low fat, 140 calories

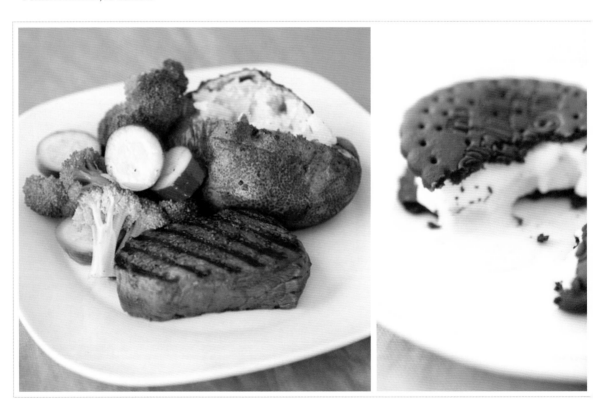

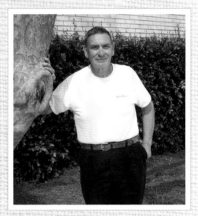

Andy NOW: November '09 / age: 64
212 lbs. / BMI 27.2

. . . .

It was late March, 2009, and I felt old. My sixty-fourth birthday was approaching and yet I felt like I was eighty. My knees hurt when I walked, my breath came in gasps at the least bit of exertion, and I had absolutely no energy. I knew what the problem was—I was fat! I could have been kind to myself and said large framed or big boned but the truth of the matter is that I was fat. My cholesterol was high, my blood pressure was high and my self-esteem low! I weighed in at just over 260 pounds and felt every one of them. I had stopped smoking about a year and a half before (about the only good thing I had done for my health) and gradually added pounds to replace nicotine.

I was finally convinced that I had to change or die. When I looked at it that way the choice was pretty obvious. I started looking for a diet. I looked at almost every single plan that there was and realized that I had done them all before: high protein, low carb, Eastern, Western, Mediterranean, low fat, fruit—not a single thing that was new. I searched the internet for food logs and found NutriMirror.

The site offered a "free" food journal, talked about lifetime weight control and nutritional balance, and was well laid out. It seemed easy to use so I joined.

I started logging what I was eating. I added my statistics and measurements, and saw my BMI (Body Mass Index) for the first time. I also saw exactly and immediately what the food choices I was making were doing for (and to) my health. The tools offered by the site were some of the most comprehensive I had seen. I logged for a few days and was hooked. I started making choices that were better for my health and my nutrition. Gradually, which everyone says is the best way to do it, I started to lose weight. My food choices improved as I learned what was best for me and how to "Go for the Green."

In five months I lost thirty-eight pounds and twelve inches from my waist. My cholesterol and blood pressure are now within normal ranges without medication and I feel better than I have in ages. I walk three to four miles on a daily basis and have even started jogging again. The biggest change, however, has been in the positive approach that I now take to each day. I enjoy getting up in anticipation of what the future holds for me.

. . . .

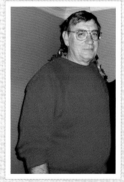

Andy THEN: April '09
. . . .
261 lbs. / BMI 33.5

"I PURPOSELY TOOK THE WORDS *TRY* AND *HOPE* OUT OF MY VOCABULARY."

username: deeishealthy / *first name:* Dee / *location:* Maple Ridge, BC Canada

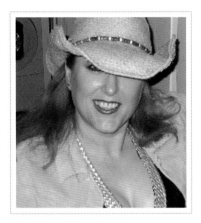

Dee NOW: August '09 / age: 41
153 lbs. / BMI 28 / waist 33″

I've never ever been a yo-yo dieter. I had never tried losing weight, and was always very happy in my own skin. What bothered me at 5′2″ and 208 pounds was that I could feel my neck when I was lying down. I wore size 22 pants. When I went shopping, I had to make sure they had an elastic waist in case I got, yep, fatter. Shame finally hit me when I was diagnosed with fatty liver disease. I couldn't even bring myself to tell my husband. I mean, after all, if he knew I had FLD, he'd know I was fat. The HORROR!! My sister lovingly referred me to a weight loss program that had been successful for her. She had done the program successfully and knew that it would be a fit for me. I decided I would do it. I followed that program and ate within its guidelines. I was eating clean. Over a two year period I lost sixty-three pounds. I did it slowly, and I did it smartly. And I did it my way.

I purposefully took the words *try* and *hope* out of my vocabulary. I didn't try to lose weight, and I didn't hope I could do it. I firmly believe that when you use those words, you are giving yourself permission to fail. I decided that I was accountable and responsible for my decisions and actions, no matter what they were.

One thing that worked well for me (not advocated by anybody) is that I took off one day a week from the program. When I drove by McDonald's on Wednesday and craved a Big Mac, I'd promise myself that if I still wanted it on Sunday, I'd have it. Every Sunday during that first year I was enjoying that Big Mac!

I noticed my taste buds started changing. I'll never forget the last time I had fish and chips. It was not worth it to me to consume all those calories only to feel disgusted and sick to my stomach afterwards. A similar thing happened with movie popcorn.

My body felt healthier eating clean. My skin, hair, and nails, and everything else, were healthier. I lost forty pounds during the first year, and twenty-three more the second year.

I began tracking my food on homemade Excel sheets. I could no longer afford to pay for the

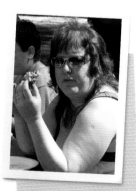

Dee THEN: Feburary '07
208 lbs. / BMI 38 / waist 45″

program I had been using, but I needed to stay accountable for everything I put in my mouth. I tried not tracking, and just relied on my body to tell me when I was satisfied. But that remained a struggle that I just couldn't win.

I started really noticing how different foods were affecting my body. At 208 pounds, not much seemed to affect me. But at 147 pounds, a cup of coffee at 8 P.M. and I'd be up all night. Sodium bloated me. I started reading online forums and shadowing blogs. I could see common themes and threads. There seemed to be more to this eating thing than just weight. People watched levels. I began searching for a free program because I could afford free.

I used online search engines. I tried four different programs. They were all good, but they each lacked something that I was looking for. I would get settled and into a new program, when a new (or, I should say, new to me) focus was introduced. I began to realize that there is more to eating healthy than I knew. There's this thing called "balance." I didn't know how people managed to eat a balanced diet.

While browsing the Diet Forum on Craigslist, I saw a mention of NutriMirror. I Googled it and found our beloved website. (Insert choir music here.) I took the time to go through the tutorial. Wow. I was impressed. It seemed to cover everything. But then, so had the others. I had invested hours and hours in the others but had not been satisfied.

I have been with NutriMirror for eight months as of this writing. It has every single feature that I need. Nothing is missing.

Since using this site, my doctor has told me that I'm done with my weight loss journey. I wanted to be healthy, and I am achieving it.

Nothing is scarier than being told you are done. For two years, I had been successful, but was afraid of maintenance. People fail on maintenance, but I have NutriMirror which continues to help and guide me. I simply adjusted my goals so they didn't include losing weight. My calories were all adjusted for me. I budget my food to reflect "green" in all the categories. I exercise to earn more calories if I want to indulge. Nothing has really changed except that I have more room to juggle all my good clean nutritious choices. I am not done. I have to track my intake for the rest of my life. That is my reality. The good news is that with NutriMirror, I am not only tracking my food, I'm educating myself, too. Using NutriMirror, I know that my body is as healthy as I can make it.

I set exercise goals, and I meet them. I plan and stay within my calorie budget, and I shoot for green daily (98% of the time). If I do indulge and reflect "red" on any given day, I know I can look to my Home Page long-term trend scoring to learn if I'm still in balance. Focusing on the long-term balance trend keeps me from being crazy with my choices on any single day. I'm not perfect, but I know that I'm living a healthy lifestyle.

MY PHYSICAL ACTIVITY

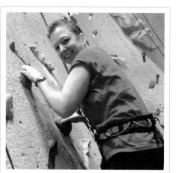

In my world, exercise is a bad word. Always has been. But sadly (for me) in order to get to and to maintain a healthy, happy body, exercise is necessary.

I started out with walking around the block three times a week. It took me thirty-five minutes and pretty much almost killed me. I signed up for a Vancouver Sun Run, which is a 10km run, and did a "couch to ten kilometer" training module.

I discovered that I need variety. An exercise session that I enjoy today, I will dread next week. However, this has led to an active lifestyle that allows me to do such things as knee boarding and hiking on a regular basis. And, occasionally, you can even find me wall climbing. These are things I couldn't do when I was unhealthy. NutriMirror shows me the fuel I need to consume after exercising, and has taught me what works and does not work for my body.

DEE'S *GREEN* DAY

- Calories Expended: **2,096**
- Calories Eaten: **1,678**
- Net Calorie Balance: 418

Green days are so GREAT! When I turn off my computer at the end of the day, with my account all in the green, I feel like I have accomplished something wonderful. And I have. I've accomplished taking care of ME. I've done the very best I can on this day to ensure that I remain healthy and have longevity. By being green I am giving myself a wondrous gift—a life that is happy and worth living. In this new life I can do anything I set my mind to, without the physical limitations of being unhealthy. How great is that?

MY GREEN DAY NUTRITIONAL FACTS

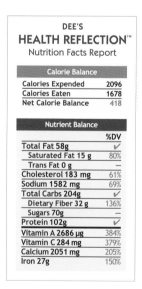

DEE'S
HEALTH REFLECTION™
Nutrition Facts Report

Calorie Balance	
Calories Expended	2096
Calories Eaten	1678
Net Calorie Balance	418

Nutrient Balance	
	%DV
Total Fat 58g	✔
Saturated Fat 15 g	80%
Trans Fat 0 g	—
Cholesterol 183 mg	61%
Sodium 1582 mg	69%
Total Carbs 204g	✔
Dietary Fiber 32 g	136%
Sugars 70g	—
Protein 102g	✔
Vitamin A 2686 µg	384%
Vitamin C 284 mg	379%
Calcium 2051 mg	205%
Iron 27g	150%

MY BREAKFAST –393 calories

I always start my day with a healthy breakfast. It revs my body up and prepares me for a healthy day. When I start the day off right, I tend to continue it that way. I lean towards something fairly heavy that will sustain me for a few hours until lunch. Oatmeal is one I turn to a lot. Egg white omelets are another favorite. As long as it's healthy and tasty, I'm a happy lady!

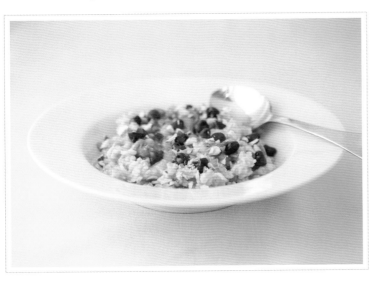

CEREAL WITH MILK AND FRUIT, NUTS AND VITAMINS
- 1/3 cup porridge oats (oat flakes, oat bran, wheat bran, flax), 120 calories
- 2 tbsp. craisins, sweetened, 16 calories
- 1 tbsp. almonds, 31 calories
- 1 cup milk, nonfat, 86 calories
- 1/4 banana, 26 calories
- B-50 with choline and Inositol, 0 calories
- Calcium with vitamin D, 0 calories
- 1 tbsp. PB2 powdered peanut butter, 27 calories
- 1/3 cup Almond Breeze beverage, unsweetened, 13 calories
- Salmon & fish oil blend, 40 calories
- One-A-Day women's vitamin, 0 calories
- 1 tbsp. chocolate chips, 34 calories

MY SNACKS
–455 calories

I live for snacks. I was never a snacker in my former life. Oh, except for those middle-of-the-night forages into the fridge. Now I have afternoon snacks to hold me over to dinner. Most of the time they are healthy, but once in a while I indulge in a treat. Ordering a special coffee from Starbucks and allowing the calories for a cookie… that's a super indulgence. It's these little pleasures that make the journey sustainable. I have treats and still manage a completely Green Day!

STARBUCKS AND COOKIE
- Starbucks' Grande Skinny Caramel Café Americano Misto, 55 calories
- Molasses cookie, 400 calories

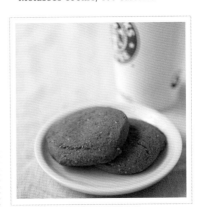

MY LUNCH–309 calories

By the time lunch hits, my breakfast has worn off and I am hungry. I often used to eat fast-food for lunch. Now I find that a half sandwich and some carrot sticks satisfy me and keep me full longer than a burger and fries (which is twice as much food!) does. The secret is marvelous bread, full of fiber. It amazes me how eating healthy fuels the body!

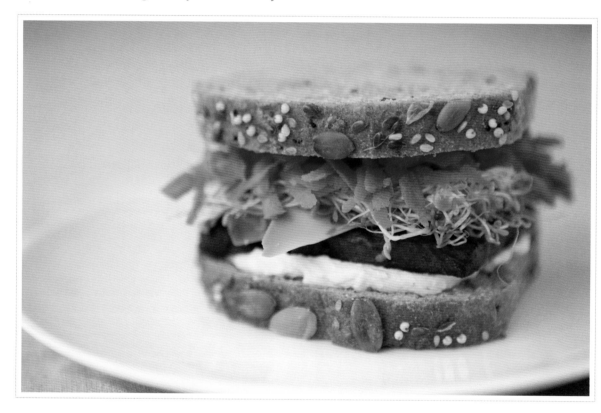

SANDWICH WITH TOFU, CREAM CHEESE, AND VEGETABLES
- 1/4 avocado, 80 calories
- 1/2 oz. alfalfa seeds, sprouted, 5 calories
- 1 cup carrots, 52 calories
- 1 tsp. cream cheese, nonfat, 5 calories
- 1.4 oz. tofu, organic, extra firm, 47 calories
- 1 piece flax bread, whole grain, 120 calories

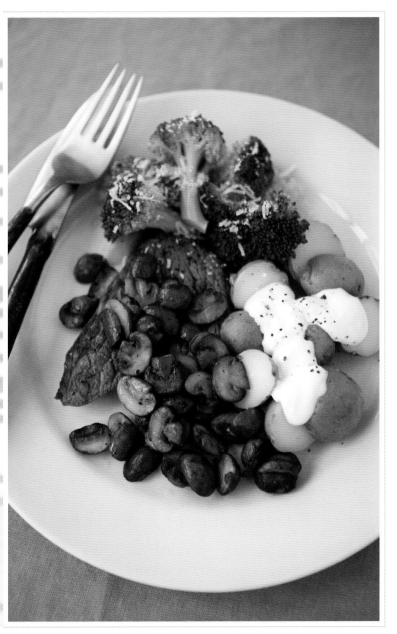

MY DINNER
−521 calories

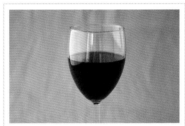

Dinner for me is always the biggest meal of the day. I've read that lunch actually should be, but I just can't seem to break my mind and body into accepting that. Dinner needs to be satisfying and filling. And it has to be lean meat accompanied by good quality, nutrient-rich vegetables, or else I feel deprived. What I've learned though, is that it doesn't have to be swimming in gravy or sauces! Food actually has great flavour if you don't smother it.

MEAT, SALAD, VEGETABLES, YOGURT, POTATOES, AND WINE

- 2 TBL plain yogurt, 16 calories
- 2 cups broccoli, cooked, 109 calories
- 3 large mushrooms, fresh, 15 calories
- 5 oz. beef round, broiled, 270 calories
- 1 oz. red wine, 25 calories
- 1 tbsp. Romano cheese, shredded, 18 calories
- 5 oz. baby new potatoes, fresh, 68 calories

"I'VE DISCOVERED LATE IN LIFE THAT I AM A FIGHTER. AND MY ENEMY IS FATHER TIME."

username: Gouldthorp / *first name:* David / *location:* Eastern Tennessee

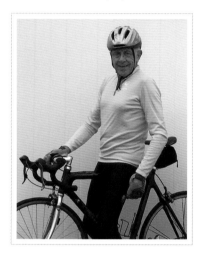

David NOW: July '09 / age: 65
145 lbs. / BMI 22.4 / waist 33˝

I have another oxymoron to add to the likes of Military Intelligence and Jumbo Shrimp: Aging Gracefully.

There's nothing graceful about the body's process of gradual decay. Things stop working, stuff wears out. Bits and pieces droop and sag. Some parts eventually just fall off or get misplaced, like my memory. But it seems that as much as we want to postpone this process of decay for as long as possible, the modern world doesn't necessarily want to go along.

I remember the exact day I turned forty-nine years and 358 days old. How come? That was the day an unsolicited AARP membership kit dropped into my mailbox. Had the Age Police ratted me out? I was horrified; mortified even. My son was amused. "Hey Dad," he beamed, full of teenage testosterone and know-it-all-ness, "you're gonna hit the big five-oh in a week. Man, that's *old*."

Old? Fifty was the new thirty, wasn't it? I ran. I cycled. I coached track and cross-country at the local high school. I ate healthy and I even took aerobics classes. Old? I thought I was the poster boy for middle age, for Heaven's sake. I was cool. I was hot, dig?

But not for too much longer, sad to say, because it *happened*. I can't say exactly how, where or when it happened, but it *happened*—a missed run, a shortened bike ride, a skipped workout, chili-cheese fries, cans of Coke, beer in front of the television, an imperfect spinal

fusion and, worst of all, for shame, I fell off the nicotine wagon. In short, over the course of a dozen short years, my get up and go simply got up and went.

Fast forward to my first day of retirement, which was truly superb: the alarm did *not* go off at 4:00 A.M., I finished my second cup of coffee in the early morning sun on my deck before tending to my small vegetable patch. Lunch was leisurely with a glass of wine followed by a long overdue nap and supper, a repeat of lunch. I remember thinking contentedly, "So this is retirement." Six months later

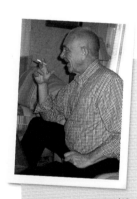

David THEN: November '08
170 lbs. / BMI 27.0 / waist 38˝

my thinking was, "So *this* is retirement?" I was bored stiff, unmotivated, and feeling like the end was at hand.

The hours were becoming increasingly more difficult to fill, but I love to cook and I love to eat; so I cooked and I ate. And ate. I didn't consider myself particularly overweight—a little gravitationally challenged perhaps or equatorially expansive maybe. But fat? No.

Then something happened which changed my thinking in a hurry—one day I foolishly decided on the spur of the moment to go for a long bike ride just like I did in the old (read: slim, fit, younger, non-smoking) days. I didn't even make it up the gentle slope out of the parking lot. I was crushed. Reality won. I had to face it; I was fat.

On the drive home, I decided that some 'C' change was needed in my life. But where to go? Where to start? Over time, my only source of exercise had become long periods of wandering aimlessly around the Internet. And then, one day, either through Divine Intervention or an accidental mouse click, I found a site that determines an individual's virtual physical age and calculates their life expectancy based on their lifestyle—just what the doctor ordered, if you'll pardon the pun. So what the heck—just click on the little boxes, right? Smoke? Check. Drink? Check. Exercise? Nyet. Lifestyle? Couch potato. Outlook? Grim. Etcetera, etcetara, etcetera. Press [Enter] and *what????* Virtual age: plus fifteen. Life expectancy: less than five years. I couldn't believe my eyes. Sixty's the new forty, right? With all of the recent advances in medicine, I was still (technically) in my prime, right? Life expectancy was increasing, right? Well, I guess for me, the answers were: wrong, wrong and (almost dead) wrong.

I sat at my computer trying to wrap my mind around this pending death sentence—one which, if I'd have been paying even the slightest bit of attention, would not have come as a complete surprise.

Was it too late to lose some weight, quit smoking, get back in shape, live healthy, and maybe find peace with my inner demons? No it wasn't too late. Let me restate that; *hell no*, it wasn't too late.

I don't remember what I Googled but the top search result was NutriMirror and the rest is history. While logging my food intakes was easy, the process made me painfully aware of the necessity to change my lifestyle from "I cook therefore I must eat" to "I eat therefore I must cook." And, I have to add, "and exercise."

I thought the gym at the local Seniors' Center would be an ideal place to start, but boy was I wrong. Normally, when I greet someone and ask, "How are you?" I expect the reply, "Fine." I do not, repeat, do not want to know about the problems you're having with Medicare over reimbursement for your pacemaker batteries. I know you love your wife, but come on, fella, some things should be kept private and no, I don't want to read your newspaper clipping about the latest advances in hemorrhoid surgery.

Eventually, as a group, they wore me out—drained me flatter than a flashlight left on in a kitchen drawer. I needed to move on and eventually found a gym that, while offering special rates to the long-in-the-tooth group, didn't offer special treatment in their workouts. It's a lean, mean, get-sweaty-or-go-home kind of place. I love the attitude there and, even better, I love that it works!

Exercising on a regular basis, combined with the tools that NutriMirror provides has given me a new lease on life—my weight is down twenty-five pounds, my cholesterol is down from the mid-200s to 156, my resting heart rate has dropped from 72 to 40 beats per minute, and best of all, I finally went on that long bike ride and made it all the way.

So what's next for this old Boomer? Who knows? I'm a walking, talking work in progress, truly happy in my skin and eager to turn the page on the next chapter of this very special journey.

I am determined that I will not bow willingly to the ravages of time. I will not age gracefully. I will age defiantly. I will not go out with a tube up my nose or a monitor beeping in my ear. No. I want to be remembered for when my parachute doesn't open, sky-diving on my hundredth birthday. Or maybe getting shot in the rear by some other old geezer for making goo-goo eyes at his moll at the Tuesday afternoon bingo game.

Even better, maybe I'll just wait for the nurses to eject me from the Shady Pines Nursing Home for putting whoopee cushions under all the chairs in the television room, and simply expire from an excess of glee.

I've discovered, late in life, that I'm a fighter. And my enemy is Father Time. I will look him in the eye until, knowing that he will never blink, I must submit, but not a moment before I have to.

It's said that a person doesn't die as long as their name or words are spoken down through time. And so, for as long as someone, anyone, passes on to another my belief that there is no such thing as aging gracefully, then my journey will surely have been worth it.

Do I hear an "Amen?"

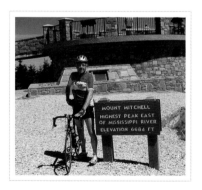

MY PHYSICAL ACTIVITY

My only 'before' exercise was frequent trips from my couch to the refrigerator. Now, I take a spin class at my local gym four or five times a week. A one hour, high intensity class burns around 1,000 calories. Additionally I'm fortunate enough to live reasonably close to the Blue Ridge Parkway, so when the weather forecast is good, I cycle to the summit of Mount Mitchell, the highest point in the East. It's a forty-two-mile round trip that burns around 2,500 calories. The breathtaking views from the summit as well as the enormous sense of accomplishment make this my perfect day out.

DAVID'S *GREEN* DAY

- Calories Expended: **2,637**
- Calories Eaten: **2,184**
- Net Calorie Balance: **453**

While retirement was a welcome change to almost fifty years of work, the one-two punches of a complete lack of exercise and my love of cooking (and eating) had me down for the count at over 170 pounds. My journey back to overall well-being, while not always easy, has been simple—the combination of a regular exercise regimen and well thought-out food choices.

I'm careful to monitor my daily exercise energy expenditure as well as everything that I eat. With the aid of NutriMirror, keeping these two variables in balance has helped me attain my weight goal of 145 pounds.

The meals and snacks that I now consume are balanced, healthy, and, most importantly, highly enjoyable.

MY GREEN DAY NUTRITIONAL FACTS

DAVID'S
HEALTH REFLECTION™
Nutrition Facts Report

Calorie Balance	
Calories Expended	2637
Calories Eaten	2184
Net Calorie Balance	453

Nutrient Balance	
	%DV
Total Fat 55g	✔
Saturated Fat 15 g	62%
Trans Fat 0 g	—
Cholesterol 141 mg	47%
Sodium 2007 mg	87%
Total Carbs 337g	✔
Dietary Fiber 41 g	134%
Sugars 137g	—
Protein 103g	✔
Vitamin A 2148 µg	239%
Vitamin C 387 mg	430%
Calcium 2454 mg	205%
Iron 60 mg	750%

MY BREAKFAST–336 calories

Breakfast used to be an Egg McMuffin (sometimes two) or something equally lethal from one of the local fast-food outlets, accompanied by a deep-fried side dish. NutriMirror quickly made me realize that the saturated fat, sodium, and cholesterol content of a meal such as that were not doing me any nutritional good whatsoever. Now, I typically start my day with some simple cereal and reduced fat milk. The bulk of the Grape-Nuts keeps me full until lunch time.

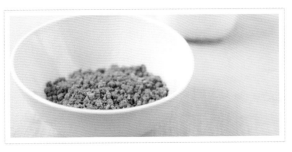

CEREAL WITH MILK AND VITAMINS
- 3/4 cup milk, reduced fat, 103 calories
- 1/2 cup Grape-Nuts cereal, 200 calories
- 2 tsp. sugar, 33 calories
- OneSource supplement, 0 calories
- Calcium 600 + D, 2, 0 calories

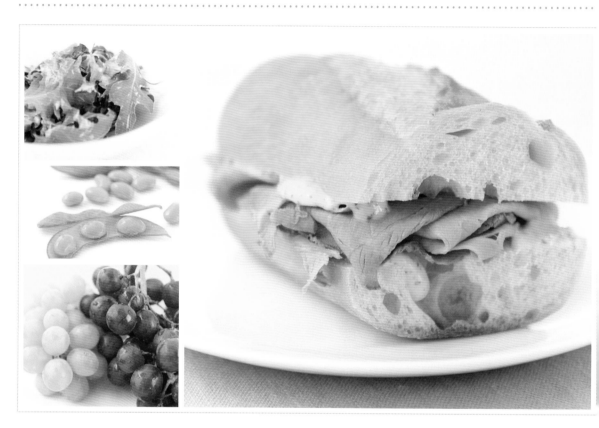

MY LUNCH–915 calories

Lunch is now my main meal of the day—a well-balanced combination of nutritious foods necessary to fuel me through my late afternoon spinning workout without 'hitting the wall' or feeling too full. The crustiness and texture of my home-baked artisan bread has a wonderful chewiness; it's quick, easy to prepare, and leaves supermarket baked products in the dust.

SANDWICH, SALAD WITH DRESSING, AND FRUIT
- 2 oz. roast beef, 80 calories
- 1 tsp. horseradish, 2 calories
- 3/4 tbsp. margarine, made with yogurt, 34 calories
- 2 pieces artisan bread (see recipe), 126 calories
- 25 grapes, 86 calories
- 2 oranges, 173 calories
- 1 cup soybeans (edamame), cooked, 254 calories
- 1 tbsp. blue cheese dressing, 40 calories
- Side salad, 120 calories

ARTISAN BREAD

Adapted from Jeff Hertzberg and Zoë François' Artisan Bread in Five Minutes A Day. Makes six small loaves, or can be formed into a round loaf or Italian bread shape and baked on a pizza stone. I also use it for pizza crust.

INGREDIENTS

3 cups lukewarm water (about 100°F)
1 1/2 tbsp. granulated yeast (2 packets)
1 1/2 tsp. kosher salt
6 1/2 cups unbleached all-purpose flour, plus a little extra for dusting
Sprinkle of cornmeal

PREPARATION

1. In a large, resealable plastic container, mix the yeast and salt into the water. Using a large spoon, stir in the flour until the mixture is uniformly moist with no dry patches. Do not knead. The dough will be wet and loose enough to conform to the shape of the container. Cover, but not with an airtight lid.

2. Rest the dough at room temperature. It should rise until it begins to flatten on top or collapse (2–5 hours). At this point, the dough can be refrigerated up to 2 weeks. Refrigerated dough is easier to work with than room temperature dough, so the authors recommend that first-time bakers refrigerate the dough for at least 3 hours, or preferably overnight.

3. When ready to bake, sprinkle cornmeal on a pizza peel. Place a broiler pan on the bottom rack of the oven. Place a baking stone on the middle rack, and preheat the oven to 450°F, heating the stone for at least 20 minutes.

4. Sprinkle a little flour on the dough and on your hands. Pull the dough up and use a serrated knife to cut off a grapefruit-sized piece (about 1 pound). Working for 30–60 seconds, turn the dough in your hands, gently stretching the surface of the dough, rotating the ball a quarter turn as you go to create a rounded top and bunched bottom. As you work the dough, add flour as needed to keep your hands from sticking. Most of this dusting should fall off and not be incorporated into the dough.

5. Place the shaped dough on the prepared pizza peel and let it rest, uncovered, for 40 minutes. Repeat with the remaining dough or refrigerate it in lidded containers. (Even a single day's storage improves the texture and flavor of the bread. The dough can also be frozen in one-pound portions in airtight containers, and defrosted overnight in the refrigerator prior to baking day.)

6. Using a serrated knife, slash the top of the dough in three parallel, 1/4-inch deep cuts (or in a tic-tac-toe pattern). Slide the dough onto the preheated baking stone. Pour one cup of hot tap water into the broiler pan and quickly close the oven door to trap the steam. Bake until the crust is well-browned and firm to the touch, about 30 minutes. Remove from the oven to a wire rack and cool completely.

MY DINNER–483 calories

After a good workout it's time to recharge the batteries, and a plate of Moroccan lamb is just the ticket. Lamb is a wonderful, tasty alternative to beef and when properly trimmed, it's lower in fat too. The cumin and cinnamon add an Eastern undertone to the dish and the crushed dried chilies add a little heat. Of course, if you like it hot, go ahead with the chili jar and shake, shake, shake!

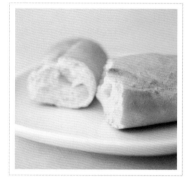

LAMB, BREAD WITH SPREAD
- 1 serving Moroccan lamb (see recipe), 323 calories
- 3/4 tbsp. margarine, made with yogurt, 34 calories
- 2 pieces artisan bread (see recipe), 126 calories

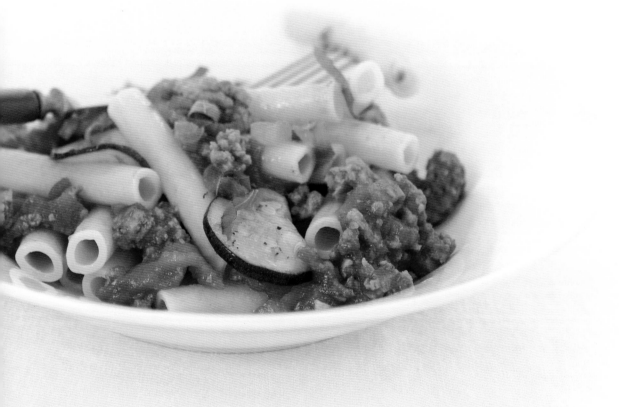

MOROCCAN LAMB

This recipe was adapted from a page torn from an old magazine, possibly Ladies Home Journal. It looks a little challenging, but if you have the spices on hand it isn't any more complicated than making a spaghetti sauce with ground hamburger. Leftovers (if any!) store well in the fridge for a couple of days. Makes five servings.

INGREDIENTS

2 tsp. oil
1 small onion, chopped
15 oz. ground lamb
1 clove garlic, chopped
1/4 tsp. red pepper flakes
1 tsp. cumin
1/8 tsp. cinnamon
1 can unsalted stewed tomatoes
4 oz. dried pasta
1 medium zucchini, peeled and sliced
Sprig of fresh mint, chopped

PREPARATION

1. Heat water for pasta, bringing it to a boil as you follow steps 2 through 5.
2. Meanwhile, heat the oil in a separate skillet.
3. Add the chopped onion to the skillet and cook for 2 minutes.
4. Add the ground lamb to the onions and cook until the juices run clear (about 5 minutes). Drain the fat.
5. Add the garlic, red pepper, cumin, and cinnamon to the lamb mixture. Cook for 15 seconds, then add the stewed tomatoes. Simmer gently, stirring occasionally.
6. Add the pasta to the boiling water.
7. When pasta has about four minutes remaining, add the zucchini to the lamb mixture.
8. Drain the pasta when it's ready, stir in the chopped mint, and toss with the lamb and zucchini mixture.

MY SNACKS
−450 calories

The well-balanced meals that I enjoy during the day keep my energy levels high and stop my stomach constantly complaining that it's being ignored. Gone are the Snickers bars, chips, sodas, and endless evening round-trips to the snack cupboard. An apple is not only a good source of fiber; it also keeps the hunger pangs at bay. And if I still have the "nibblies," I find that a 100-calorie pack of Oreos mid-afternoon and maybe another in the evening, along with a glass of soy milk, are sufficient to tame the chocolate monster.

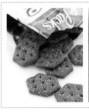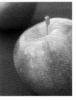

FRUIT, MILK, AND COOKIES
• 1 apple, 110 calories
• 2 servings Oreo Thin Crisps, 100-calorie pack, 200 calories
• 1 cup chocolate soy milk, 140 calories

"BEN AND JERRY ... I THOUGHT YOU LOVED ME!"

username: blazinmomma / *first name:* Jessica / *location:* Federal Way, WA

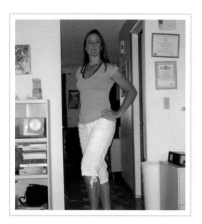

Jessica NOW: September '09 / age: 44
168 lbs. / BMI 24.1 / waist 30.5˝

I never had a weight problem growing up. I was brought up at the Berkeley Co-op on whole foods, the bulk section, fresh fruits and veggies, and I was only allowed to go to McDonald's when I was playing over at a friend's house. If I wanted sweet cereal (Cap'n Crunch), I had to earn the money and take myself to the store on my bike and buy it.

Although I was a very popular girl and dated many guys, I could never seem to keep a boyfriend. My relationships always failed, me having

played a part, of course. By looking for my absent father's love in all the wrong places I was always left terribly broken-hearted. By the age of thirty-two I had had only two serious relationships, neither lasting more than a couple of years. I earned my court-reporting license and moved for my first job to a small town east of the Cascades. Court reporting is a wonderful profession, but it leaves you very secluded and makes it hard to make friends in a new town. I was overworked and lonely, and became very good at attracting the wrong guys. My last relationship left me a broken-hearted new mom in a small town. I had no friends or family nearby.

Heavy from the pregnancy weight, I decided it would be the last failed relationship. Food became my friend. I would have a pint or two of Ben & Jerry's on the couch in front of the television after getting my son to bed. At least Ben and Jerry would never break my heart! I

figured (subconsciously) if I ate enough and fattened myself up enough, it would drive away any man remotely interested. Eating would pad me from the pain I inevitably would face. I put all of my attention into being a single mom, taking care of my son. I lost sight of myself and gained sixty-five pounds.

After hearing concerns from my father, of all people, and seeing pictures of me in shorts and a tank top looking pretty hefty, I decided it was time to change. I joined Weight Watchers for a year and lost

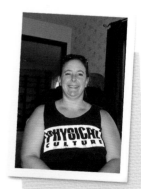

Jessica THEN: August '05

230 lbs. / BMI 28.9 / size 20

fifty-six pounds. But as soon as life's pressures came down on me, the weight gain started creeping back. I hadn't learned enough from Weight Watchers about how food affects me, how to balance my diet, and portion control. I weighed 198 pounds and worried I'd go over the 200 mark again, so I joined a Biggest Loser contest at my gym. I knew I would need to reduce my calories, so I went online searching for a computer food log and found NutriMirror. I had always been good at exercise, but not so good at being aware of how much food I was actually eating.

When I first started NutriMirror, I was impressed with how easily I could balance the nutrients in my diet. What was a shock was to really realize how much I was actually eating. My recommended weight loss calorie amount was so much lower. At first I was very hungry all the time, but I soon figured out that if I ate every couple of hours, I didn't feel so hungry. I also realized that by choosing certain calorie friendly items I could actually eat more volume.

But the biggest thing the site has taught me is portion control. I have really been able to get portion sizes set in my mind and my stomach has adapted. Now, I can easily recognize when I am full. I have learned to enjoy and manage smaller portions of sweets and I have been able to build my willpower over this period of time by just sticking to NutriMirror's golden rule—*go for green!*—which is now a habit.

The other thing I've learned is that I have a choice in what I eat. I have become acutely aware of how foods affect me both in calorie amounts and physically. I can't eat fast-food anymore. It makes me feel sick. I don't want diet soda anymore, and as soon as I stopped drinking it, my cravings for sweets virtually went away. Though I only treat myself to Ben & Jerry's on rare occasions now, I simply love my sixty-calorie lime Popsicle. If I want my favorite bowl of cereal in front of the television at night, I log it in advance in the morning so I know what I have to work with before I get to the end of the day when I'm tired

and have the least amount of willpower.

Through this process of actually paying attention to my health, I discovered myself again. Yes, I am an individual person, a proud mother, someone who enjoys her healthy food choices and looks forward to working out every day. I am worth the effort it takes to become and remain in shape. I look and feel great and I live each day knowing I am doing the right thing.

MY PHYSICAL ACTIVITY

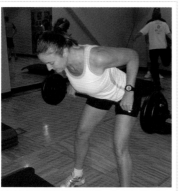

I have never had a problem exercising. I have always done it to keep active and relieve stress. I am one of those intense exercisers who burns a lot of calories and sweats.

I belong to the local community center gym, which offers everything you could ever want in choices of exercise, my preference being group exercise. I like it because there is camaraderie, it hits most all areas of the body, and you also know exactly when it is going to be over. I take Kickboxing, Zumba—which is Latin dance—and Group Power (a weightlifting class set to music).

JESSICA'S *GREEN* DAY

- Calories Expended: **2,664**
- Calories Eaten: **2,134**
- Net Calorie Balance: **530**

Since I have always been a rather healthy eater, my main focus has been on changing portion sizes. Also, I'm learning that food is for fueling and nourishing my body, not for emotional comforting.

In learning the healthy portion sizes, I also had to learn to eat more often during the day. I needed to spread my allotted calories throughout my waking hours so that I could keep my blood sugar steady and not feel hungry. I have total control over what and how much goes into my mouth.

The idea and the challenge of being "green" have really helped to curb the emotional eating. No longer do I choose to have pints of B&J in my freezer.

MY GREEN DAY NUTRITIONAL FACTS

JESSICA'S
HEALTH REFLECTION™
Nutrition Facts Report

Calorie Balance	
Calories Expended	2664
Calories Eaten	2134
Net Calorie Balance	530

Nutrient Balance	
	%DV
Total Fat 68 g	✔
Saturated Fat 14 g	59%
Trans Fat 0 g	—
Cholesterol 170 mg	57%
Sodium 1629 mg	71%
Total Carbs 279 g	✔
Dietary Fiber 46 g	154%
Sugars 117 g	—
Protein 116 g	✔
Vitamin A 1652 µg	236%
Vitamin C 128 mg	171%
Calcium 1279 mg	128%
Iron 29 g	161%

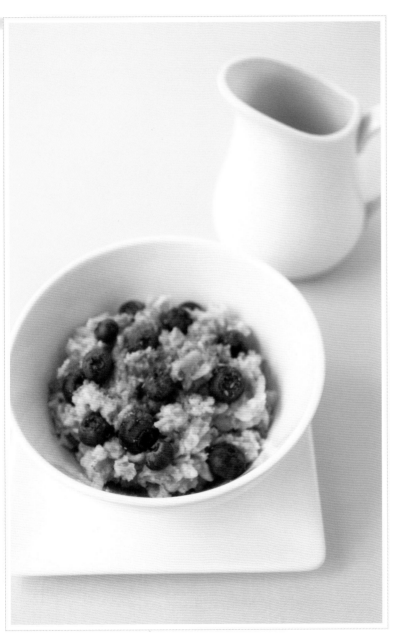

MY BREAKFAST
—312 calories

I am a creature of habit and when I find filling foods I like and foods that fuel me, I stick with them. That is why I eat oatmeal every day. The difference in my oatmeal before and my oatmeal now is that before I was eating double the serving size with butter, brown sugar, and a bunch of milk. Now, I eat the normal serving size with blueberries, ground flax seed and just a little 1% milk.

CEREAL WITH MILK, FRUIT, AND CINNAMON; COFFEE
- 1 serving oatmeal, 150 calories
- 1/2 tsp. ground cinnamon, 3 calories
- 1/4 cup blueberries, 21 calories
- 3/4 cup milk, low fat, 76 calories
- 2 tbsp. ground flax seed, 60 calories
- 6 oz. coffee, 2 calories

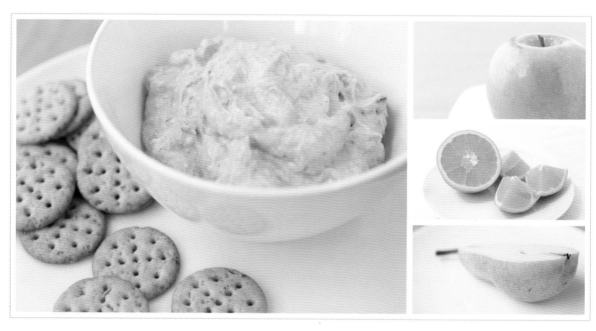

MY SNACKS–994 calories

My list is usually long because I sometimes eat up to five snacks in a day, particularly if I have exercised. Because I am fueling my body to have workout energy, to keep my blood sugar steady, and to stave off hunger, most of my snacks are combinations of a complex carbohydrate and some protein. A pre-workout snack I really love is a half cup of nonfat vanilla yogurt with a quarter of an apple, one quarter cup homemade granola, and a tablespoon of pumpkin seeds. There's lots of fuel in that one!

CRACKERS WITH TOFU DIP
- 8 12-grain mini snack crackers, 51 calories
- 2 tbsp. tofu and curry dip (see recipe), 61 calories

YOGURT SNACK
- 1/4 apple, 17 calories
- 1/4 cup vanilla yogurt, 45 calories
- 1 oz. pumpkin seeds, 125 calories
- 1/4 cup granola (see recipe), 142 calories

MILK AND CEREAL
- 2 cups milk, low fat, 204 calories
- 2 cups Joe's O's toasted whole grain cereal, 220 calories

MORE SNACKS
- 1 orange, 45 calories
- 1/2 pear, 48 calories
- 6 oz. coffee, 2 calories
- 6 oz. tea, 2 calories
- 1 tsp. sugar, 15 calories
- 1 egg white, hardboiled, 17 calories

GRANOLA

Adapted from **The Eat-Clean Diet Cookbook**. *Makes seven 1-cup servings.*

DRY INGREDIENTS
1 cup rye flakes
1 cup rolled oats
1 cup Kamut flakes
1 cup wheat flakes
1 cup raw, sliced almonds (unsalted)
1/2 cup sunflower seeds (unsalted)
1/4 cup sesame seeds

FOR COATING MIXTURE
1/2 cup Sucanat (unrefined cane sugar) or rapadura (dried sugarcane juice)
Pinch sea salt
1/2 tsp. cinnamon
1/4 cup canola oil
1 tsp. vanilla
1/4 cup honey

OPTIONAL
1/2 cup raisins
1/2 cup dried cranberries

PREPARATION
1. Preheat oven to 350°F. Mix dry ingredients in a large bowl.
2. Place all ingredients for coating mixture in a saucepan. Warm gently and stir to dissolve honey.
3. Pour coating mixture over dry ingredients and mix well
4. Line a large cookie sheet with parchment paper, then spread granola mixture onto it.
5. Bake for forty minutes, watching carefully and stirring occasionally to make sure everything is evenly toasted.
6. Set baking sheet out to cool. Add optional raisins and cranberries. When cool, transfer to an airtight container. Keeps for one week, or it can be frozen.

TOFU AND CURRY DIP

Adapted from **The Eat-Clean Diet Cookbook**.
Makes twelve 1-tablespoon servings.

DRY INGREDIENTS
6 oz. tofu
1 1/2 tbsp. lemon juice
2 tbsp. extra virgin olive oil
1/4 tsp. sea salt
2 tbsp. chopped green onion
1/2 tsp. curry powder
1 tbsp. parsley
2 cloves garlic, minced

PREPARATION
Combine all ingredients in a food processor. Pulse to combine, being careful not to over-process. Refrigerate covered.

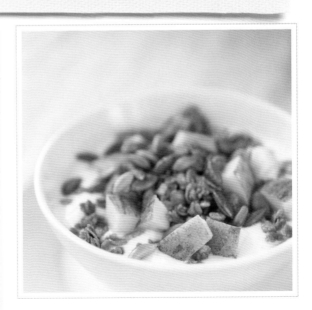

MY LUNCH–457 calories

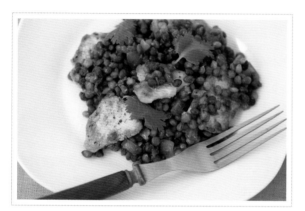

I used to eat a sandwich, potato chips, diet soda and a cookie for lunch all the time. I was not only eating too much, I was falling asleep by 2 P.M. Now I enjoy making large recipes that I can enjoy more than once during the week, like this Moroccan chicken and lentils dish from my favorite cookbook. I control the ingredients and keep the sodium and saturated fat low. I also save money by not eating out every day. I almost always add a salad at lunch now. I can even enjoy my favorite salad dressing in moderation.

MOROCCAN CHICKEN WITH LENTILS, SALAD, DESSERT

- 1 serving Moroccan chicken and lentils (see recipe), 305 calories
- 1 1/2 cup red leaf lettuce, 7 calories
- 1 beet, cooked, 22 calories
- 1 carrot, 25 calories
- 1 red ripe tomato, 20 calories
- 1/4 cup red cabbage, 6 calories
- 1 tsp. balsamic vinaigrette, 12 calories
- Trader Joe's fat-free Fruit Floes, lime, 60 calories

MORROCAN CHICKEN WITH LENTILS

Adapted from **The Eat-Clean Diet Cookbook.**
Makes six 2/3-cup servings.

INGREDIENTS
8 cups water
1 1/2 tsp. salt (divided)
8 oz. dried lentils, rinsed, drained, picked over
2 tbsp. + 1 tbsp. extra virgin olive oil
1/4 cup red wine vinegar
1 tbsp. + 1/2 tbsp. ground cumin
1 tbsp. + 1 tsp. chili powder
2 cloves garlic, peeled and minced
1 cup chopped onion
1.25 lb. skinless, boneless chicken breast, thinly sliced
1/4 tsp. cinnamon
1/2 cup cilantro

PREPARATION
1. Pour water into stock pot and add 1/2 tsp. salt. Add lentils and bring to a boil. Cover, reduce heat, and simmer 20–25 minutes until lentils are soft. Drain and rinse lentils under cold water. Set aside in large bowl.

2. In a small bowl, combine 2 tbsp. olive oil, vinegar, 1 tbsp. cumin, 1 tbsp. chili powder, garlic, and 1/2 tsp. salt. Pour this mixture over lentils and toss gently.

3. Heat 1 tbsp. olive oil in a large skillet. Add onion and sauté until dark brown and soft, about five minutes. Add chicken, 1/2 tsp. salt, 1/2 tbsp. cumin, 1 tsp. chili powder, and cinnamon. Sauté until chicken is cooked.

4. Arrange lentils on a serving platter and arrange cooked chicken mixture on top of lentils. Sprinkle with cilantro. Serve at room temperature.

MY DINNER—371 calories

My quick-to-prepare dinners usually include a protein of either fish or chicken that I bake with basic seasonings and some sort of vegetable. This veggie dish is a favorite that I make enough of to last through the week. I used to eat lots of crusty bread and corn with dinner, which not only meant I ate too many calories, but also led to big swings in my energy levels.

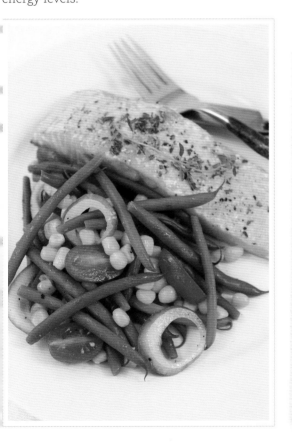

FISH
- 3 oz. salmon, cooked, 196 calories

GREEN BEANS, CORN, AND TOMATO SALAD
Makes six servings of 175 calories each.
- 3 ears corn, husk and silk removed
- 1 1/2 lb. green beans
- 3 cloves garlic, 3 cloves, peeled and smashed
- 4 tbsp. extra virgin olive oil
- 3 tbsp. red wine vinegar
- 1/2 cup sweet purple onion, thinly sliced
- 1 medium tomato
- 2 cups cherry tomatoes
- Sea salt and ground pepper to taste

BAKED SALMON

INGREDIENTS
Cooking spray
Fresh salmon
2 tbsp. lemon juice
Salt and pepper to taste
3 green onions, trimmed and cleaned
Sprig fresh rosemary
Sprig fresh thyme

PREPARATION

1. Preheat oven to 350°F. Spray baking dish with cooking spray and lay salmon on it.

2. Pour lemon juice on salmon and sprinkle with salt and pepper.

3. Place whole green onions on top of salmon.

4. Bake for 10 minutes.

5. Remove onions and sprinkle with herbs.

"I WILL SPARE YOU THE DETAILS OF HOW I ENDED UP IN A MENTAL HOSPITAL."

username: jwarren / *first name:* Joey / *location:* Crimora, VA

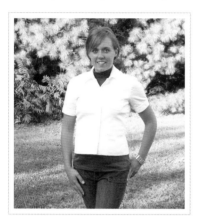

Joey NOW: September '09 / age: 29
129 lbs. / BMI 22 / waist 28˝

Saying I have battled with food issues all my life is an absolute understatement. My fight began long before I was even conceived. It was passed down my family line like a treasured heirloom given from mother to daughter, from one generation to the next. I have heard the word diet more times in my life than I care to recall, so it is no surprise that I grew up with the understanding that fat is completely unacceptable. Although I maintained a healthy weight throughout my childhood, I was constantly worried about getting fat. I dieted recreationally throughout elementary school and into early middle school. It was not until the end of seventh grade that I became serious about losing weight.

I remember watching a movie in which a girl was suffering with bulimia. Somewhere in my young mind I thought it was a great idea. I wondered why I hadn't tried that before. I learned enough from watching that movie to know how to conceal my efforts from my family. I started out slowly, and felt empowered as I learned new tricks of the trade. I decided that the best way to handle the situation was to plan ahead, which lessened the chance of suspicion. I tried to keep things in perspective. I didn't want to be one of those sickly looking girls that everyone could tell was anorexic. I just wanted to be thin. The problem was that I had no idea what that meant. I didn't know where to stop or how.

Food, or lack thereof, cannot bring happiness. I will spare you the details of how I ended up in a mental hospital. It took me four years and a myriad of toxic endeavors to get there. I was hospitalized for two months. I left with a new perspective on life, and a few psychiatrists. I stayed in therapy throughout high school. Although I still had issues, my fear of fat seemed to dissipate. I started eating like a normal teenager, meaning I ate nothing but junk food. This caused me no problems at first because I ran five miles every day and played soccer eight months out of the year. It wasn't until I was

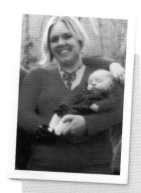

Joey THEN: November '07

195 lbs. / BMI 33.3

idelined by an ankle surgery that I began to notice some major changes.

My weight crept up slowly after the surgery, so I never really noticed it. I learned that I needed to eat, but I was never taught how to eat. By the time I graduated, I was already up to 130 pounds. This is by no means overweight for a 5´4″ person, but it was just the beginning. I managed to turn the dreaded "freshman fifteen" into a nice round thirty. I remember stepping on the scale for the first time in months and thinking that it was impossible for me to weigh 160 pounds. I started thinking of ways to lose weight, which is when I came up with the brilliant idea of using drugs to facilitate weight loss.

I spent my entire life watching the women of my family take appetite suppressants. Truthfully, I could not find any real difference between those pills and their illegal counterparts. Both options came with the possibility of addiction and horrible side effects. I was able to shed twenty pounds in just a few

months. Heavy drinking kept me from losing more. I spent the next few years in and out of stupors. My body looked flabby and bloated from excessive partying and horrific diet. None of this seemed out of the ordinary to me because everyone I surrounded myself with was in the same state. I wound myself in and out of relationships, looking for someone to pull me up off the floor. It slowly occurred to me that I was the only person who could do that. I realized that I didn't like who I was. I kicked one bad habit at a time, and in the process learned who my real friends were. When my final bad relationship ended, I called on a childhood friend to console me. We now have two beautiful children together, which is what brings me here.

I gained sixty pounds during each of my pregnancies. Most of the weight came off easily after my first pregnancy. However, the second one was very different. I left the hospital weighing 210 pounds, and four months later still weighed 180 pounds.

That is when my resolution kicked in. I was driven to find a new me, someone I could be proud of. I returned to college to finish my final year, and began searching my soul to find the healthy me within. At first, the hurried walk from one class to the next was enough to get me winded, but I enjoyed the exercise. By the time I was finished with my first semester, I could practically run to class. I also began counting my calories, and limiting my intake of unhealthy foods. I felt wonderful, but the scale would not budge below 160 pounds. The following semester, I started biking to and from campus. My exercise regime was really shaping up, but my eating habits were slipping because I got tired of the work involved in counting calories. I needed an easier way to hold myself accountable for my decisions. I finally found NutriMirror.

Since my heavist weight in November 2007 I've lost sixty-six pounds. Having an easily accessible visual aid has helped motivate me to watch my portion size. My diet is by no means perfect, but I have found a balance of food and exercise that makes me happy. I started running and playing soccer again. These two things once seemed like lofty dreams, but are now reality. I am back to the same weight I was when I graduated high school, but I am much healthier now than I was then. I have reached my ultimate goal and I love my bod

MY PHYSICAL ACTIVITY

Initially, my exercise program consisted of small amounts of activity worked into my daily life. I parked at the back of parking lots, used the stairs, etc. When I returned to college, I considered it exercise walking to and from class. I gradually incorporated running into my days, starting with 1/10 mile. I have now finished two 5 km runs, and am currently training for my first half-marathon. I generally run four days a week at an average pace of 6.0 mph for about forty minutes, which burns 389 calories per session. I do one long run every Sunday, adding one mile each week. I also returned to playing soccer this spring, which was my ultimate exercise goal. I trade two days of running for soccer games during the season, because fifty minutes of playing time burns 488 calories. My next aim is to add weight training to my regimen in order to balance my cardio workouts.

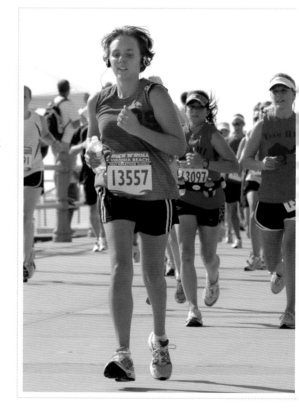

JOEY'S *GREEN* DAY

- Calories Expended: **2,133**
- Calories Eaten: **1,621**
- Net Calorie Balance: 512

I have never had a problem enjoying healthy food. My problems have largely been about controlling portion sizes. Over the span of my lifetime, I have oscillated between eating too little and eating too much. I have recently begun understanding the impact of portion control on my body. Too little food and I feel weak because I am not getting the proper nutrition. Too much food and I pack on pounds.

I feel that this time I have the necessary tools for long term success. I have learned to listen to that voice in the back of my head that says, "Hey girl, you're overdoing it." It was there all along, but I am now prepared to listen.

MY GREEN DAY NUTRITIONAL FACTS

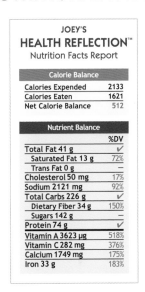

JOEY'S HEALTH REFLECTION™
Nutrition Facts Report

Calorie Balance	
Calories Expended	2133
Calories Eaten	1621
Net Calorie Balance	512

Nutrient Balance		
		%DV
Total Fat 41 g		✔
Saturated Fat 13 g		72%
Trans Fat 0 g		–
Cholesterol 50 mg		17%
Sodium 2121 mg		92%
Total Carbs 226 g		✔
Dietary Fiber 34 g		150%
Sugars 142 g		–
Protein 74 g		✔
Vitamin A 3623 µg		518%
Vitamin C 282 mg		376%
Calcium 1749 mg		175%
Iron 33 g		183%

MY BREAKFAST–289 calories

look forward to my morning cereal, so I don't ver get too creative with breakfast. Fiber rich ereals have been my favorite since I was a child. have learned to measure my portions in order to ut down on calories. I also added the flax in order o boost my fiber and iron intake. Overall, I have ot made many changes to this area of my diet.

CEREAL WITH FLAX SEED AND MILK, AND COFFEE
- 1 cup milk, low fat, 101 calories
- 1 tsp. flax seed, 16 calories
- 12 oz. coffee, 4 calories
- 1 cup Shredded Wheat with strawberries, 168 calories

MY LUNCH–237 calories

This is a pretty unusual lunch for me as I tend to stick with steamed veggies. But since I eat what is offered in the dining hall at work I sometimes end up pulling together whatever's available, which can be tough since I'm a vegetarian. This meal isn't ideal, but it is an example of working with what's available.

SANDWICH AND FRUIT
- 1 tbsp. margarine-lite spread, 17 calories
- 1/2 slice white bread, 20 calories
- 5 oz. Mandarin orange cup, 80 calories
- 1/2 riblet with sauce, 120 calories

MY SNACKS–672 calories

I love snacks. In fact, I may enjoy them more than my meals. I keep both my office and my home stocked with quick, easy to enjoy food. My favorite snacks are fruits and nuts. I also love sweets, so I treat myself to something sugary once a day. The trick is not to go overboard. One fun size bar usually curbs the cravings, especially if you switch milk chocolate for dark chocolate.

CEREAL, MILK, FRUIT, YOGURT, JUICE, CANDY, AND VITAMIN
- 1/2 cup milk, low fat, 51 calories
- 1 large apple, 110 calories
- 6 strawberries, fresh, 34 calories
- 12 almonds, 83 calories
- 1/2 Milky Way dark bar, 40 calories
- One-A-Day women's vitamin, 0 calories
- 8 oz. V8 juice, 50 calories
- 1 1/2 oz. prunes, pitted, 100 calories
- 6 oz. Greek yogurt, blueberry, 120 calories
- 1/2 cup Shredded Wheat with strawberries, 84 calories

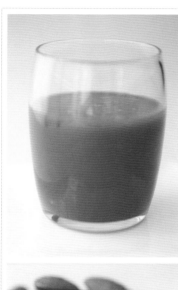
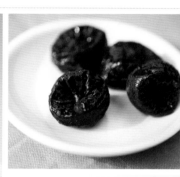
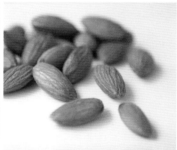
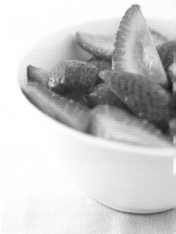
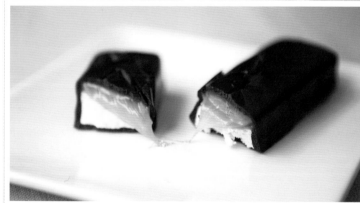

MY DINNER—423 calories

Dinner means family time for me. This is the time that I use to emphasize fun, healthy foods with my children. I like to incorporate different menu selections all the time, and especially enjoy ethnic foods. Whether I make tacos, a stir fry, eggplant bahartha, or sashimi, I am never afraid to try something new. Plus, I love seeing my husband's face when I say, "Just trust me."

VEGGIE TACOS
- 4 tsp. sour cream, fat free, 58 calories
- 1/4 cup red ripe tomatoes, chopped, 8 calories
- 3/4 oz. taco shells, baked, 101 calories
- 1/2 cup Burger Crumbles, 116 calories
- 2 cup mixed baby greens, 15 calories
- 1 oz. pepper jack cheese, 110 calories
- 2 tsp. taco seasoning, 15 calories

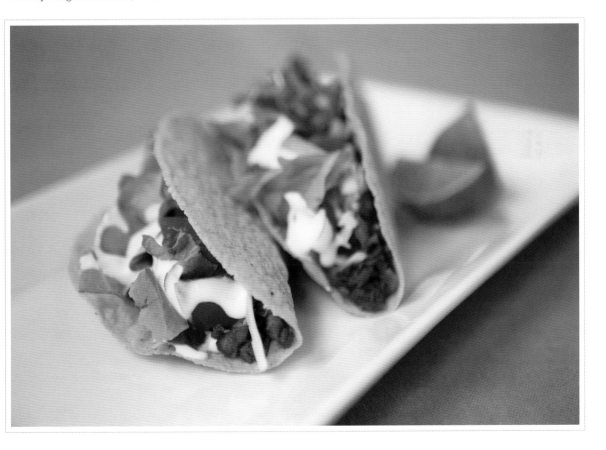

"WE WERE JUST EATING TO EAT. OUR STOMACHS WERE GETTING FULL, BUT WE WEREN'T NURTURING OUR BODIES."

username: PamelaAnn / *first name:* Pam / *location:* Fallbrook, CA

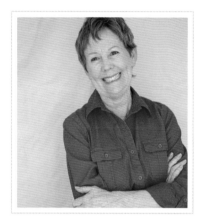

Pam NOW: October '09 / age: 66
114 lbs. / BMI 20.2 / waist 27˝

Over the years I've gone to nutritionists and taken mountains of vitamins, spending hundreds of dollars a month in the process. I exercised regularly by walking and playing tennis. I even trained to walk a marathon by walking several hours a day over a three-month period. And I walked that marathon plus an extra mile for good measure. Mostly, I've been at a healthy weight.

However, during my menopause years I gained about fifteen unwanted pounds and just couldn't seem to lose it. I was told that in addition to the hot-flashes that accompany menopause a woman will typically gain weight. So, I just thought *this is it.*

Fifteen pounds is not that much, but I'm only 5´3˝ tall and it was enough to make me uncomfortable.

Then my husband, Jim, developed a health issue that demanded quick action. He had hypertension and was told to cut down on sodium and lose weight. These orders came from his physician with an ominous warning.

Jim had embarked on various diets over the years, but only to lose weight. He never thought about his health. This time was different. He realized he had to do something but sodium was everywhere.

He searched the Internet looking for an answer. There were a lot of websites, but none really answered his questions. He wanted something easy and fast—something that let him see everything he needed in a single glance.

Enter our son, Michael. Together, Jim and Michael, after intensive research on the matter, developed NutriMirror. During this period they needed testers—people who would put the system to the test, follow their directions, and answer questions.

So I volunteered to be one of the testers. I started by logging my food. I didn't look that closely at the reports. After all, this was for my husband, not me. I was only

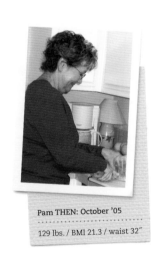

Pam THEN: October '05

129 lbs. / BMI 21.3 / waist 32˝

helping with the development.

I'm not sure when it happened but as the site developed and I started using it more I noticed warning signals in "red." I thought, I don't eat poorly so there must be "bugs" in the system. It's new and it's being worked on all the time, right? It couldn't be me.

However, denial doesn't last long when the facts stare you in the face. I started checking things more closely—sodium, fat, and protein. I was either getting too much or not enough. My vitamins needed a boost across the board. I noticed there were days I didn't meet my calorie recommendations. I saw the foods I ate that were causing the problems; and I discovered I was a sporadic eater. I almost never ate breakfast. By the time lunch rolled around I would be starving. I would eat a huge lunch and still eat dinner later on. Over the last couple of years I've learned I was either eating an entire day's worth of calories in one sitting or not eating enough.

NutriMirror is teaching me "how" to eat. It calculates my needs. I enter my choices and it tells me how those choices will affect me, such as if I need more protein or less carbohydrate. I also learned I needed to cut down on sodium. Jim and I ate a lot of fast-food. We never took lunch to work and there's a McDonald's on every corner. Here again, by only eating the kids' meal, we were fooling ourselves. We also ate well at nice restaurants—usually with rich desserts included. The only thing we shared was, "you can have half of my dessert if I can have half of yours." Most times we would leave feeling stuffed and uncomfortable.

While using NutriMirror, I have learned:

1. It is possible to lose those pesky fifteen pounds and keep them off.
2. Breakfast is good.
3. I haven't given up anything I really like.
4. I can eat all day long.
5. I can still go to nice restaurants.

All these things are possible because I have learned to plan ahead. I have favorite foods that are nutrient-dense and are now part of my regular diet. I have developed "snack" foods I know my body needs. My body stays fueled all day. There is never a time I sit down to eat that I'm starved. This makes eating more enjoyable. If a serving size is too big I will divide it before I start eating. Fast food is a thing of the past and it isn't missed. I always bring snacks to work. Jim and I have discovered a new love of fruit. Never a day passes without an apple or orange or both. Carrots are also eaten most every day.

None of these things would have been possible without NutriMirror. All the nutritionists I've consulted, all the reading I've done, and all the supplements I've taken never made me feel the way I do now. And they never gave me the personal control over the health of my body that I now enjoy. I am responsible for what happens to my body and I now have the tool that shows me what I'm doing, and that keeps me in control.

I am not a cook and I'm always willing to go out to eat. My husband and I took the easy (restaurant) way for too many years. But now I have learned I can whip up good tasting food! Fresh veggies and fruits, whole grains, and lean protein are at the center of our meals. Fast-food, though convenient and momentarily gratifying, was ruining our bodies. Nice restaurants are great and we still go out. But we've learned how to order tasty foods without creating imbalances.

We both knew we weren't really eating wisely. We were just eating to eat.

Our stomachs were getting full, but we weren't nurturing our bodies. We were enabling each other. NutriMirror opened our eyes. I learned if I'm responsible for feeding my family and I make the wrong choices it affects the ones I love, not just me.

I've talked a lot about Jim in my story. This has been a family affair. I would like to pass this observation on to others: if you are unhealthy and you have a family, your family is probably unhealthy too. My advice? Provide your family with good foods and be a healthy example. If enough of us do that, we can make the world a healthier place

MY PHYSICAL ACTIVITY

Walking. This is my exercise choice. It's free, it doesn't require expensive equipment and, living where I do, I can do it just about whenever I want; during breaks at work, after work, or during lunch time. Just take off and let your mind wander. I can walk at a fairly good pace (about 4 mph), but, I still enjoy the scenery. And, I sometimes take a camera and photograph things along the way. Exercise has become an outing, not a chore.

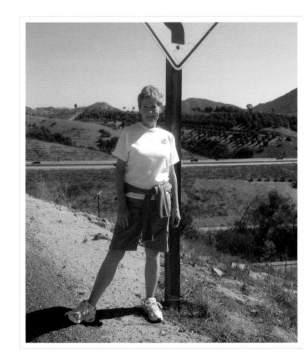

PAM'S *GREEN* DAY 1

- Calories Expended: **1,659**
- Calories Eaten: **1,570**
- Net Calorie Balance: **90**

Nutrition comes in all forms. It doesn't have to be three sit-down meals and a snack each day. The day I've chosen has a lot of small items that give me the nutrition I need. There are twenty-nine items and most can be eaten alone. This means I eat all day long so I'm never starving for anything.

PAM'S NUTRITION FACTS, GREEN DAY 1

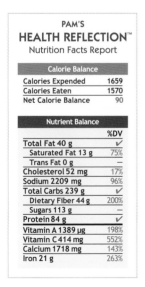

PAM'S
HEALTH REFLECTION™
Nutrition Facts Report

Calorie Balance	
Calories Expended	1659
Calories Eaten	1570
Net Calorie Balance	90

Nutrient Balance	
	%DV
Total Fat 40 g	✔
Saturated Fat 13 g	75%
Trans Fat 0 g	—
Cholesterol 52 mg	17%
Sodium 2209 mg	96%
Total Carbs 239 g	✔
Dietary Fiber 44 g	200%
Sugars 113 g	—
Protein 84 g	✔
Vitamin A 1389 µg	198%
Vitamin C 414 mg	552%
Calcium 1718 mg	143%
Iron 21 g	263%

MY BREAKFAST—251 calories

My old breakfast would have been sixteen ounces of coffee in a travel mug. I might also have had a bagel with cream cheese or a donut once in a while, but normally I didn't eat breakfast. But I've learned that my body needs "nutrition." Now I plan breakfast: fruit, cereal, yogurt, toast—whatever I can pack and take to work.

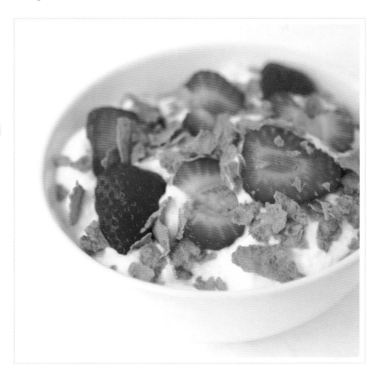

MY GO-TO BREAKFAST
- 1/2 container plain yogurt, nonfat, 63 calories
- 1/2 cup strawberries, fresh, 26 calories
- 1/2 cup Total cereal, 67 calories
- 16 oz. coffee, 5 calories
- 1 tsp. Coffee-mate, 10 calories
- 1 piece sprouted grain bread, low sodium, 80 calories

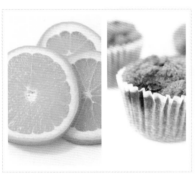

MY LUNCH–315 calories

A quick trip to McDonald's or some other fast-food joint was the old lunch. I'm more nutritionally balanced now. I usually eat at my desk, so I take simple items that don't need a lot of prep time.

SNACKS FOR LUNCH
- 1 cup orange slices, 85 calories
- 1 cup milk, nonfat, lactose free, 90 calories
- 1 oz. string cheese, light, 60 calories
- Blueberry fiber mini cake, 80 calories

MY SNACKS–676 calories

This is the most important thing I have learned —eat often! My snack packs assure I will do that. I always include fruit, vegetables, and protein snacks that are portable and easy to pack. I have found if I eat often I never sit down to a meal starving. This means I never overeat and my body's metabolism is always firing.

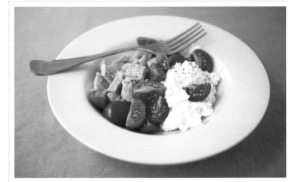

KEEP ON EATING
- 1/2 cup cottage cheese, nonfat, 62 calories
- 2 oz. tuna, solid white, 70 calories
- 3 oz. red ripe tomatoes, 15 calories
- 4 oz. apple, 58 calories
- 2 tbsp. peanut butter, 200 calories
- 3 oz. carrots, 35 calories
- 1 oz. sweet green peppers, 6 calories
- 1 oz. sweet red peppers, 7 calories
- 1 oz. sweet yellow peppers, 8 calories
- 1 piece Swiss cheese, light, 35 calories
- Chips Ahoy Thin Crisps, 100-calorie pack, 100 calories
- 2 tbsp. fresh salsa, 10 calories
- 2 pieces Wasa Crispbread, 70 calories

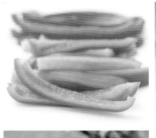

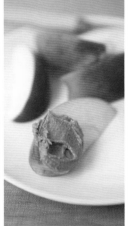

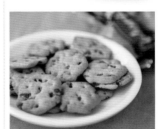

MY DINNER
—328 calories

My old dinner was usually good, and large enough for two people. Because breakfast and lunch weren't supplying me with the support I needed I would go overboard at dinner. I thought mostly about taste and I finished everything on my plate. Now that I've learned what my body needs, I've made the necessary changes. I know portion sizes, calorie needs, nutritional requirements, and how to manage these in ways that provide both health and pleasure.

FRUIT, CRACKERS, AND DESSERT
- 1/2 cup cantaloupe cubes, 27 calories
- 1/2 cup honeydew melon cubes, 31 calories
- 1/2 cup pineapple, diced, 37 calories
- 1/2 cup watermelon, diced, 23 calories
- Cheese Nips Thin Crisps, 100-calorie pack, 100 calories
- English Toffee Crunch ice cream bar, low fat, 110 calories

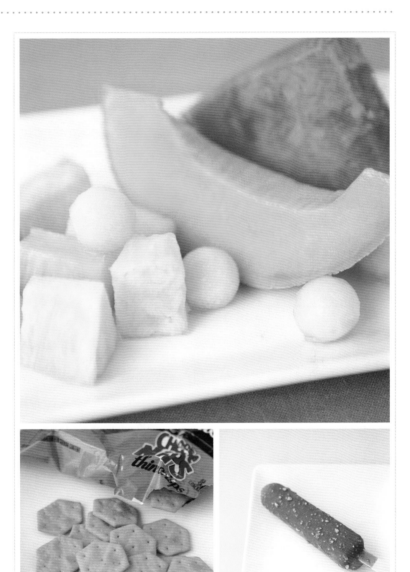

PAM'S NUTRITION FACTS, GREEN DAY 2

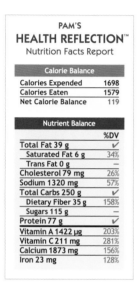

MY BREAKFAST—330 calories

- 1 breakfast bar (see recipe), 99 calories
- 1 cup apples, sliced, 55 calories
- 1 cup yogurt, 160 calories
- 16 oz. coffee with Coffee-mate, 16 calories

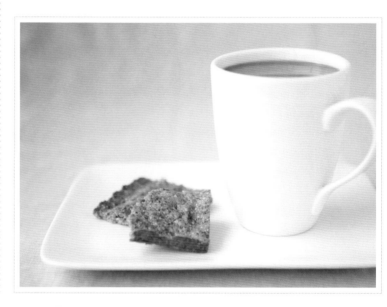

BREAKFAST BAR   *Adapted from Ellie Krieger's* **The Food You Crave**. *Makes 24 bars.*

INGREDIENTS

Cooking spray
1 cup quick rolled oats
1/2 cup shelled raw sunflower
   seeds (unsalted)
1/2 cup toasted wheat germ

1/4 cup whole wheat flour
1/2 cup dried apricots
1/2 cup raw almonds
1/2 cup raisins
1/2 cup pitted dried dates

1/2 cup nonfat dry milk
1/2 teaspoon ground cinnamon
1/3 cup pure maple syrup
2 large eggs

PREPARATION

Preheat oven to 350°F. Coat 9-inch by 13-inch pan with cooking spray. Add oats, sunflower seeds, wheat germ, flour, apricots, almonds, raisins, dates, dry milk, an cinnamon to a food processor. Pulse until finely chopped. Add maple syrup and eggs. Pulse until mixture is well combined and resembles coarse paste. Transfer to the pan and spread evenly to cover bottom. Bake for about 20 minutes, or until lightly browned. Cool 15 minutes, then cut into 24 pieces. Store in air-tight container at room temperature. May be wrapped and frozen for up to three months.

MY LUNCH—336 calories

SANDWICH
- 2.4 oz. Chicken breast, 112 calories
- 1/2 oz. apples, chopped, 7 calories
- 1/4 oz celery, chopped, 1 calorie
- 1/2 tbsp. cranberries, dried, 11 calories
- 1/2 tbsp. mayonnaise, 45 calories
- 2 pieces sprouted grain Ezekiel bread, 160 calories

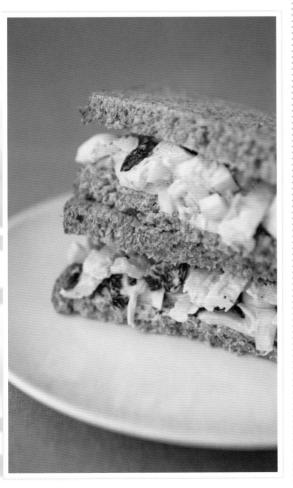

MY SNACKS—568 calories

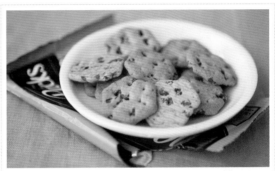

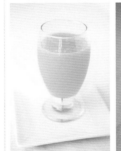

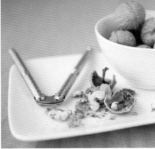

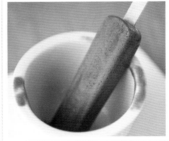

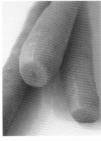

- 3 oz. carrots, 35 calories
- Fudgsicle, no sugar added, 44 calories
- Chips Ahoy Thin Crisps, 100-calorie pack, 100 calories
- 8 oz. orange juice, 110 calories
- 1/2 cup Total cereal, 67 calories
- 1/4 cup milk, nonfat, 23 calories
- 1 oz. walnuts, 189 calories

MY DINNER—345 calories

TUSCAN VEGETABLE SOUP (MAKES SIX 158-CALORIE SERVINGS)

1/4 tsp. black pepper, 1 calorie
1/2 tsp. dried sage, 0 calories
1 tbsp. fresh thyme, 2 calories
1/2 cup chopped carrots, 26 calories
1/2 cup chopped celery, 7 calories
1 tsp. fresh garlic, 4 calories
1 cup chopped onions, 67 calories
1 1/2 cup chopped zucchini, 30 calories
16 oz. can white beans, 531 calories

4 cups chicken broth, 99% fat free, 60 calories
1 tbsp. extra virgin olive oil, 120 calories
15 oz. can diced tomatoes, 84 calories
2 oz. baby spinach, 17 calories

SERVED WITH
2 pieces Wasa crispbread, 90 calories
3 oz. tomato slices, 97 calories

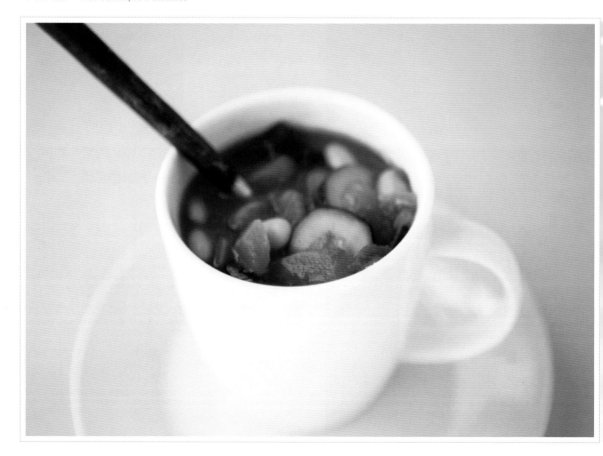

PAM'S NUTRITION FACTS, GREEN DAY 3

PAM'S
HEALTH REFLECTION™
Nutrition Facts Report

Calorie Balance	
Calories Expended	1673
Calories Eaten	1479
Net Calorie Balance	194

Nutrient Balance	
	%DV
Total Fat 45 g	✔
Saturated Fat 13 g	79%
Trans Fat 0 g	—
Cholesterol 34 mg	11%
Sodium 1322 mg	57%
Total Carbs 220 g	✔
Dietary Fiber 33 g	159%
Sugars 109 g	—
Protein 64 g	✔
Vitamin A 3215 µg	459%
Vitamin C 373 mg	497%
Calcium 2047 mg	171%
Iron 21 mg	117%

MY BREAKFAST—334 calories

SMOOTHIE
- 2 oz. banana, 50 calories
- 2 oz. blueberries, 32 calories
- 2 oz. strawberries, 18 calories
- 2 oz. orange juice, 27 calories
- 2 oz. plain yogurt, nonfat, 27 calories

ON THE SIDE
- 1 slice sprouted grain Ezekiel bread, 80 calories
- 1 tbsp. peanut butter, 100 calories

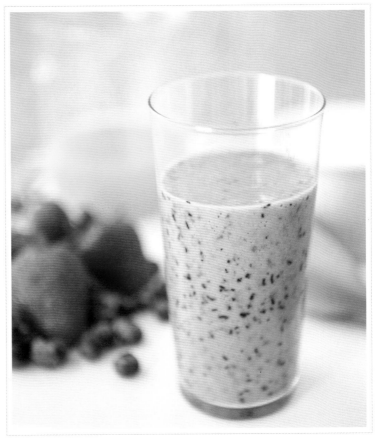

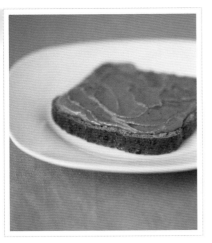

MY LUNCH–247 calories

- Banana, 90 calories
- 1/2 cup Total cereal, 67 calories
- 1 cup milk, nonfat, 90 calories

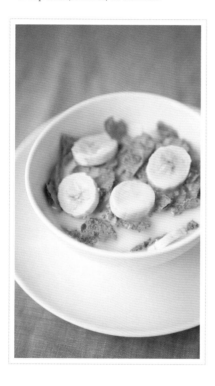

MY SNACKS–482 calories

- 1 cup sliced apples, 57 calories
- 1 tbsp. peanut butter, 100 calories
- 3 oz. carrots, 35 calories
- 8 oz. orange juice, 110 calories
- English toffee crunch ice cream bar, 110 calories
- 1 piece string cheese, 70 calories

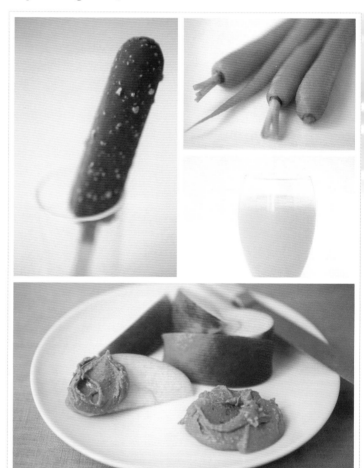

MY DINNER—416 calories

ISH STEW
Makes seven 260-calorie servings.
1 1/2 cup chicken broth, 99% fat free
1 cup carrots, chopped
1 cup celery, chopped
White potato, small
13.7 oz. orange roughy
1 15-oz. can chickpeas
(garbanzo beans)
1 28-oz. can tomatoes, diced,
no salt added

SALAD
2 cups mixed baby greens, 15 calories
1 oz. each green, red, and yellow
peppers, 21 calories
1 tbsp. extra virgin olive oil,
120 calories

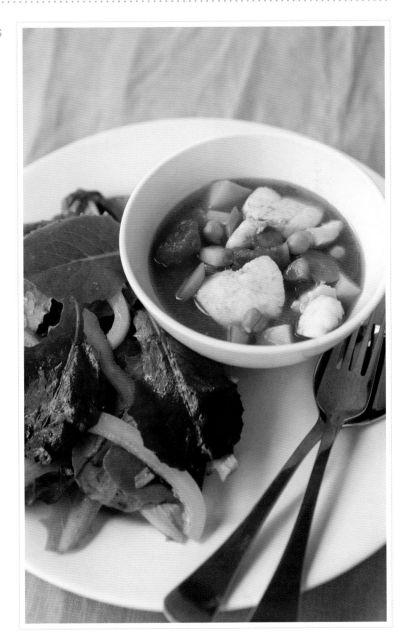

"WHEN I LOOK BACK I SEE MY FAILURES WERE BECAUSE I DIDN'T KNOW WHAT I WAS DOING."

username: jessica30 / *first name:* Jessica / *location:* San Diego

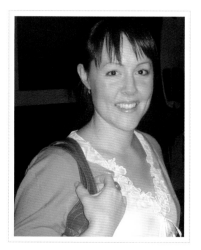

Jessica NOW: October '09 / age: 30
158.5 lbs. / BMI 24.2 / waist 29.25˝

There really wasn't one big thing that made me decide to start losing weight. I guess a little bit of everything happened all at once. I got engaged, I turned thirty years old, and I started a new job.

I was just tired of the way I looked in the mirror and the way that I felt about myself. I didn't want to leave the house. I hated all of my clothes because of the way I appeared in them. Every picture I saw of myself just made me more depressed. Now, some of those

pictures shock me. I knew how much I weighed, I had the number in my head, but I really didn't think I looked that big!

I finally just got tired of it. I didn't want to feel sorry for myself anymore. I had tried to lose weight many times before but I felt like I couldn't do it on my own. I thought that if everyone around me was eating poorly, then I had to also.

If everyone at work was going out to get a sandwich and potato chips then I had to go too. At first work was tough; it still is. I work in a typical office environment. People with good intentions bring snacks all the time and it's hard not to partake when the tender morsels are tempting you. Well, I had to get over that one.

I didn't think I would have the time or energy to exercise when I got home from work. I had to get over that too. I used to work ten-hour days and I knew I couldn't exercise before work since I am not a morning person. I had to figure out

something else. The only other choice I had was to exercise when I got home from work. Since I am tired when I get home, that would be difficult. I really had to motivate myself to put gym clothes on and start my exercise DVD. But once I got started I just couldn't help but keep the momentum going. Only the getting started part was, and can still be, challenging.

Next, I had to work on my eating habits. In the past, I had tried a few different diets that I thought would help break some

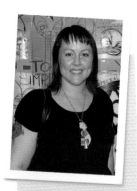

Jessica THEN: September '09
214 lbs. / BMI 32.4 / waist 37˝

of my bad habits. They usually worked for a few weeks, but then I would break down and eat something that wasn't in the plan. Later I would have a really hard time getting back on track. Most times I would go back to eating junk foods until I got grossed out with myself. Then I would try another crazy diet. No carbs. No fruit. No sugar. There were all sorts of foods that I cut out of my diet; and a lot of them were not bad foods for me. Following one particularly crazy diet, I lost seventeen pounds in two weeks. Within two months, the weight was back.

I learned then that when weight is lost during an intense diet— where you lose a lot of weight in a short period of time—it always seems to come back. I had to make permanent changes. I had to stop thinking about what other people around me were eating. I had to eat for myself. I really had to pay attention and remember what I was eating throughout the day.

I remember logging my food on one of my first days with NutriMirror. I couldn't believe how much food I'd eaten! If I didn't take the time to think about the whole day, I would have forgotten half of the things I had eaten. It really helped me realize how important GOOD food is. Now when I see something that I want to eat, or I'm getting ready to order something at a restaurant, I remember what I have already eaten and what I plan on eating later in the day.

NutriMirror really helps me with meal planning. It gives me the knowledge to make much better choices. Even when I weighed less, I really wasn't healthy. I wasn't exercising and was nutritionally imbalanced because I was eating poorly.

I had gained weight gradually for most of my life but had always thought that it would be too hard to change to a healthier way of living. I could never keep myself motivated. When I look back, I see my failures were because I didn't know what I was doing. I never had the information I needed to consistently make the choices my body wanted and needed.

I have come a long way and I still have a ways to go before I reach my goal, but for the first time in my life I am on track and feel like I am in control. I know where I want to go and how to get there. There is no quick fix for getting healthy. But knowing that I have been working hard makes me feel better about myself. I am proud of myself and happy. I did this because I want to look good when I get married, but I also want to look and feel good everyday. I am far more educated on the food that I eat, and now my body is thanking me because I am, finally, doing the things it has always expected, wanted, and needed from me.

MY PHYSICAL ACTIVITY

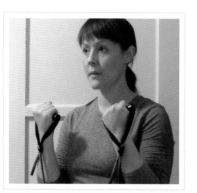

I had never been too active on my own so getting started on an exercise plan took a little bit of getting used to. I started with Power 90. Three days a week you have the "sweat" routine and the other three days you have the "sculpt" routine for a total of six days a week. Once I felt comfortable that I could do everything just as they do it in the video, I knew I was ready for the next step. I bought P90X. This program gives you a lot of choices to find the workout that is best for you. I chose the "Lean" program which is for those who want to slim down and not gain a lot of muscle mass. I am still doing my lean routine six days a week.

JESSICA'S *GREEN* DAY

- Calories Expended: **2,372**
- Calories Eaten: **1,439**
- Net Calorie Balance: **933**

I had never put much thought into what I ate on a daily basis before joining NutriMirror. I didn't know the nutritional value of any of the foods I was eating. I just ate them because I liked them. I just assumed that all of the healthy foods that I should be eating would take too much time and work to prepare. I even thought that I couldn't afford to eat healthy! Now I am saving money, I can make dinner in ten minutes and I enjoy every meal I eat. When I started entering the foods I routinely ate into the NutriMirror food log I was so surprised at how bad some of those favorite foods were for me. Now I know what to eat. I have set up my favorite healthy meals in my short-cut storage areas like Custom Menus and Favorites and Custom Recipes so they are super easy to log. Because of the knowledge I have gained and the pleasure I experience in healthy foods and physical activity, there is no desire or need to ever go back to the old habits.

MY GREEN DAY NUTRITIONAL FACTS

JESSICA'S
HEALTH REFLECTION™
Nutrition Facts Report

Calorie Balance	
Calories Expended	2372
Calories Eaten	1439
Net Calorie Balance	933

Nutrient Balance	
	%DV
Total Fat 38g	✔
Saturated Fat 13 g	81%
Trans Fat 0 g	—
Cholesterol 131 mg	44%
Sodium 2113 mg	92%
Total Carbs 215g	✔
Dietary Fiber 27 g	134%
Sugars 65g	—
Protein 75g	✔
Vitamin A 1582 µg	226%
Vitamin C 266 mg	355%
Calcium 1107 mg	111%
Iron 42g	233%

MY BREAKFAST—409 calories

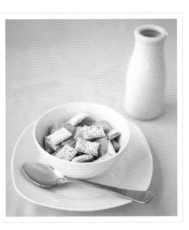

I used to go to the coffee shop or the bagel place close to work for my breakfast. My favorites were bagels and cream cheese, or the chocolate chip muffin. I thought because they were heavy and filling that I would feel satisfied and full until lunch time.

I really felt like I a had a rock in my stomach. I wanted to fall asleep by lunch time. The bagels and muffins were delicious, but they didn't do anything to satisfy the needs of my body. I usually don't have much time in the morning to make anything for breakfast so cereal is my number one choice. One of my favorites is Fiber One Frosted Mini Wheats. It is super delicious, quick to get ready and it fills me up for the morning.

CEREAL, MILK, AND COFFEE
- 14 oz. milk, 2% milkfat, 205 calories
- 12 oz. coffee, 4 calories
- 1 cup Fiber One Frosted Mini Wheats, 200 calories

MY SNACKS—380 calories

I used to try not eating between meals, but after starving myself, I would just eat more at my main meals. Having a snack keeps my appetite in check so I don't overeat at meal time. Plus, I always have a multivitamin once a day to ensure I get enough vitamins and minerals. On this day I had a good calorie balance at the end of the day so I treated myself to a Peppermint Pattie. To my knowledge, they are one of the lowest calorie candies available. It satisfied my craving and I still managed a totally Green Day!

FIBER BAR, MINT PATTIE AND VITAMIN
- York Peppermint Pattie, 160 calories
- Multivitamin, 10 calories
- Oatmeal bar, high fiber, 210 calories

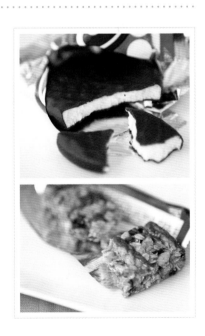

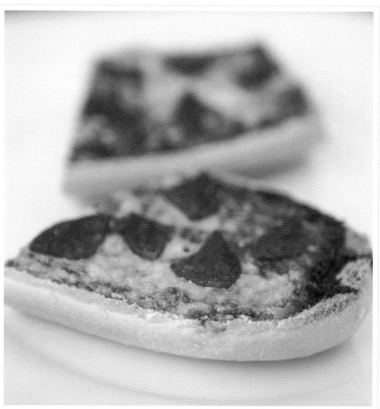

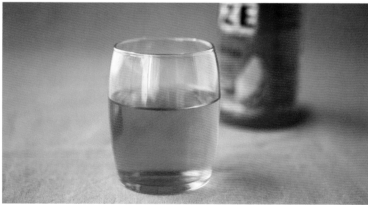

MY LUNCH–460 calories

I stay at work for my lunches and I always try to bring something good to eat. In the past I went out for lunch almost every day, spending too much money and eating whatever sounded the tastiest. I sometimes still go out for lunch but having an idea of the calorie content of most foods, I now chose more wisely. On this day the neighborhood Starbucks brought us samples of their new sandwich. Even though it was a tiny sample I still added it to my log! On most days I will have some sort of frozen meal and a drink. Lean Cuisine makes some pretty good meals that are not very expensive. So whenever I don't have much time to prepare something the night before, these work well.

PIZZA, 1/2 SANDWICH, AND DRINK
- Pepperoni French bread pizza (Lean Cuisine), 290 calories
- 1/2 serving roast turkey & Swiss cheese sandwich (Starbuck's), 160 calories
- 16 oz. Fuze tropical punch, 10 calories

MY DINNER—190 calories

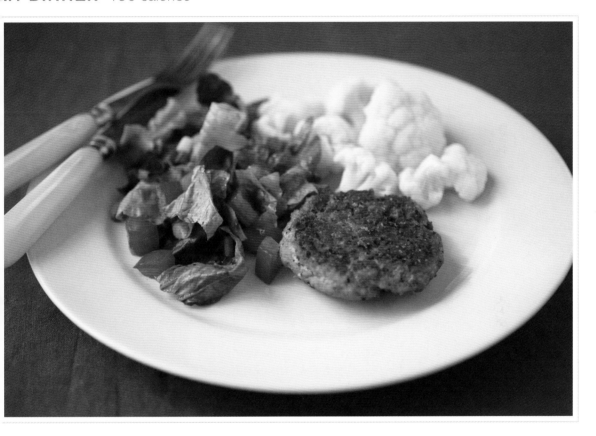

After I finish my workout it is time to relax and enjoy a really good meal. No more ordering pizza, breadsticks, and buffalo wings. Now I have learned that the dinners I once ate used up all my allowable calories for the entire day. The dinners that I make now always include a salad, a vegetable (in this case steamed cauliflower), and some sort of protein like the extra lean ground turkey I had on this day. I don't drink soda much these days, but on this day I treated myself to a diet Coke.

PROTEIN, VEGETABLE, AND SALAD WITH A DIET COKE
- 8 flowerets cauliflower, cooked, 32 calories
- 1 cup red leaf lettuce, shredded, 5 calories
- Spring onion/scallion, 2 calories
- 1/2 medium red ripe tomato, 11 calories
- 12 oz. diet Coke, 0 calories
- 3 oz. ground turkey breast, extra lean, 90 calories
- 2 tbsp. balsamic & bail vinaigrette, 50 calories

"SUGAR IN ALL FORMS WAS DELICIOUS, AND AS A CHILD I WANTED IT. NO, I NEEDED IT."

username: stra2612 / *first name:* Kelly / *location:* TC

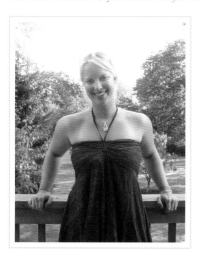

Kelly NOW: September '09 / age: 23
149 lbs. / BMI 24 / waist 27.5˝

I like sugar. I like cake. I like homemade cake, cake from a box, store-bought cakes. I like the colorful sweet frosting flowers that are so perfect for scooping from the corner-piece and raising to my lips. I like cookies. I like soft cookies with big chocolate chips that are perfect for extracting when the cookie is crumbled for maximum cookie bliss. I especially like candy. I like sweet and sour and crunchy and chewy. I like the colorful, crinkly packages and the sparkling sugar diamonds drizzled on top. Sugar, in all its forms, was delicious, and as a child, I wanted it. No, I needed it.

I spent hours hovering over the computer in the family room adjoining the kitchen. I watched the kitchen, waiting for my mother to leave so I could snatch packages from the treasure trove that was in the left cupboard, and then chow down the contents as quickly as possible. I never thought about my weight until my sophomore high school year when I traded up my size 29 jeans for a size 30. I was 5´5˝ and weighed 145 pounds. I was a three-sport varsity athlete. I was the second fastest girl when running lines in the basketball program. I worried I was too big. But those were the days I could eat anything—a bag or two of Sour Patch Kids after a Ranch drizzled salad and bowl of clam chowder for lunch. Sometimes I would have a Pop Tart on the bus ride to a sports game and still stay fit. Exercise is an absolute necessity for a sugar addict.

It wasn't until my sophomore year of college that my eating habits began to overtake my activity level. I was a catcher on a softball scholarship to a college where sports ruled. At least forty hours each week were taken up with softball activities. I was constantly active, but paid no attention to what I ate. The softball girls and I would often go out for Chinese food after practice, grab pizza while doing homework, and cook extravagant post-game Italian dinners.

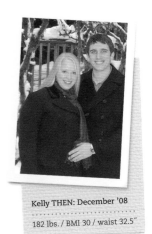

Kelly THEN: December '08
182 lbs. / BMI 30 / waist 32.5˝

My weight crept up and up without me realizing it, until I stepped on the scale one day in March and was stunned by the number. I weighed 167 pounds. This number was totally unacceptable and I made huge changes in my diet and exercise. This set off the first of several yo-yo diet cycles, which always included tons of exercise and meager amounts of food. I always felt like I was in a race to lose weight.

I spent every summer of college working as a river guide on the Salmon River in Idaho. I based a lot of my self-worth on what my stomach looked like in photos. Showing up to the river in shape became my sole obsession beginning every March. The job was hard work. I rowed rafts twenty miles a day on the river. There was heavy lifting involved before and after the trips. All of the work involved wearing a swimsuit. To me, looking good on the river was of great importance. Each subsequent spring, the scale crept up a few pounds more than the year before. I weighed 155 the first year, 165 the second,

167 the third, 170 the fourth. I'd work hard each summer to lose weight. I would feel fabulous by August, and then slowly regain the weight (and a little more) each winter. During the winter of 2008, I gained more weight than I ever had before. I spent a lot of nights on dates in fancy restaurants with my boyfriend. We sipped cocktails, had dessert, and I did not work out. My clothes fit tighter and tighter, until I had to buy bigger sizes.

I considered visiting river guide friends over the Christmas break, but was ashamed of how much weight I had gained. I didn't go. I didn't know exactly how much weight I had gained until I went to the doctor in February. I stepped on the scale, making sure to first remove my shoes, so I wouldn't get a skewed reading. I wanted to die when I saw the number. I weighed 182 pounds.

This was ten pounds more than the heaviest I'd ever been. On the BMI chart, I was considered obese. I was obese and miserable. A week later, I stumbled upon NutriMirror

while searching the Internet for weight loss advice. I browsed the site and liked what I saw. It seemed like a straightforward, logical solution to my problems. It reduced weight loss and gain to numbers instead of magical pills or wild diets. I was shocked to see that what I thought was a relatively healthy day of eating was actually a totally unbalanced diet. I was intrigued.

I logged everything I ate meticulously, and lost ten pounds in the first month. I continued to log my food intake meticulously, and lost three pounds the second month. Perhaps it was not as easy as I first thought. But I was really enjoying the diet I had adopted—and when I use the word diet, I mean the foods that I was choosing to eat, not the foods that I was restricted to.

While eating a balanced diet, I had more energy, slept better at night, recovered faster from intense workouts, and was generally a happier person. It was not easy to give up sweets and bad foods, but logging my food intake led me to realize it's possible to mix sugary treats with my healthier food choices and still achieve balance.

Logging made me realize that I often ate out of boredom rather than hunger—a habit that was detrimental to my weight loss attempts. Since I've started logging, I've lost thirty-three pounds through eating a green, balanced diet and working out hard. My BMI indicates that I'm at a healthy weight for my height. The trick will be maintaining this weight loss.

I am now armed with the information to be healthy. I know I can't always be as active as I am while working on the river in the summer, or as I was while playing college sports, but that doesn't mean I am doomed to gain weight either. Fitness, a balanced diet, and a healthy body are all tied together in life. I am excited to see how logging my food intake and exercise will help me maintain my weight, and I am very optimistic. I finally have created a lifestyle plan I can stick to that makes perfect sense to me, and for that I am very happy.

MY PHYSICAL ACTIVITY

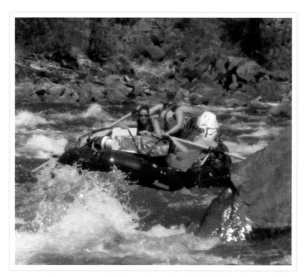

My favorite way to exercise is through outdoor activities. I love to snowboard, and I especially love whitewater rafting. They are both activities that I can do all day long, and they are so much fun that I don't even realize that I'm burning over a thousand calories. I've also started running and completed my first 5 km race. (I didn't have to walk a single step!)

All these activities are a great way to keep my weight in check without having to spend so much time at the gym.

KELLY'S *GREEN* DAY

- Calories Expended: **2,400**
- Calories Eaten: **1,760**
- Net Calorie Balance: **640**

I've come to realize that I don't need to consume as many calories as I thought. Eating 1,700 calories of high-nutrition food is much more filling than eating 2,500 calories of junk. Even though I'm eating fewer calories, I'm eating much more food than before! I try to plan meals and snacks so that I am eating throughout the day. I don't like to wait until I get hungry, because then it becomes more difficult to make smart decisions.

MY GREEN DAY NUTRITIONAL FACTS

KELLY'S
HEALTH REFLECTION™
Nutrition Facts Report

Calorie Balance	
Calories Expended	2400
Calories Eaten	1760
Net Calorie Balance	640

Nutrient Balance	
	%DV
Total Fat 42 g	✔
Saturated Fat 10 g	51%
Trans Fat 0 g	—
Cholesterol 192 mg	64%
Sodium 1880 mg	82%
Total Carbs 270 g	✔
Dietary Fiber 50 g	203%
Sugars 123 g	—
Protein 103 g	✔
Vitamin A 2164 µg	309%
Vitamin C 217 mg	289%
Calcium 1830 mg	183%
Iron 30 g	167%

MY BREAKFAST–419 calories

If I don't eat a nutritious breakfast, it's hard for me to stay green the rest of the day. I try to get as much fiber as I can in the mornings, mostly through cereal, oatmeal, fruit, and flax. This keeps me going until lunch without any problems. I also usually include a latte in my daily plan. I always choose skim milk and go very light on the flavoring. I love coffee, and a latte is a treat for me, a tasty way to get some calcium. I keep thinking that I should give them up, but when I plan for them, I don't have to!

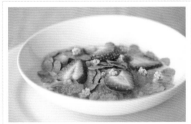 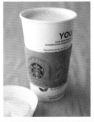

CEREAL, FRUIT, AND A LATTE
- 1/2 cup milk, nonfat, 43 calories
- 1/2 cup strawberries, 26 calories
- 1 cup Fiber One Honey Clusters, 160 calories
- 2 tbsp. flax seed meal, whole ground, 60 calories
- Skinny vanilla latte grande, nonfat, 130 calories

MY LUNCH–562 calories

I've never liked sandwiches—too much bread, too many condiment choices, and too many calories. I find pitas, though similar in many ways to bread, much more enjoyable. In this meal, I drizzle a small amount of olive oil onto a pita, top with favorite spices, bake it, and add veggies. It's very filling (especially when dipped in hummus) and incredibly delicious. I finish lunch with an apple and peanut butter for a sweet and nutritious ending to my meal.

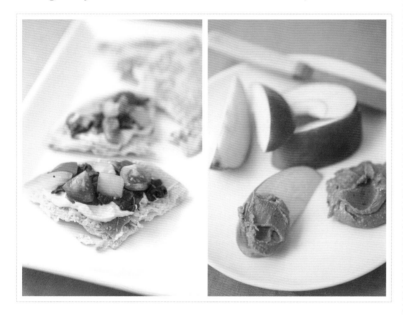

PITA WITH HUMMUS DIP; APPLE AND PEANUT BUTTER
- 2 tbsp. parmesan cheese, grated, 42 calories
- 2 cloves garlic, 9 calories
- 1 cup cooked spinach, 41 calories
- 3 tbsp. hummus, 80 calories
- 1 large pita bread, whole wheat, 153 calories
- 1 1/2 tsp. extra virgin olive oil, 60 calories
- 3 tsp. peanut butter, 105 calories
- Apple, 72 calories

MY SNACKS
–451 calories

Fruit is my favorite snack to reach for. I'm not picky at all. Berries, apples, oranges, bananas, or melon—they're all sweet and filling. And my snack selections help me get green for the day. If I need more calcium, I may have a piece of cheese, or if I'm low on carbs, I might make a smoothie. Other favorite snack foods are Luna bars or Clif bars. These give me energy for a run; they have lots of fiber and vitamins, and don't contain any scary ingredients I can't pronounce.

FRUIT, CHEESE, AND ENERGY BAR
- 2 cups watermelon, diced, 91 calories
- Iced oatmeal-raisin Luna bar, 180 calories
- 8 oz. original superfood juice (Odwalla), 130 calories
- Mini Baybel light cheese, 50 calories

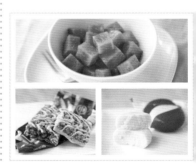

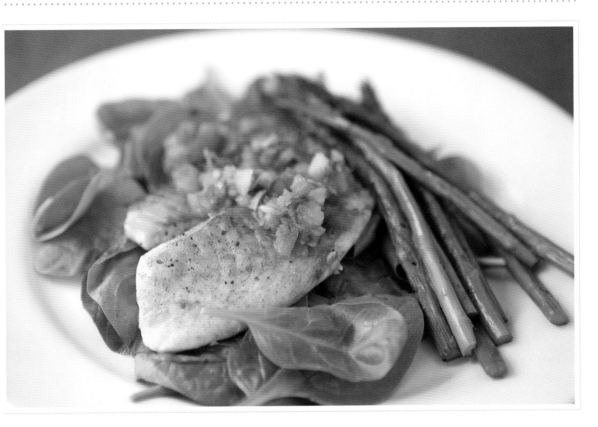

MY DINNER–328 calories

My dinners are rarely repeats of each other, but they always share the same characteristics: lean protein, lots and lots of veggies, and something chocolate at the end. I love grilled chicken breasts, shrimp fajitas (with my own seasonings so I can control the sodium), or southwest tilapia fillets. I like to use spices to add flavor to my food instead of fats (oils and butter).

PROTEIN, VEGGIES, AND CHOCOLATE
- 6 oz. tilapia filets, 136 calories
- 2 cups spinach, fresh, 14 calories
- 2 tbsp. pico de gallo salsa, 10 calories
- 6 oz. asparagus, roasted, 48 calories
- Fudge brownie, 120 calories

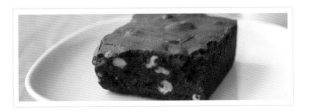

TAKING CHARGE: "NO MORE SELF-PITY, NO MORE EXCUSES."

username: kristalFriberg / *first name:* Kristal / *location:* Twin Cities, MN

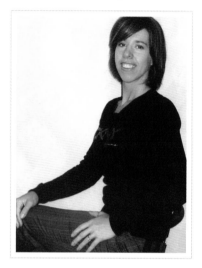

Kristal NOW: August '09 / age: 31
129 lbs. / BMI 22.2 / waist 27.75˝

My lifestyle, until now, was never balanced. My weight in particular has been up and down since I was a kid. I was heavy and was teased about it. Healthy eating and a balanced lifestyle were not part of the theme growing up in my household.

I turned to food whenever I was bored, lonely, or stressed. I remember that my Mom would always complain about "just wanting to lose 15 pounds." She would then go on the cabbage

soup diet, the liquid diet, the grapefruit diet or whatever the fad was at the moment. It was always something temporary. Weight control was a painful thing that you did for a little while until you fit into those pants in the back of the closet. Exercise was something that accidentally happened when you had to run into the grocery store because it was raining. It was never about living a lifestyle that was balanced. My mother's lifestyle was so unhealthy, that it led to her death at the age of thirty-eight. I should have learned a lesson.

In my twenties, I didn't really care about my health at all either. When I turned thirty, I started taking a serious look at all facets of my life, and was struggling with a lot of changes. My health in particular had become a real frustration for me. I was feeling miserable, both physically and mentally.

I was used to my weight going up and down, but this time I knew I was in trouble. I was

to the point of eating a whole pizza in one sitting, and inhaling a candy bar when no one was looking. I was so tired at work that I could barely keep my eyes open without chugging four cans of diet Mountain Dew. As the scale crept up and my energy levels sank, I knew I wasn't headed anywhere good. I tried to justify the weight and would make up excuses.

Once the size 12 pants I had bought the previous month started getting tight, I figured at the very least I should try to lose a couple of pounds so I wouldn't have to buy new clothes again.

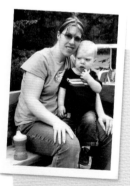

Kristal THEN: June '05
168 lbs. / BMI 28.7 / waist 32.5˝

I was trying to find a cheaper alternative to Weight Watchers when a coworker told me about NutriMirror. I was immediately amazed and overwhelmed. I was afraid to take a look at what I was really eating. I was confronting some ugly truths that I wasn't sure I was ready for. I logged all my food for a week. I logged everything I ate. I nearly cried when I saw what I was putting in my mouth. I was a long, long way from balance.

I decided enough was enough. No more self-pity. No more excuses. I knew that I had been blessed with a body that was capable of so much more. I knew that in order to make the changes necessary I was going to have to get to the root of the behavior, as painful as that might be. I started paying attention to when I ate, but more importantly I started paying attention to why I ate. I discovered that I was a stress eater. I was also a boredom eater and a lonely eater too. I realized that for me to become truly healthy it was going to require more than just a diet, it was going to require an entire

behavior modification effort. I knew that if I couldn't find a way to incorporate exercise and healthy eating into my everyday routine, I wouldn't stick with it. I also needed to put value on myself.

In order to stay accountable for the food part of it, I started logging my food everyday on NutriMirror. Every time I went to grab a snack, I literally stood there and evaluated why I wanted to eat. I decided that if I was feeling stressed, I would work out instead of eat. Sometimes I would walk for just five minutes. I was amazed at how good exercise made me feel. It not only curbed my munchies, but it got my energy level up. I started treating myself to a quiet bath after the kids went to bed. It was very relaxing and left me feeling much better than any pizza ever did.

I started exercising two or three days a week. I invested in a couple of DVDs that I really liked and started doing some resistance training as well as cardio. I made sure that I stayed within my calories for the day.

I made major changes to the types of food I was eating. I realized that I could get so much more out of whole foods than the boxed junk. Making the switch was relatively painless. It was easier to hit my goals of "going green" as well. As I put better food in my body, I started feeling better too, which was all I needed to be hooked.

I now exercise six days a week for forty-five to ninety minutes depending on the day. It is as much a part of my day as getting dressed, brushing my teeth, or doing my devotions. I am stronger than I have ever been. I am healthier than I have ever been. I feel better about myself not because of how I look, but because of what I have accomplished.

A nice perk to my new lifestyle is that I lost thirty-nine pounds, 17.25 inches, and my BMI has gone from 28.7 to 22.2.

MY PHYSICAL ACTIVITY

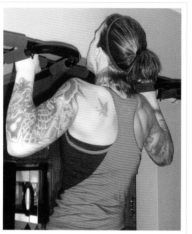

Being active is a crucial part of my lifestyle. When I started Nutrimirror I would just walk for thirty minutes on the treadmill and use DVDs to do Pilates and weights another day or two a week. I found that I love the extra energy that working out gives me. And I love that I can do push-ups and pull-ups now! I've increased my workouts gradually and now I work out five to six days a week, for fifty to seventy minutes a day. I get bored easily so I do a variety of things to keep it interesting: weight training, core work, biking, walking/jogging, and my personal favorite, the elliptical. I set my goals and log both my exercise and my food every day. It's great to be able to see the progress I have made and to continually set new goals for myself. Not only is the exercise beneficial for me, but my kids have shown a huge interest in being active since I have started working out.

KRISTAL'S *GREEN* DAY

- Calories Expended: **1,923**
- Calories Eaten: **1,438**
- Net Calorie Balance: **485**

Like many people I have a a busy schedule. I don't usually spend a lot of time on cooking dinner unless it is the weekend. I like to keep my meals simple and keep lots of fresh items on hand that can be thrown together to make a healthy dinner. I used to be the "box meal" queen, but now I've learned that a meal doesn't have to come from a box or a fast-food restaurant to be quick!

We always keep plenty of our favorite staples on hand, and since I've saved my custom menus and recipes in NutriMirror, logging our frequently eaten meals is a snap. This day in particular I used what I had on hand, and came out green with no problem.

MY GREEN DAY NUTRITIONAL FACTS

KRISTAL'S
HEALTH REFLECTION™
Nutrition Facts Report

Calorie Balance	
Calories Expended	1923
Calories Eaten	1438
Net Calorie Balance	485

Nutrient Balance	
	%DV
Total Fat 33 g	✔
Saturated Fat 6 g	38%
Trans Fat 0 g	—
Cholesterol 186 mg	62%
Sodium 1005 mg	44%
Total Carbs 203 g	✔
Dietary Fiber 31 g	154%
Sugars 92 g	—
Protein 100 g	✔
Vitamin A 2470 µg	353%
Vitamin C 208 mg	277%
Calcium 1070 mg	107%
Iron 51 g	283%

MY BREAKFAST
–401 calories

Breakfast is my favorite meal of the day. I've always been a cereal lover so it's great to eat a cereal that isn't loaded with sugar and that helps meet some of my daily nutritional requirements. I always make sure to eat breakfast because I like to work out early in the day and it keeps me going right until the end.

CEREAL, COFFEE, FRUIT, AND VITAMIN
- 3/4 cup milk, nonfat, 64 calories
- Banana, 121 calories
- 12 oz. coffee, 4 calories
- 3 tbsp. no-dairy creamer, 45 calories
- Chewable multivitamin, 0 calories
- Calcium chews, 20 calories
- 1 cup bran flakes cereal, 147 calories

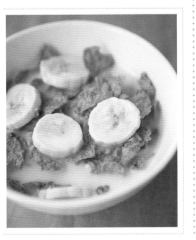

MY LUNCH–245 calories

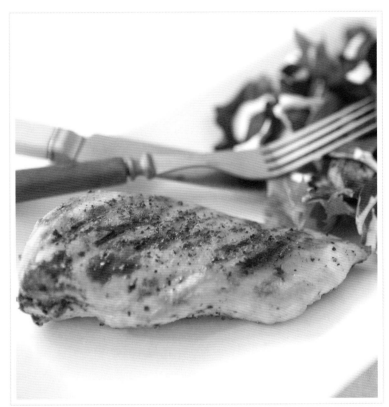

This lunch was literally just put together by grabbing what was in the fridge. I usually keep my lunch light and simple. I've found that by packing lunch for work I save money and it is much less frustrating than trying to figure out what the "healthiest" item is at the local drive-thru.

CHICKEN, SPINACH, DRESSING, AND CROUTONS
- 5 oz. grilled chicken breast, boneless, skinless, 148 calories
- 1 cup spinach, fresh, 7 calories
- 1 tbsp. ranch dressing, light, 40 calories
- 10 cheese and garlic croutons, 50 calories

MY SNACKS–429 calories

I snack frequently. I rarely go more than a couple of hours without eating, so I focus on easy items that can be eaten on the go and that will help fill in any of the nutritional gaps from my main meals. I love the smells, tastes, and textures of whole foods like fruits and vegetables, but I wanted a little bit of dark chocolate on this day too.

FRUIT, PEANUT BUTTER, FIBER BAR, AND CANDY
- 1 cup sliced apple, 53 calories
- 1/2 cup blackberries, 31 calories
- 1/2 cup grapes, 55 calories
- 1/2 oz. M&M's dark, 70 calories
- Fiber Plus bar, chocolate chip, 120 calories
- 1 tbsp. peanut butter, 100 calories

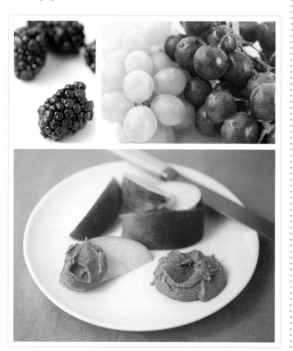

MY DINNER–363 calories

This is our "family meal." I like to try new recipes for everyone in the house, so that they can give their feedback on what is and isn't liked about them. This process helps me determine what makes it into the recipes and custom menus I store on NutriMirror. My husband is a "steak and potatoes" kind of guy, so dinner on this day was perfect for him—and it still contributed to my Green Day!

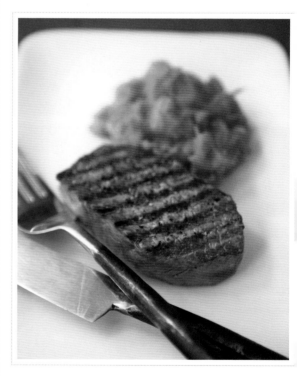

MEAT AND POTATO
- 5 oz. sweet potato, baked, 108 calories
- 5 oz. London broil, 255 calories

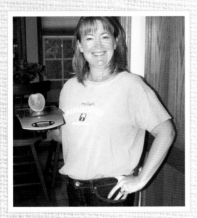

Lori NOW: November '09 / age: 45
117 lbs. / BMI 21.5 / waist 29″

. . . .

In February 2009, I started another "diet," trying to lose a few pounds before my forty-fifth birthday six months away. I struggled for four months on my own, eating less and less every day and working out more. I constantly wondered why I was such a failure at losing weight. After I lost the first few pounds, the scale wouldn't budge. I gave up for several weeks and just ate what I wanted. What did it matter? I was a failure. Then a coworker suggested that all of us in the office participate in a Biggest Loser competition. Everyone was enthusiastic … except me. I'd been trying for months and felt that there was something wrong with me. My state of mind was that I would be overweight forever, but I didn't feel that I could say no to the contest. So I signed up reluctantly.

I Googled "food log" and found NutriMirror. After logging my food for just a few days, I discovered that I wasn't eating nearly enough food. I was literally starving myself, sometimes eating only 800 calories a day. I read the logs of other participants who asked, "Why can't I lose weight?" I kept seeing the word EAT! Eat at least 1,200 calories a day! I began increasing my caloric intake and over the next twelve weeks the pounds began to drop. I won that Biggest Loser contest! And I did it by eating, not starving!

As of today, I'm 38 pounds lighter; down from 155 pounds. My starting BMI was 29.3 and I'm now at a healthy 21.5. My waist measurement went from 37 inches to 29 inches and I dropped four pants sizes. I feel so much better physically. I have more energy and love how I look. I never knew how poorly I was eating until I started logging and getting measured feedback. I have learned about the proper balance of calories in/calories out. I have become more focused on getting the right amount of protein, fat, and carbohydrates while watching my intake of sodium, fiber, and calcium. I'm able to do so many things that I couldn't do before. For example, I am now an avid exerciser and run daily. I'm much more confident in myself and am even contemplating running a 5K.

Over the course of this journey, I have discovered that keeping my logs green every day is the key to living a happy and healthy life—a life not ruled by feelings of inadequacy. I am in control my body and my health.

. . . .

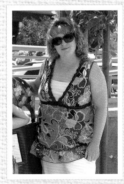

Lori THEN: June '09
155 lbs. / BMI 29.3 / waist 37″

"I FEEL BETTER AND I AM HAPPIER. WHAT MORE COULD I WANT?"

username: threem2361 / *first name:* Marna / *location:* Tipton, MO

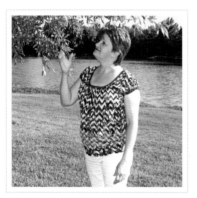

Marna NOW: October '09 / age: 48
182 lbs. / BMI 27.6 / waist 36˝

Have you ever thought to yourself, "look at that skinny thing, she needs to eat." Well that was me for the first thirty-five years of my life. I could eat anything twenty-four hours a day and not gain a pound. I loved to eat breads and cheese, and drank lots and lots of soda. At age thirty-two, I gave birth to my third child. Within three months, I was back down to 145 pounds, no problem. Then the winter after my thirty-fifth birthday I gained 35 pounds. Holy cow, what happened? At 5´8˝ and 175 pounds, I didn't think I looked that bad; I still had some curves.

Okay, so I had gained some weight. But I felt good and looked good so I did nothing to change my eating habits. The next thing I knew it was ten years later and I was carrying an additional 30 pounds.

February 28, 2006, my husband and I quit smoking. Two days later I found out my Dad had pancreatic cancer. The next week I found out my husband had melanoma and had to have surgery. Luckily the cancer had not spread into his lymph glands and he did not require chemo. Six weeks into quitting smoking, just when my husband got the all-clear from his doctor, my father passed away. The stress and depression brought on another fifteen pounds. I could not walk one block, or play with my grandchild without getting light-headed and out of breath. I thought to myself, that is why I quit smoking, but now the weight was bringing me down.

My digestive system was a mess and the doctor diagnosed me with Irritable Bowel Syndrome

(IBS). He prescribed medication that helped some symptoms but was not a cure. I did not want to live with IBS so I started omitting foods to determine what was causing my problems. First, I omitted wheat and gluten but that did not seem to help, so I then moved on to dairy products and found that they were the cause of most of the gas and bloating. Once I cut them out, my bloated stomach started to shrink and I could lean over again. Now I eat dairy in moderation, and have turned, instead, to some soy products.

That single change gave me the incentive to eat healthier,

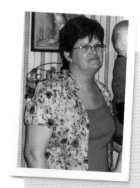

Marna THEN: April '06
220 lbs. / BMI 33.3 / waist 46˝

exercise, and begin a new chapter in my life. I also wanted to track not only my food intake but also my vitamins and minerals. I went online to find a food journal. I found NutriMirror and started logging. I soon realized that there was too much fat and not enough fruit and vegetables in my diet (which is crazy because I love both). Now, I try to stay away from processed and fried foods.

The other day I went to get the shortening out and realized it had gone rancid. So I threw it out. I remember when I used to buy a tub a month. Most of my meat today is grilled or broiled and if it is "fried" I use cooking spray and chicken or vegetable broth.

Most of my shopping is done on the outside edges of the store, stocking up on fresh fruit and vegetables as much I can. My family hates that I announce how many calories are in everything we eat, but I think it is sinking in a little.

My toy poodle is my jogging coach. I take her for walks which never seem to be long enough—she wants more. When we started out I could only jog about one hundred feet and would have to slow down to a walk. Now I can jog much greater distances. Then The Coach will make me run some more. She is a good dog with very short legs, thank goodness. Other than jogging, my exercise has been very spotty. I have some exercise tapes that I do here and there but without any real regimen.

When I get home from the office I hardly ever sit down. I am always cooking or cleaning. But my favorite activity is working in the yard and garden.

I have two teenage daughters that keep me on the run, and my son and his wife bring my four-year-old grandson over to thoroughly wear me out. They are my inspiration to stay healthy. I want to be here for them so I can play with them and be part of their lives.

Now I count my calories and try to stay between 1,200 and 1,400 a day. I log every bite and watch my sodium, fat, sugar, vitamins, and minerals. I don't think of my new eating habits as a diet but

relearning what I already knew— the things my mother taught me, that had been lost somewhere down through the years.

I still have about twenty-two pounds to go. But, this is not a do-or-die quest for me. It is more of a life journey of self improvement. I feel better and I am happier. What more could I want?

MY PHYSICAL ACTIVITY

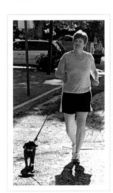

I love to exercise but have not set a regular routine. One thing I do get done is walking my toy poodle. She loves it when I kick it up and jog with her on our walks. We will walk/jog one or two miles three times a week. It did not come easy at first. Walking around the block was a chore. But I just kept pushing; now I am jogging across town.

MARNA'S *GREEN* DAY

- Calories Expended: **2,205**
- Calories Eaten: **1,239**
- Net Calorie Balance: **966**

Since joining NutriMirror I have learned how to balance my meals. I have created several different snack choices that help me get many of my vitamins and minerals while still letting me have the calories to eat a good meal. Best of all I stay full all day, which helps me overcome those late night munchies.

Every day I am finding new and better choices to add to my cupboard of goodies. Now when I head for a snack I look at the calories and if they fit into my day then I see if they're worth it or just empty calories. Six months ago I would have just eaten whatever and then felt sick the rest of the day, cancelling any thoughts of exercise. Now my diet gives my body the fuel to keep on going.

MY GREEN DAY NUTRITIONAL FACTS

MARNA'S
HEALTH REFLECTION™
Nutrition Facts Report

Calorie Balance	
Calories Expended	2205
Calories Eaten	1239
Net Calorie Balance	966

Nutrient Balance		
		%DV
Total Fat 35 g		✔
Saturated Fat 6 g		44%
Trans Fat 0 g		—
Cholesterol 47 mg		16%
Sodium 2258 mg		98%
Total Carbs 178 g		✔
Dietary Fiber 45 g		260%
Sugars 77 g		—
Protein 87 g		✔
Vitamin A 3219 µg		460%
Vitamin C 208 mg		277%
Calcium 1713 mg		171%
Iron 28 g		156%

MY BREAKFAST—264 calories

I love eggs, so changing this was going to be hard. Now I just eat the whites and add spring onions and mushrooms to add flavor, but giving up my bacon grease that I fry them in is not an option right now. I have changed to whole wheat bread and three pumps of spray butter instead of butter and jelly. Since milk does not settle well with me, I now drink vanilla soy milk. Grapefruit tops off my breakfast. I also eat strawberries, blueberries, peaches, or blackberries—whatever is in season.

EGG WHITES, VEGGIES, FRUIT, MILK, AND BREAD
- 2 large egg whites, 34 calories
- 1/4 tsp. bacon grease, 10 calories
- 1/2 grapefruit, 32 calories
- 1 tbsp. chopped onion, 4 calories
- 1 cup vanilla soy milk, light, 80 calories
- 1/2 oz. portobello mushroom, 4 calories
- 2 pieces 100% whole wheat bread, 100 calories

MY LUNCH–219 calories

Some days I am just on the run and this was one of them. When I got home for lunch there was nothing that looked good in the fridge so I headed for the freezer and I grabbed a Boca burger. When you top one with romaine lettuce and just a touch of ketchup and mustard it makes for a satisfying lunch. I added a little cooked spinach to this healthy sandwich, not only for color but also for its vitamin A and K content.

BOCA BURGER WITH VEGETABLES
- 1 Boca burger, 90 calories
- 1 tsp. mustard, 3 calories
- 1 leaf romaine lettuce, 5 calories
- 1 1/4 cups spinach, cooked, 51 calories
- 1 piece 100% whole wheat bread, 50 calories
- 1 tbsp. ketchup, no salt, 20 calories

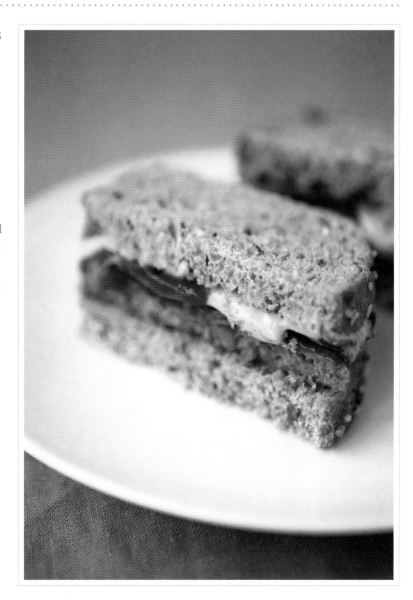

MY SNACKS–444 calories

My snacks change from day to day but I always have almonds and carrots. I try to get my one or two servings of fruit and I am a pushover for crunchy foods. So this day I had Special K wheat crackers in the afternoon and popcorn in the evening. My snacks keep me from overeating at lunch and dinner time.

NUTS, CRACKERS, FRUIT, CARROTS, POPCORN, AND MILK

- 1 apple, 70 calories
- 5 strawberries, 29 calories
- 9 baby carrots, 32 calories
- 16 almonds, raw, 111 calories
- 1 cup popcorn, 20 calories
- 1 1/2 cups vanilla soy milk, 150 calories
- 6 Special K multigrain crackers, 32 calories

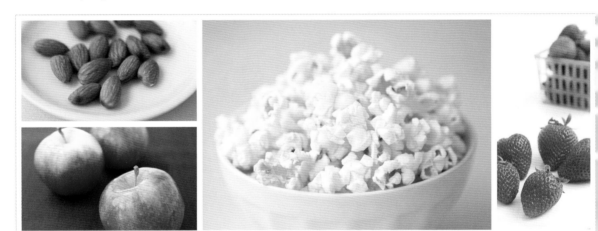

MY DINNER–312 calories

I chopped up some leftover chicken breast and tossed it in the skillet with some zucchini and summer squash. I filled a tortilla with the heated mixture and topped it off with a little leftover spaghetti sauce. Being an ex-smoker I still have this "I need an end to my meal" mentality so I finished off my meal with a Blueberry Vita Muffin. Believe me, it tasted a lot better than a cigarette.

CHICKEN, ZUCCHINI, TORTILLA, SAUCE, AND BRAN MUFFIN

- Tortilla, whole wheat, 50 calories
- 1 1/2 oz. chicken breasts, 47 calories
- 1/4 serving spaghetti sauce, 20 calories
- 2 servings grilled zucchini & summer squash, 95 calories
- Blueberry Vita Muffin, 100 calories

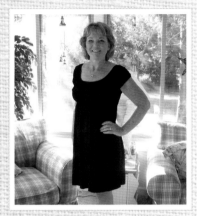

Cynthia NOW: November '09 / age: 50
174 lbs. / BMI 26.4 / waist 32″

. . . .

"You're big!" That's what an eight-year-old boy told me when I was in the third grade. That was over forty years ago, but I can still hear those words ringing in my head.

With my history of being a chubby child, an overweight teen, and eventually an obese adult, losing weight seemed just a dream—a dream that I would always wake up from, only to find that I was still that same overweight person. I knew that the right way to lose weight was by limiting the number of calories I ate. This began a thirty-year quest to find the easiest way to do just that.

I made several attempts at drastically limiting my calories and losing weight: buying expensive pre-packaged foods, joining costly diet clinics, taking experimental diet pills, low-carb and low-fat diets, hand-written food journals, and hypnosis. A couple of these worked for a short time, but eventually I would revert to my old habits.

I eventually decided that I was destined to be overweight, and I should just live with it. Then in October of 2008, my granddaughter was diagnosed with leukemia. For three months, the only comfort I could find was in food. I was in self-destruct mode. Supported and sustained by the strength of my faith in God, knowing that He is in control, I was able to place her in His hands.

In January of 2009 I was introduced to NutriMirror, the answer I had been looking for my whole life—the connection between healthy eating and losing weight.

Since becoming a member, I've lost forty-one pounds. I'm amazed at how easy it was. And believe me, I mean easy. As the pounds come off, my self esteem is increasing. What used to be an obsession with losing weight has now become a desire to be healthy. Don't get me wrong, losing the pounds is important and reaching my ideal weight is my ultimate goal, but somewhere along this fabulous journey, I realized that incorporating healthy food choices and physical activity were the answers to my thirty-year quest. They are now part of who I am.

And whenever someone notices the difference in me now, I happily share with them how I've gained control over the choices that make me healthy.

. . . .

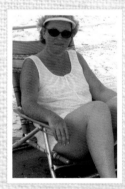

Cynthia THEN: January '09
. . . .
215 lbs. / BMI 32.6 / waist 40″

MANAGING BALANCE AFTER GASTRIC BYPASS SURGERY.

username: kelbeaudoin / *first name:* Kel / *location:* St Paul, MN

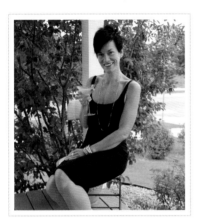

Kel NOW: August '09 / age: 43
148 lbs. / BMI 22.4 / waist 28.5˝

I once thought it was easier to find love than to find a healthy relationship with food. Had I placed an advertisement on a dating service for food, I would have been matched up with NutriMirror. This website has been a tremendous tool in helping me develop a happy and healthy relationship with food.

I won't take you through the years of dieting—dieting that started when I was very young. Years of dieting took me from a 160-pound eighth grader to a 270-pound thirty-eight-year-old. It had to stop.

In November of 2003, I sought a permanent and final change in my tumultuous relationship with food. I was looking for what I thought was the only way I could make this change. I researched gastric bypass surgery on the Internet. I found a weight loss surgery clinic in my area, scheduled a consultation with the surgeon, and started the process.

In May 2004, I underwent gastric bypass surgery. I had some complications that left me with a four-inch scar down my abdomen and another scar that I call my "second belly button." My surgery was a success. I was the ideal patient, following the prescribed regimen of six small meals a day. I ate primarily protein, and I worked out at least five days a week. A year later, I reached my goal weight of 140 pounds and I felt great.

Some time later, I was working out with a personal trainer. I gained good, strong muscle and seven pounds. I didn't worry

about it. I was working hard and was not going to be an "after the after" story.

But I watched in horror as one by one, thirteen additional pounds came back. I didn't think I ate much. A new man in my life, rich dinners, and wine could account for some of the weight gain; the rest I blamed on my workouts. I was walking thirty minutes a day, four days a week, and strength training twice a week. I blamed the exercise for part of the weight gain.

One of my dear friends got engaged and her wedding was

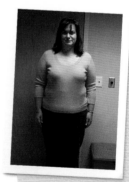

Kel THEN: December '03
267.1 lbs. / BMI 41 / waist 41˝

the perfect reason to get back to my fighting weight. I had had success before in weight loss using a food journal. So I searched the Internet for "food journals" and saw the word free." I was there.

I started with NutriMirror in October of 2008. My weight was 160 pounds, and my size four clothes no longer fit. I wondered how I had gotten back "there." I was back to a number that I thought I would not see on the scale again. Using NutriMirror, it did not take me long before I realized how it had happened. I was eating terribly. I entered my foods, and the program showed me exactly what was going wrong. For example, my morning oatmeal from the office café exceeded 500 calories. I was great at drinking water loaded with packets of crystals of sweetness and gobs of artificial sweeteners. By ten o'clock in the morning I would dip into the candy jar on my desk. I remember adding Tootsie Pops and Smarties candies to the NutriMirror database. I helped myself to the community M&M's. When I

looked at the amount of empty calories I consumed every day, I saw how and why the weight had come back.

I began using NutriMirror to look at calories in and calories out. With this site, the physics of weight loss are easy to understand. When more calories are consumed than expended, weight is gained. For quite some time I used the program only for evaluating calories. Once I felt comfortable with the calorie balance, I started to delve deeper into the nutritional analysis information I was receiving. My diet was lacking fiber, calcium, iron, and key vitamins. As a gastric bypass patient, I had committed to a lifetime of vitamin supplements, but I was not taking them. This was one explanation why I was constantly getting kicked out of my company blood drives. The other explanation was my poor choices.

Sodium. It was everywhere. Everything I ate had tons of sodium. I began to evaluate my food choices. I couldn't believe it.

Instant oatmeal had 310 mg of sodium. I could make my own at home, and add my own dried fruits. Lunch—the frozen food entrées were deadly; time to pick better choices. Raw almonds arrived on the scene, as well as Greek yogurt sweetened with honey, high fiber breads with peanut butter, and fruits and veggies dipped in peanut butter or hummus. Who says you can't have peanut butter and lose weight?

I ate small, healthy, clean meals every two and a half to three hours. I increased my exercise to five to six days a week. I increased the intensity of my workouts, transitioning from walking to running intervals. I was down to 153 pounds, 7 pounds less than when I started NutriMirror. I had a new hurdle to overcome—the "toxic" packets I was using to flavor my water. I had done enough research on the Internet to be convinced that these little bundles of sweetness were responsible for my sugar cravings—those gnaw-your-arm-off needs for carbohydrates that kept me reaching into my candy jar, and keeping me away from my 147 pounds. I cut back gradually. I replaced one flavor packet with plain water until eventually it was all water. As if by magic, the cravings for sweets were gone. Over time, those extra pounds simply went away!

One of the things I have learned is that making healthy food choices does not equate to food that is lacking in taste or comfort. I love all of my food choices. Otherwise, I would not be eating them. There is something truly comforting about a warm bowl of oatmeal, or a chicken burger piled high with avocado, tomato and hummus, and some grilled asparagus on the side. I still bake and enjoy cookies and treats. I can still eat anything I want, but what I *want* to eat has changed.

MY PHYSICAL ACTIVITY

I never dreamt that I would be a person who LOVES exercise! I work out five to six days a week, and choose a variety of different types of exercise to keep my body guessing! Weather permitting, I take my workouts outdoors, running three to five miles or cycling for twenty to thirty-five miles. I typically strength train three days a week at the gym. I do cardio on those days as well, preferring the treadmill. On this particular day, it was a fast paced walk on an incline and then a variety of strength moves for the legs, with an ab workout thrown in for fun! I use a foam roller to really work my core during my ab exercises. I had some errands to run later in the day, so I chose to walk to the store and back. Every bit counts!

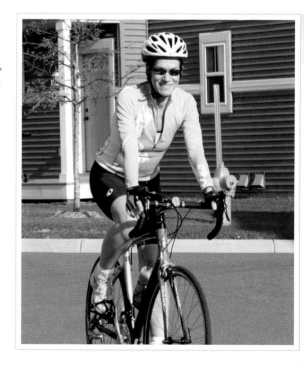

KEL'S *GREEN* DAY

- Calories Expended: **2,299** • Calories Eaten: **2,273** • Net Calorie Balance: **20**

Being aware of your food choices means so much more than how many calories you can consume. I can choose to eat a high-fat, high-calorie fast-food meal for 2,200 calories, or I can choose a day like this one. I eat these foods not only because they meet my daily nutritional requirements, but also because they taste good! Success at weight loss, and then weight maintenance, means that you love the food you are eating, and get pleasure from it. There were many weight loss programs on which I succeeded, but eventually I gained the weight back because I could not maintain their regimens. These are my choices, and I love every last calorie!

MY GREEN DAY NUTRITIONAL FACTS

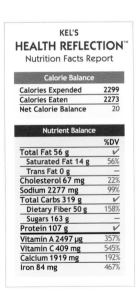

KEL'S
HEALTH REFLECTION™
Nutrition Facts Report

Calorie Balance	
Calories Expended	2299
Calories Eaten	2273
Net Calorie Balance	20

Nutrient Balance	
	%DV
Total Fat 56 g	✔
Saturated Fat 14 g	56%
Trans Fat 0 g	—
Cholesterol 67 mg	22%
Sodium 2277 mg	99%
Total Carbs 319 g	✔
Dietary Fiber 50 g	158%
Sugars 163 g	—
Protein 107 g	✔
Vitamin A 2497 µg	357%
Vitamin C 409 mg	545%
Calcium 1919 mg	192%
Iron 84 mg	467%

MY BREAKFAST—292 calories

On days I work out in the morning, it is important for me to fuel both before and after the workout. I try to keep it simple, and something that will be easy to digest. Cinnamon raisin toast with Better'n Peanut Butter and a banana fits that need, and is delicious! I eat breakfast every day, breaking it into smaller meals. I often start with a smoothie or toast, and then have oatmeal or cereal and fruit. Because of my surgery, I run the risk of not properly absorbing my vitamins, so I take supplements, but strive for green (balance) without them.

COFFEE WITH CREAM, CEREAL, MILK, AND FRUIT, TOAST, PEANUT BUTTER, AND VITAMINS

- Banana, 70 calories
- 1 slice cinnamon raisin toast, 80 calories
- 1 tbsp. Better'n Peanut Butter, 50 calories
- 1 tbsp. half and half, 20 calories
- 1 tbsp. half and half, nonfat, 9 calories
- 2 oz. coffee, 8 calories
- Iron supplement, 0 calories
- Calcium chews, 40 calories
- Flintstones Gummies, 15 calories

MY LUNCH–463 calories

I have made this tuna salad different ways, with whatever ingredients are handy. The addition of egg whites bumps up the protein. The toasted almonds and celery add crunch, and the cranberries are great for color and sweetness. I love all of the wraps that are now available at the store, and choose one based usually on the fiber content and the price! This day I chose a soft taco as the wrap for my salad. I add sliced apple for dessert, and that contributes to my fiber total for the day. The chocolate was my REAL dessert. I have chocolate almost every day!

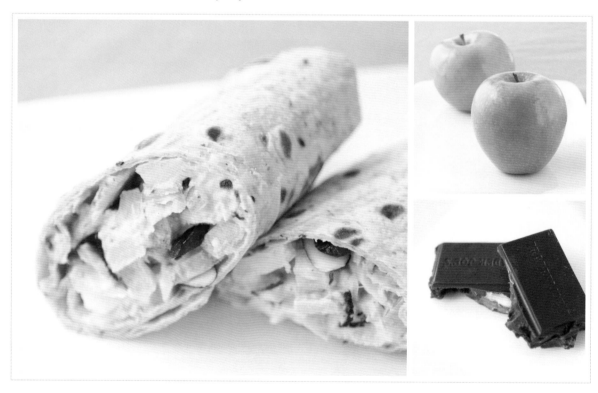

SALAD, WRAP, FRUIT, AND DESSERT
- 1 serving tuna and egg salad (see recipe), 237 calories
- 1 cup apple slices, 58 calories
- 1/3 oz. spinach, 2 calories
- 2 pieces dark chocolate with raisins and pecans, 85 calories
- 1 tortilla, low carb, low fat, 81 calories

TUNA AND EGG SALAD

Makes four 1/2-cup servings.

INGREDIENTS

3 tbsp. slivered almonds

3 large eggs, hardboiled

6 oz. albacore tuna, packed in water, drained

5 tbsp. mayonnaise (regular, low fat, or a combination of both)

3 stalks celery, diced

1 oz. dried cranberries

PREPARATION

1. Toast the almonds in a sauté pan over medium heat.

2. Remove and discard the yolks from the hardboiled eggs. Chop the whites.

3. In a large bowl, combine the almonds, egg whites, tuna, mayonnaise, celery, cranberries, and almonds. Mix well.

4. Serve on your favorite bread, cracker, wrap, or fork!

MY SNACKS–635 calories

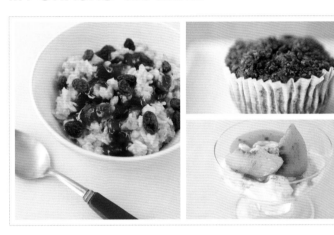

After a workout, I get some protein from egg whites and a delicious bowl of oatmeal with raisins and strawberry jam for energy. An afternoon trip to Trader Joe's means a snack of their high fiber pomegranate cranberry muffins. One of my favorite snacks is fat-free Greek yogurt with agave for sweetening, and frozen peaches. Delicious! Sometimes my "snack" is simply a piece of fruit or a small salad; other times it may be a homemade chocolate chip cookie, or an iced soy latte. All, in the right combination, can be considered healthy and contribute to a "green" day!

EGG WHITES, CEREAL, FRUIT, AND MUFFIN
- 1 serving oatmeal, 150 calories
- 1/4 tsp. cinnamon, 2 calories
- 1 1/8 oz. raisins, 90 calories
- 1 tbsp. strawberry preserves, 50 calories
- 2 large egg whites, 33 calories
- 1 cup Greek yogurt, nonfat, 120 calories
- 2 tsp. raw agave nectar, 40 calories
- 2/3 cup peach slices, fresh frozen, 50 calories
- Pomegranate-cranberry-bran muffin, 100 calories

MY DINNER–883 calories

I love to cook, and get several magazines that give me great ideas. I adore mangos, so I was quite excited to find this recipe for grilled halibut with mango salsa. It is high in protein, and very low in fat. The roasted beets and a salad of grilled romaine were delicious. I still love bread with dinner, and a garlic naan fit in nicely. I also love red wine, and enjoyed a glass as I prepared dinner. Dessert? Of course! I baked eggless lemon snaps earlier in the day—crisp, yet chewy, and a great end to the meal.

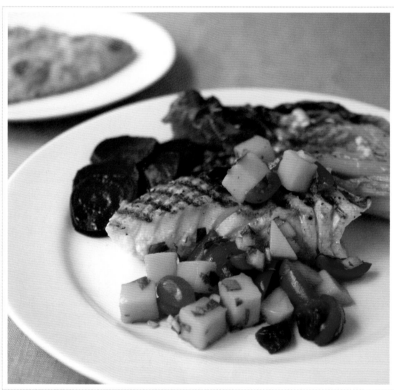
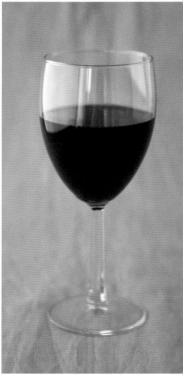

FISH, SALAD, NAAN, WINE, SOY MILK, AND DESSERT

- 1 serving grilled halibut w/mango salsa (see recipe), 190 calories
- 1 beet, cooked, 22 calories
- 6 oz. red wine, 150 calories
- 1 cup vanilla soy milk, light, 80 calories
- 1/2 piece tandoori garlic naan, 120 calories
- 1 tbsp. Champagne pear vinaigrette with gorgonzola, 23 calories
- 1 serving grilled romaine (see recipe), 114 calories
- 3 serving eggless lemon snaps (see recipe), 184 calories

GRILLED HALIBUT WITH MANGO SALSA

Makes four servings.

SALSA
1 cup diced mango
1/4 cup diced tomato
2 tbsp. diced red onion
3 tbsp. dried cherries
1 1/2 tbsp. chopped fresh cilantro
1/2 tbsp. chopped fresh mint leaves
1/2 tbsp. red wine vinegar
1/2 tbsp. raspberry vinegar
1/2 tsp. minced garlic

HALIBUT
1 lb. halibut, cut into 4 pieces
1/2 tsp. sea salt
1/4 tsp. black pepper

PREPARATION:

1. Mix together to mango, tomato, dried cherries, onion, cilantro, mint, red wine vinegar, raspberry vinegar, and garlic. Place in refrigerator. Can be made ahead.

2. Season both sides of fish with salt and pepper.

3. Grill each side of fish 3–4 minutes, or until done.

4. Serve each piece of fish topped with 1/4 cup of the mango salsa.

GRILLED ROMAINE

I serve this with a Champagne pear vinaigrette from Trader Joe's, but it is just as delicious drizzled with some good quality balsamic vinegar.

Makes two servings.

INGREDIENTS
1 head romaine lettuce
Extra virgin olive oil
Salt and pepper

PREPARATION:

1. Remove and discard just the outer leaves of the intact head of lettuce. Do not remove the bottom of the head; you need this to keep it together on the grill.

2. Slice the head of lettuce in half, drizzling the halves with one tablespoon of olive oil. Turn to coat both sides. Season with salt and pepper.

3. Heat the grill (either an outdoor grill or an indoor grill pan).

4. Place the lettuce cut-side down on the grill for about 30 seconds, then turn the lettuce over for another 30 seconds.

5. Lettuce is done when the outer leaves are slightly wilted and brown.

6. Before serving, cut off the bottom of the head to separate the leaves.

EGGLESS LEMON SNAPS

Makes thirty cookies.

INGREDIENTS

1 cup white all-purpose flour
1/4 cup almond meal
3/4 cup white sugar
1 tsp. baking soda
Pinch of salt
1 1/2 tbsp. lemon zest
6 tbsp. butter, melted
1/4 cup lemon juice
1 tsp. vanilla extract

PREPARATION

1. Preheat oven to 350°F.

2. Line a cookie sheet with parchment paper.

3. Stir together flour, almond meal, sugar, baking soda, salt, and lemon zest in a medium bowl.

4. In a separate bowl, mix together the butter, lemon juice, and vanilla extract.

5. Create a well in the dry ingredients, then pour the wet mixture into it. Stir together. Dough will be quite sticky.

6. Scoop small spoonfuls onto the prepared cookie sheet. Leave lots of room, as the dough spreads!

7. Bake 10–12 minutes, just until the edges start to brown.

8. Cool for 5 minutes on the cookie sheet, then transfer to a cooling rack. Once cooled, store in an airtight container.

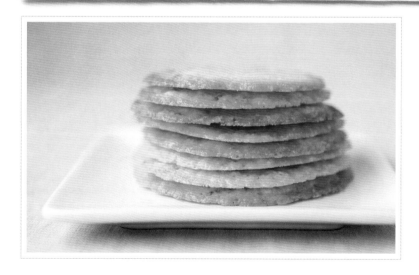

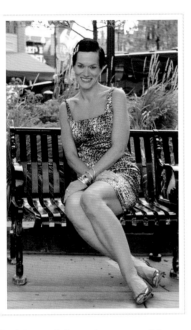

Kel Beaudoin writes a weekly lifestyle column for NutriMirror called *TGIF with Kel*. Each Friday Kel uses her own experiences of overcoming personal challenges to inspire her readers to strive for lives in balance. As her story on the previous pages tells us, at one time Kel weighed 270 pounds—122 pounds heavier than she is today.

A realization that she was living only half of the life she was destined for, and a shortened one at that, led her to seek assistance in her battle to control her weight and enjoy better health. Kel knows too well that striving for happiness through food only leads to an unhealthy, unhappy life. Choosing to fill emotional voids by suppressing feelings with comfort food, and a too sedentary lifestyle, led Kel to the brink of a health disaster. Today, she is winning the battle. Kel has a newfound passion for life, happiness, and health that motivates her to bring others back from that same brink. Now, her goal each week is to use her gifts of effective communication and humor to educate and inspire others. Through her weekly column, she provides readers with insights into their lives and the guidance they may need to be successful at self-managing the behaviors that make them healthy and happy. We invite you to meet her at *NutriMirror.com/people/ TGIFwithKel* every Friday.

She has also agreed to write a Health Reflection™ book. Kel will share tips from her successful transformation to better health and discuss the benefits of laughter, healthy eating, and exercise. She aims to help her readers achieve their dreams to live fuller, happier lives.

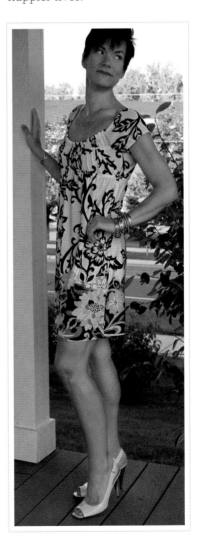

"I VOWED TO BETTER MYSELF THROUGH PROPER NUTRITION AND FITNESS FOR LIFE."

username: MelissaEileen / *first name:* Melissa / *location:* Seattle, WA

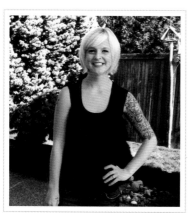

Melissa NOW: October '09 / age: 25
114 lbs. / BMI 19.5 / waist 26˝

"But you're not fat!" That is what a friend said when I told her about NutriMirror. She told me that she couldn't understand why I was using a diet website if I didn't need to lose weight. Of course, I promptly explained to her that NutriMirror is not a diet. It's about learning how to live in balance and to maintain a healthy lifestyle. It is not just another temporary wellness fix, like many diet plans tend to be.

My goal was, and is, to become more aware of what is truly good for my body. I want to learn how to manage a lifetime of healthy habits to keep me in balance. So when I realized that the site was about gaining practical knowledge on how to obtain and manage balance throughout your entire life, I was instantly intrigued. I plan on living a long and active life.

Before joining, I did not eat healthy; I just thought I did. Almost all of my meals were self-proclaimed "healthy" microwave entrées or low-calorie salty snacks. In truth, my daily sodium intake was through the roof and I was consuming very little of the healthy nutrients my body required. I also rarely went near any fresh fruits or vegetables. I never drank water, only massive amounts of diet sodas.

I was not educated on the importance of a healthy diet. I often felt sluggish. I had blotchy skin, and I never truly felt satisfied after eating. Luckily, the tool I needed to change all that came into my life for the rescue. One of the first lessons that I learned was just because the package says "healthy" or "low calorie" does not necessarily mean that it's good for your body. Considering my diet at the time, this was clearly one of the most important lessons that I learned.

Although I had a weight loss goal (which I've met), my main purpose was to learn how to eat healthy, to exercise more, and to stay healthy. I was seeking practical, actionable advice about my diet and fitness goals, which didn't seem to exist in the countless "diet" articles. NutriMirror not

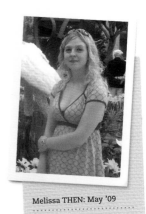

Melissa THEN: May '09
128 lbs. / BMI 21.9

nly provides its members with practical tools that they need for managing their choices, but also a journal room—an excellent place where members chat, support each other and share sound advice about this business of making better choices. I've had priceless exchanges about healthy living there.

The ever-so-honest and caring folks I've met have helped open my eyes to the fact that if I had continued to eat the way I was eating, I would have been putting myself at high risk for becoming overweight or developing a chronic lifestyle disease at some point in life. I don't feel like it is an exaggeration to say the knowledge I've gained is potentially life-saving.

I've gained a wealth of knowledge that has positively impacted my life. When I first started logging my foods (the ones that I thought were healthy), I had a rude awakening. I saw that my diet was horrific and most likely contributed to my developing gallstones at the ripe old age of twenty.

The whole process has shown me that I need to nourish my body properly in order to function well and fight off disease.

I made a vow to myself to change. I vowed to better myself through proper nutrition and fitness for life. No more temporary fixes. By logging my foods and exercise routines each day, I am confident that I will be able to accomplish my goals. Every day brings another helpful learning experience. I've learned what nutrients my body needs. I've learned how to control my sodium. I've been learning from my mistakes rather than beating myself up over them. If I had enough room to list everything that I've learned (and will learn), this book would have to be a hundred pages longer.

I've changed my diet almost entirely and have already noticed vast improvements in the way I feel. I now eat at least two fruits and vegetables daily. I've completely eliminated microwavable frozen entrées, and I've replaced diet soda with about fourteen eight-ounce glasses of water per day. I feel fantastic!

It's amazing what proper nutritional habits can do for your body in just a short period of time. In only a few months I have increased my energy, my skin has became clearer, and I can now exercise longer without feeling fatigued. I am convinced that these positive changes that I've made are why I can now run ten miles almost effortlessly. I even registered to run the Seattle Marathon later this year! I truly feel like a new person. I am a healthier person, a livelier, more energetic person, and I am determined and confident that I will be this person for life.

MY PHYSICAL ACTIVITY

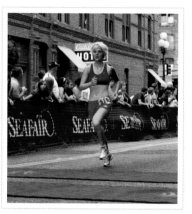

Running has become one of my favorite pastimes. I can now forget about the worries of life while I'm pounding away at the pavement. However, before I joined NutriMirror, I could only run two miles tops; any added mileage would have probably caused me to pass out. As soon as I learned that proper nutrition is a major component in building endurance, I started developing better diet habits in hopes of improving my fitness levels. It worked! When I improved my diet, my running also improved significantly. I now participate in local races almost every weekend and I'm continuing to train hard for the Seattle marathon.

Publisher's Note: Melissa has since completed her first marathon.

MELISSA'S *GREEN* DAY

- Calories Expended: **2,085**
- Calories Eaten: **1,686**
- Net Calorie Balance: **399**

At first, having an all-green day was extremely difficult. I thought it would never happen. I had a hard time keeping my sodium under control and I wasn't getting enough of the essential vitamins and minerals that my body needed. Thankfully, on the NutriMirror homepage, there are links to reports that show you at a glance exactly what your "problem foods" are. It also gives you guidance on better food options. By using this tool, I slowly began to reinvent my diet. Then, I had my first all-green day! This was probably the first time in my entire life that I had truly eaten healthy. I worked hard for that first Green Day, but the more time I spend learning on NutriMirror, the easier it is getting to stay balanced.

MY GREEN DAY NUTRITIONAL FACTS

MELISSA'S
HEALTH REFLECTION™
Nutrition Facts Report

Calorie Balance	
Calories Expended	2085
Calories Eaten	1686
Net Calorie Balance	399

Nutrient Balance	
	%DV
Total Fat 39 g	✔
Saturated Fat 7 g	37%
Trans Fat 0 g	—
Cholesterol 97 mg	32%
Sodium 1811 mg	79%
Total Carbs 273 g	✔
Dietary Fiber 51 g	216%
Sugars 131 g	—
Protein 80 g	✔
Vitamin A 3467 µg	495%
Vitamin C 455 mg	607%
Calcium 2473 mg	247%
Iron 28 g	156%

MY BREAKFAST
-410 calories

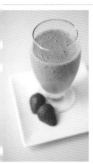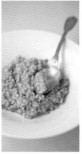

'm a gal on the go, so I like to have a quick and nutritious breakfast that will keep me fueled until my next meal. I found that instant oatmeal and a blended smoothie make the perfect combo. They provide many of my essential vitamins and minerals without the sodium that many dry cereals contain. I also take a multi-vitamin and a calcium + D supplement.

MILK, CEREAL, FRUIT, YOGURT, JUICE, AND VITAMINS
- 4 oz. milk, nonfat, 40 calories
- 2 packets apple-cinnamon instant oatmeal, 260 calories
- Calcium + D supplement, 0 calories
- 4 oz. orange juice, fortified, 55 calories
- Daily vitamin, 0 calories
- 4 oz. strawberry yogurt, nonfat, 55 calories

MY LUNCH–317 calories

I made a few simple adjustments to my turkey sandwich to make it healthier. I replaced white bread with whole grain; replaced the pickle with fresh spinach; and instead of processed I used fresh turkey meat. Now I have a sandwich that contains essential whole grains, is higher in vitamins, and lower in sodium. I also eat an apple for added fiber, which helps keep me full longer.

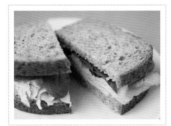

TURKEY SANDWICH AND FRUIT
- 1 tsp. mustard, 3 calories
- 1 apple, 72 calories
- 1/4 cup fresh spinach, 2 calories
- 3 pieces turkey lunch meat, oven roasted, 60 calories
- 2 pieces whole grain bread, 180 calories

MY SNACKS–604 calories

The majority of the foods that I snack on are fresh fruits and vegetables that contain the nutrients that satisfy the needs of my body. I found that if I do not consume these nutrients throughout the day, my body will crave them; therefore I'll feel hungry more often. I also allow myself a lite ice cream bar treat. I never allow myself to feel like I'm being deprived.

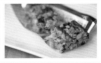

FRUIT, NUTS, FIBER BAR, AND SKINNY COW
- Banana, 121 calories
- 10 strawberries, 57 calories
- 1/4 cup almonds, dry roasted, salted, 206 calories
- Fiber One Chewy Bar, 140 calories
- Skinny Dipper vanilla ice cream, 80 calories

MY DINNER—355 calories

Since I do most of my running in the evening, I like to have a dinner that is high in protein and antioxidants. Protein helps to build muscles while antioxidants help repair some of the oxidative damage that occurs during hard workouts. This is why I choose chicken, which is high in protein, and broccoli, which is rich in vitamin C, a powerful antioxidant. Also, eating a dinner that is high in protein keeps me full longer; therefore I don't feel the need to reach for a late night snack.

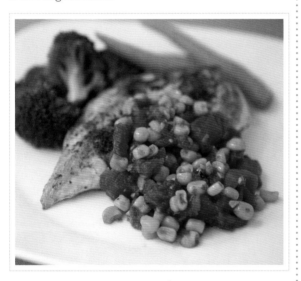

CHICKEN, FRUIT, VEGETABLES, AND TEA
- Chicken in spicy chipotle sauce (see recipe), 203 calories
- 15 grapes, 52 calories
- 4 1/2 spears broccoli, 48 calories
- 15 baby carrots, 52 calories
- 16 oz. iced green tea, 0 calories

CHICKEN IN SPICY CHIPOTLE SAUCE

Makes four servings.

INGREDIENTS
1 tbsp. olive oil
4 boneless, skinless chicken breast halves
  (about 6 oz. each)
3/4 tsp. chipotle chile powder, divided
3/4 tsp. dried oregano, divided
2 cloves garlic, slivered
1/2 cup canned crushed tomatoes
3/4 cup yellow corn kernels
2 scallions, thinly sliced
Lime wedges for serving

PREPARATION
1. Heat the oil in a skillet over medium-high heat.

2. Season chicken with 1/4 tsp. chipotle powder and 1/4 tsp. oregano. Sauté chicken until golden brown on one side, about four minutes. Turn chicken over, add garlic to pan, and continue cooking for another minute.

3. Add tomatoes, 1/3 cup water, and remaining chipotle powder. Bring to a boil.

4. Reduce heat to a simmer and cook uncovered for another five minutes or until chicken is almost done.

5. Add corn and scallions. Cook two minutes more until chicken is done and corn is heated.

6. Serve with lime wedges.

username: erinatx / *first name:* Erin

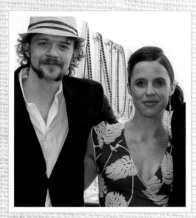

Erin NOW: November '09 / age: 28
124 lbs. / BMI 20.7 / waist 24.5˝

. . . .

After being asked to participate in two of my best friends' weddings, I was desperate to shape up when I stumbled upon NutriMirror. I had tried everything to get fit quickly—hitting the gym (but not regularly), changing my diet (zero-to-no results), taking herbal pills (enough said), and trying to keep track of my food intake in a notebook. The scales didn't cooperate.

I resigned myself to the thought that it was just my build and I was stuck with it. Things changed when I read a blurb in a fitness magazine about keeping a food journal. I searched the Internet and NutriMirror popped up. The site appealed to my organized side immediately with its charts and easy-to-understand figures. The information—and idea-rich Journal Room—connected me to many with similar goals. The people I met there were encouraging, stressing that whole foods—not diet pills or calorie-restricted menus—were key.

After familiarizing myself with the site, I started to track every bite that crossed my lips. I just sat back and watched NutriMirror chart what I was eating. And no wonder I wasn't losing weight! On some days I got triple the amount of calories my body needed; on others I was getting far too few. My sodium was high, my vitamins and fiber were low. I was all over the place—a long, long way from healthy balance.

I decided "Going for Green" (balance) was going to became my new personal mantra. Keeping track of both the food I ate and the calories I burned through exercise was a whole new form of accountability for me. For the first time in my life I set a weight loss goal and actually reached it! Can you say *empowered*? I couldn't believe I didn't feel like I was depriving myself! In fact, I felt and continue to feel so much more satisfied with the food I eat. My body has responded to the balanced lifestyle not only with weight loss but also with brighter and clearer skin, shiny hair and nails, and a lot less emotional stress. I have an overall sense of well-being.

Today I feel strong, beautiful, and completely inspired not only by my own transformation but also those of other members I've met in the Journal Room. This inspiration has manifested itself in a serious career path change. I hope to become a certified nutritionist and personal trainer within the next two years.

. . . .

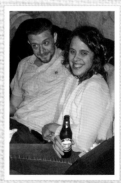

Erin THEN: April '09
. . . .
142 lbs. / BMI 23.7 / waist 28˝

DIABETES: "I CAN AND WILL DO WHAT THEY (MY PARENTS) COULDN'T OR WOULDN'T."

username: munkstir / *first name:* Molly / *location:* Fredericksburg, VA

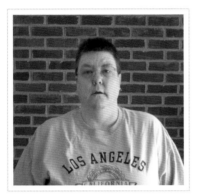

Molly NOW: August '09 / age: 49
204.6 lbs. / BMI 34.9 / waist 41.5˝

In 1968, my Pop was diagnosed with a disease that would change my life. He was forty-five years old and I was eight. That year was the beginning of my crash course in a disease known as diabetes. I learned about exchange food lists, ketones, and sugar in the urine, and what sodium did to blood pressure. I watched my father give up foods that he had once loved. I watched his life take a turn. My father accepted the challenge with little trepidation. I learned that he was an incredibly strong man and I wouldn't realize the measure of that strength for another twenty-five years.

I watched him wither away and eventually give up the fight against an enemy that he had attempted to stop too late in life. It attacked his body systematically and wreaked havoc with systems one would never imagine could be affected by diabetes. This once vibrant, witty, and unbelievably patient man (who I just knew could conquer the world) had been reduced to a deaf, blind, incontinent amputee who eventually resigned to leave it in God's hands. If only he had followed the doctor's advice to monitor the foods he ate, how they'd been prepared, and added a bit more physical activity, he might have died a less devastating and painful death. I was an observant daughter and swore that there was no way I was going to end up like that.

In 1982 my Mom, at the age of fifty-six, years was diagnosed with diabetes. I was twenty-two. My parents were now affectionately known as the Dueling Diabetics. As hard as Pop tried to save Mom by serving as an example, Mom simply ignored the doctors, and sadly she also ignored what Pop had become. What were the odds that both parents would become diabetic?

I was stationed in San Diego attempting to finish out a tour in Uncle Sam's canoe club, but I took the time to research this disease and saw an ugliness that words cannot describe except to say that diabetes isn't fickle, prejudiced, or gender-biased. The more I read, the more I feared my own future. I read that diabetes can be genetically linked. Oh man, I was playing

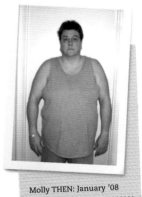

Molly THEN: January '08
230 lbs. / BMI 39.3 / waist 47˝

genetic Russian roulette and I don't like guns to begin with. I was worried enough to seek out the ship's doctor. I asked him what he thought my odds were. He told me that even though it can be genetically linked, it also had a lot to do with how well I took care of my body. He told me to eat right, exercise, and not smoke. I was physically fit and even under the standard weight for my age and frame. I thought I could quit smoking if I put my mind to it. Looked like I could dodge that bullet.

After Pop died, my Mom's health continued to deteriorate. She became labeled as a brittle diabetic (brittle diabetics can't regulate their blood sugars consistently) and continued to ignore everything she was told by her doctors and her children. She kept saying she didn't want to go on living without Pop, so she gave up. But it wasn't a quick passing. It took another sixteen years of losing her sight, her hearing, and the feeling in her hands and feet before diabetes came out the winner. She died March 19, 2009, and left us orphans. Her last hours were painful to watch and I can only imagine (though I don't want to) the pain she experienced. I'm an observant daughter and I swear that there is no way I am going to end up like that.

. . . .

"I'm going to start you on Metformin. We want to get your sugars regulated early on and you'll need to make some life changes immediately." In 2006, I was forty-six years old and became a card-carrying diabetic. I started on a new leg of my life's journey with an unwanted companion, but I knew what I had to do to keep this disease under control and made a vow to work on my own battle plan. I weighed 237 pounds when I started this reincarnation. I am 5′4″ and I looked and felt bad. I've run the gamut of emotions related to this obesity including self-loathing, desperation, anxiety, loneliness, and humor. My first priority was to lose the equivalent of a small child in weight. Not an easy task and one that I found myself daunted by, but accepted bravely.

Then a while ago, I read that keeping a food diary would help me keep my calories in check. Now I knew that in order to lose one pound of weight, I'd have to dump an average of 500 calories per day. The only thing is that I hate having to count calories, fat, cholesterol, and sodium for every single thing I eat. I spent one Saturday afternoon looking for a miracle and lo and behold, I found NutriMirror! Here was a tool that would help make that chore much easier. I could track the problem spots, make a few adjustments and share my experiences with others just like me. I knew what I needed to do, having observed my parents mishandle their diabetes.

With this wonderful tool, I can and will do what they couldn't or wouldn't. My journey as a healthier diabetic has just begun. NutriMirror provides the measured feedback to guide my choices and make this effort easier and more rewarding. With every fiber of my being, I will not go to my grave with a disease-broken body. I'm going out laughing and yelling, "Damn! What an unbelievable ride that was!"

MY PHYSICAL ACTIVITY

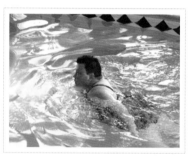

I have had to find "body-friendly" exercises as I have bad knees, back, and shoulders due to too much past living-on-the-edge and sowing wild oats in my twenties and early thirties.

Enter the recumbent bicycle. It resembles a stationary bicycle except for the seat (it looks like a chair seat) and the pedals are out in front of you. This makes it easier on my body and I manage to rack up a thirty-minute, 15 mph ride at least three days per week—right there where I work—in climate-controlled comfort!

I will also be starting water exercises. The water will provide resistance, and help keep my joints from suffering any major damage. When it's all-said-and-done, I hope to gain more flexibility and strength, so that I can tackle my next challenge—the stability ball.

MOLLY'S *GREEN* DAY

- Calories Expended: **2,062**
- Calories Eaten: **1,223**
- Net Calorie Balance: **839**

Thanks to NutriMirror, I've had an "eyes wide open" revelation as to why my dieting (and efforts to consistently lose weight) up to this point have been mostly UNsuccessful and UNheathful.

I've learned that it's MUCH more important to track the quality of my choices rather than the quantity. Not that counting calories isn't a HUGE part, it is – but it's making those calories count toward getting me "into the green" (balance) that's important. I've made numerous long-lasting changes in the areas that were consistently "red" and thereby "greened" up my day. So if I'm stayin' green, I know I'm gettin' lean !

MY GREEN DAY NUTRITIONAL FACTS

MOLLY'S
HEALTH REFLECTION™
Nutrition Facts Report

Calorie Balance	
Calories Expended	2062
Calories Eaten	1223
Net Calorie Balance	839

Nutrient Balance	
	%DV
Total Fat 31 g	✔
Saturated Fat 11 g	81%
Trans Fat 0 g	—
Cholesterol 173 mg	58%
Sodium 1063 mg	46%
Total Carbs 179 g	✔
Dietary Fiber 24 g	184%
Sugars 85 g	—
Protein 73 g	✔
Vitamin A 1988 µg	284%
Vitamin C 215 mg	287%
Calcium 1888 mg	189%
Iron 27 g	150%

MY BREAKFAST—293 calories

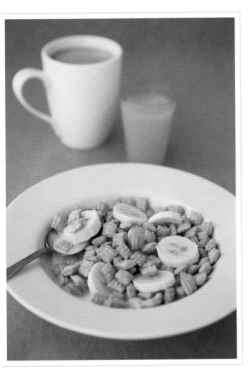

I've never really been a breakfast-type person. Then I was diagnosed as a diabetic three years ago and that all changed my attitude on "breaking the fast." I realized that in order for this machine to get properly stoked and ready for the day, it must have fuel—proper fuel. So I embarked upon finding a quick, tasty, filling, and nutritious breakfast—something that would not leave me starving an hour after eating. I researched and searched for the best combination of carbs, protein, and fiber along with lower sodium, fat, and sugar. Behold my weekday breakfast.

CEREAL WITH MILK AND FRUIT, COFFEE WITH CREAM, JUICE
- 2 tbsp. half and half, 39 calories
- 4 oz. milk, low fat, 51 calories
- Banana, 45 calories
- 10 oz. coffee, 3 calories
- 3.4 oz. orange juice, light, with calcium, 22 calories
- 1 cup Kashi Honey Sunshine high fiber cereal, 133 calories

MY SNACKS
−190 calories

Because of my diabetes, I need to keep my glucose numbers level at all times. I do this by snacking throughout the day—nothing heavy, nothing greasy, nothing salty. Usually, my snacks include a piece of fruit with some yogurt or some mini-rice cakes with some V8 low sodium juice. My evening snack is PURE indulgence on my part—frozen nonfat yogurt or Carb Smart ice cream. I am ever conscious of my past "grazing" habits so I make sure there's enough "green" room left in my day for some deceivingly healthy grazing instead.

V8, RICE SNACKS, ICE CREAM, AND VITAMINS
- 5.5 oz. V8 juice, low sodium, 30 calories
- 1/2 cup chocolate vanilla swirl ice cream, 100 calories
- Multivitamin, 0 calories
- Calcium + D supplement, 0 calories
- Carmel rice snacks, 60 calories

MY LUNCH–378 calories

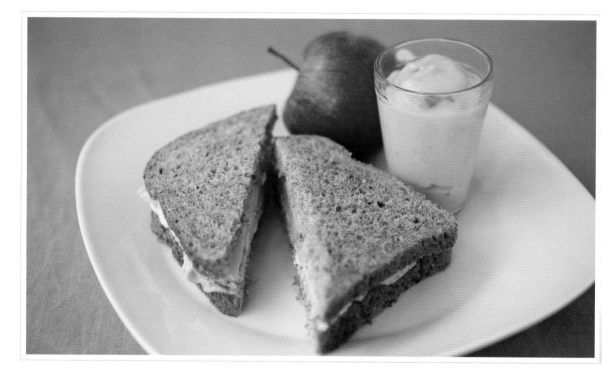

When I was a kid in school, my favorite time of the school day was lunch. Lunch is so important because it's a "re-fueling" opportunity. You've expended your breakfast and mid-morning snack calories and now it's time to stoke that engine and get it revved up so it can carry you through to the next meal. The "old me" would have either skipped lunch, grabbed something out of the vending machine, or run to the nearest fast-food joint. Nowadays I pack my lunch the night before and that way I know I'll get plenty of good stuff so that I won't be tempted by that other stuff. NO fast-

food joint can compare to a hand-crafted lunch made from home.

SANDWICH WITH MEAT, CHEESE, AND DRESSING, AND YOGURT AND FRUIT
- 1 apple, 55 calories
- 1/2 tsp. spicey brown mustard, 0 calories
- 2 pieces wheat bread, light, 80 calories
- 1/2 piece smoked Swiss cheese, 30 calories
- 2 tsp. mayonnaise dressing with extra virgin olive oil, 33 calories
- Strawberry yogurt, nonfat, 110 calories
- 2 oz. deli turkey, 70 calories

MY DINNER—362 calories

I LOVVVVVVVVVE to cook! It's a form of relaxation for me. I don't have a necessarily sophisticated palate, but I know what I like. I've recently added bulgur back into my pantry after losing touch with it for twenty-plus years; and we have a garden where beautiful squash, cucumbers, sweet peppers, and tomatoes grow. This all conjures up a host of thought-provoking combinations for dinner! I find that having new and different grains, fresh meat, and produce from the market, plus our own fresh-off-the-vines vegetables makes creating a nutritious, light—but filling—dinner so easy.

CHICKEN AND VEGETABLES AND BULGUR WHEAT
- 3/4 cup roasted chicken, dark meat, 215 calories
- 2 fresh mushrooms, 6 calories
- 2 tbsp. onions, 13 calories
- 1 cup summer squash, 36 calories
- Baby carrot, 4 calories
- 1/4 cup roasted peppers, 13 calories
- 1/8 cup bulgur wheat, 75 calories

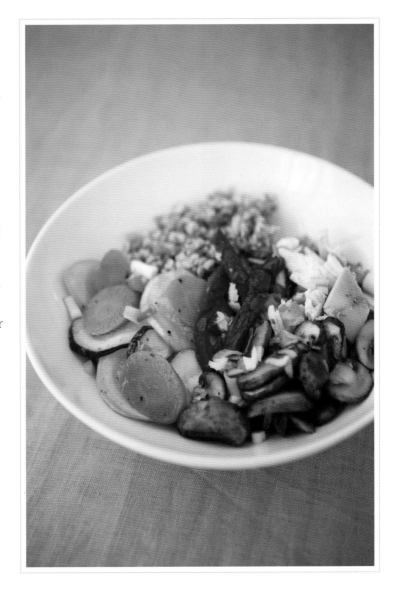

"I DO THIS FOR MYSELF, FOR THE PEOPLE I LOVE, AND IN GRATITUDE FOR THE LIFE THAT HAS BEEN GIVEN ME."

username: sulahian / *first name:* Nancy / *location:* Pasadena, CA

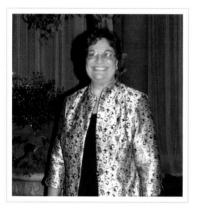

Nancy NOW: December '09 / age: 49

195 lbs. / BMI 33.3 / size 14

I went on my first diet when I was in third grade. Someone pointed out I was maybe ten pounds overweight. My mom was a little heavy too, so we dieted together. Once I was identified as fat, my body followed faithfully. I conscientiously lost weight throughout my youth, only to gain back more, repeating the cycle as so many do. In my thirties, I realized that dieting was detrimental to my health. I swore I'd never go on another diet, and I haven't.

I hit three hundred pounds at age thirty-eight. I stayed right around there for ten years. I developed serious health problems, including type 2 diabetes and bad knees. I dedicated a chunk of energy and money to sessions with a psychologist examining the fifty reasons I overeat. Eventually I gained understanding of my personal issues and felt emotionally ready for some kind of change, but didn't know what to do next. Certainly not a diet! I considered keeping a food log, but wasn't quite ready to face such a daunting challenge.

At forty-seven I was diagnosed with a rare, aggressive cancer. I had two surgeries, chemotherapy, and radiation. You'd think I might catch a break and lose a few pounds, but my medications made me ravenous. All I lost was my hair.

I wonder whether I'd have found my way to balanced eating and healthier living if not for the cancer. I may have been on the right track before, but I was taking my sweet time putting understanding into action. Life is short and I feel blessed to get another crack at it. Enlightenment and motivation can come from anywhere. Maybe if you pay closer attention, you don't have to be hit in the head.

In September of 2008, I felt sufficiently recovered (with a fairly good prognosis) to examine my healthy eating options. I was considering hand-writing a chart to log my food, when it occurred to me that there might be a website where I could plug in my food and the calories would magically appear. I did a

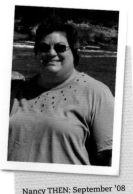

Nancy THEN: September '08

300 lbs. / BMI 51.2 / size 4X

quick search and hit the jackpot! Nutrition is about so much more than calories, and NutriMirror is a great tool that helps me quantify, own, and control all of it.

When I started logging ten months ago, I weighed 300 pounds. At first I didn't set a goal, not wanting the pressure or the feel of a "diet." Gradually, I've acquired the confidence to plug in modest, attainable weight goals, all of which I've met early. A series of those goals has led to a 105-pound loss so far.

I don't have an absolute goal weight. I'll know better as I continue to redefine my body and lifestyle what's appropriate for me. The exact number isn't a concern, since I'm not a jockey or a boxer. My true goal is good health and a rewarding life. I want my blood test numbers (glucose, cholesterol, triglycerides, etc.) to be within healthy limits. I don't want to invite heart disease, stroke, disability, or cancer. I don't want to spend my time and money on medication and doctor visits. I want to move easily, confidently, with no physical limitations

due to excess weight and lack of fitness. I want to have a chance at a long life to spend loving my people, enjoying the beauty of this world and making the best use of the gift that God has given me.

The one absolute promise I've made to myself is to log every bite I eat—looking at and owning every decision I make about food. Every time I log food and read my numbers, I'm re-learning how and why to eat. The nutrition numbers don't lie and, so far I've found that I can control those numbers. The NutriMirror logging tool lets me take decisions about food out of the emotional realm (what do I feel like eating?) and place them in the intellectual realm (what do I need to keep my nutrition balanced?).

I could write volumes about how great I feel, tell you about all the medication I no longer need, and boast about my lab results. My body feels and acts twenty years younger. I find great joy in walking, swimming, and riding my bike. Activities that I long ago crossed off my list are making their way back

into my life. Maybe I'll backpack again, or ski. I'm not dreading the next time I get on a plane. I can expect to be around to see the young people in my life grow up. I can participate fully in my own life.

It takes love and care for us to change habits and adjust attitudes. It's part of a gentle process of learning about ourselves and shaping our decisions. Consider, notice, realize, learn, and try something different. These are the kind words that build me up and make me stronger. Negative words that I've heard and used against myself for years are damaging and counterproductive.

I'm certainly not on a diet. I'm not depriving myself of anything. Can I sustain this way of eating for life? I believe so. Could I gain the weight back? Certainly. However, I intend to guard my new eating habits as carefully as a mother watches a child who has already once been abducted. Turn my head for a second and it can be all over. That's not to say I don't enjoy the flexibility of indulging from time to time; I just know I have to pay attention and own the truth, or the old ways will be back.

Here's my plan for this journey. I will engage in reasonable physical activities that I can sustain for life, not for fast weight loss. I will concentrate on eating very well, not on losing weight. I will be honest and forthright with myself about the quality and quantity of food I eat. I will respect food as nutrition and art and blessing, not using it for cheap, short-lived thrills. I will guard and hone new practices and attitudes about food each day. I will be patient and honorable to myself to the best of my ability. I do this for myself, for the people I love, and in gratitude for the life that has been given to me.

MY PHYSICAL ACTIVITY

I could no more sustain unpleasant exercise for many years than I could deprive myself of food! At first, water exercise was best for me. I walked in the pool, paddled around, then gradually moved to swimming easy laps. I don't count laps, as that feels like a chore. Rather I take in the pleasure of the stretch and the feel of gliding with less effort as my body changes. My primary exercise focus is to enjoy it so I want to do it again the next day. Sometimes I do less, sometimes more. Walking is a great activity to incorporate as it requires little preparation, expense or equipment. I can do it anywhere with whatever time or energy I have. Realizing I'm not out to conquer the world makes it easier to start any movement. I only have to commit to the first five minutes and the rest follows naturally.

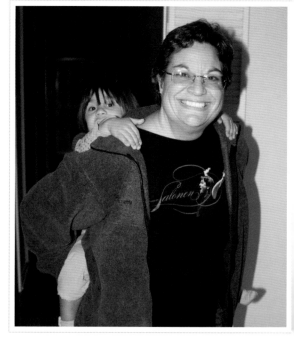

"Toting the little ones I love is my favorite exercise"

NANCY'S *GREEN* DAY

- Calories Expended: **2,305** • Calories Eaten: **1,780** • Net Calorie Balance: **525**

I've been delighted to discover for myself that eating quality food frequently and in reasonable amounts gives so much more satisfaction than eating massive amounts of low-value foods. I'm almost never hungry and I'm never stuffed. I seldom eat purely out of emotion or desperation. My eating isn't "perfect" and I constantly have to make peace with that, but overall I'm happy with my choices. It's the big picture that counts.

As I consciously practice balance in eating, I find I have more control and balance in other areas of my life. I sleep better, keep more regular hours, am naturally more energetic and active, and truly enjoy life. These changes didn't just start after the weight came off; it happened quickly as I let go of poor eating and started feeding myself what I needed.

MY GREEN DAY NUTRITIONAL FACTS

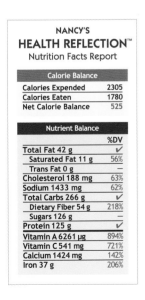

NANCY'S
HEALTH REFLECTION™
Nutrition Facts Report

Calorie Balance	
Calories Expended	2305
Calories Eaten	1780
Net Calorie Balance	525

Nutrient Balance	
	%DV
Total Fat 42 g	✔
Saturated Fat 11 g	56%
Trans Fat 0 g	—
Cholesterol 188 mg	63%
Sodium 1433 mg	62%
Total Carbs 266 g	✔
Dietary Fiber 54 g	218%
Sugars 126 g	—
Protein 125 g	✔
Vitamin A 6261 µg	894%
Vitamin C 541 mg	721%
Calcium 1424 mg	142%
Iron 37 g	206%

MY BREAKFAST—372 calories

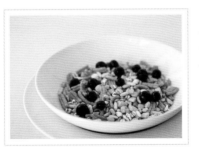

I never used to eat breakfast or lunch, and then was ravenous in the late afternoon, when I'd eat anything and everything. Now breakfast is a simple routine that reminds me first thing in the morning that this is a day to take care of myself. I usually get a chunk of my fiber and calcium needs met with a quick cereal or yogurt breakfast. Usually only the fruit changes. I take a multivitamin, but mostly as insurance.

FRUIT, CEREAL, MILK, COFFEE, AND VITAMINS
- 2 oz. blueberries, 32 calories
- 12 oz. coffee, 4 calories
- 1 cup Kashi Golean cereal, 140 calories
- Daily multivitamin, 0 calories
- 1 1/2 cups milk, low fat, 196 calories

MY LUNCH–464 calories

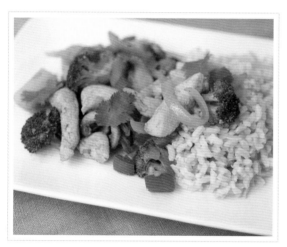

I do this kind of one-pan meal often and base it on the veggies, beans, fruit, nuts, seeds, and meat on hand. Sometimes it turns out great, sometimes it's just okay. But it's fast, satisfying, and always healthy, and I keep learning how to cook in the process. It's also great for cleaning out the fridge before a shopping trip. I make enough for two servings, either to share or keep for tomorrow's lunch. I don't like the veggies done too much; I like the bright colors, the crunch, and the chew.

MY ONE PAN MEAL
- 1/2 tsp. curry powder, 3 calories
- 3/4 tsp. olive oil, 30 calories
- 1 grapefruit, 82 calories
- 2 oz. pineapple, 27 calories
- 4 oz. broccoli, 40 calories
- 1/4 oz. cilantro, 2 calories
- 1/5 oz. garlic, 8 calories
- 1/4 oz. fresh ginger, 6 calories
- 1 1/2 oz. mushrooms, 13 calories
- 2 oz. onions, 25 calories
- 2 1/2 oz. sweet red peppers, 18 calories
- 1/2 jalapeño pepper, 2 calories
- 1/2 cup brown rice, 108 calories
- 4 oz. chicken breast, boneless, skinless, 100 calories

MY SNACKS–343 calories

Fruit is my favorite easy snack. If I add a little protein and good fat, the satisfied feeling and energy last longer. I want my snacks to be as healthy as my meals, so I plan ahead and take things with me when I go out. I never want to be caught having to choose between being hungry or eating fast-food. I love being in control of my food!

EASY SNACKS
- 1 tsp. cinnamon, 6 calories
- 1 apple, 72 calories
- 1 banana, 105 calories
- 1 apple-cranberry fiber cake, 80 calories
- Greek style plain yogurt, nonfat, 80 calories

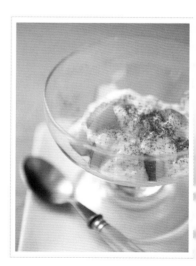

MY DINNER—601 calories

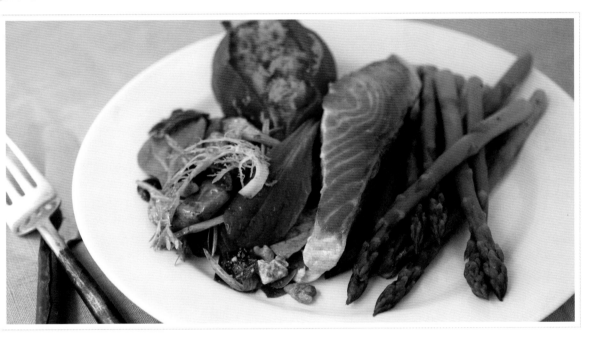

I've found that a medium-sized piece of meat or fish is tastier than a big one, and that those white carbs like white rice and potatoes just don't give much nutrition for the calories. While I'm not big on fussy food, I have enjoyed making salads special, even the center of attention, by using more exotic greens, fruit, toasted nuts, and a little funky cheese. I get plenty of taste from the salad ingredients and so don't need much dressing. This salad also works as a stand-alone meal if you throw in some diced chicken breast (or any leftover meat, hot or cold). I might like it even better when I take it for lunch and the greens get wilty and the flavors meld.

SALAD WITH PROTEIN
- 0.6 oz. feta cheese, 45 calories
- Dash of black pepper
- Dash of salt
- 1 tsp. olive oil, 40 calories
- 1/2 oz. cranberries, dried, sweetened, 44 calories
- 4 oz. asparagus, 25 calories
- 4 oz. sweet potato, baked in skin, 102 calories
- 1 tbsp. balsamic vinegar, 10 calories
- Salmon, marinated, 245 calories
- 1/3 oz. walnuts, 62 calories
- 2 cups fresh spinach, 13 calories
- 2 cups mixed baby greens, 15 calories

"MY LIFE IS NOW GOLDEN … THERE IS NO GOING BACK."

username: PraiseGodImFit / *first name:* Ola / *location:* Grand Rapids, Mi

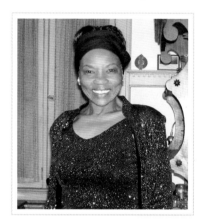

Ola NOW: October '09 / age: 55
165 lbs. / BMI 27.5 / waist 27.5˝

Wednesday, July 19, 2006
Today is my first day. I weigh 269
pounds. My goal is 200 pounds by
February 11, 2007. I will work on
losing fifty more pounds from there.

This was my first journal entry on the first day of my brand new life. I had just received my MBA and was starting my own business. A few days before my first appointment, I realized that all of my business suits were too small. I had one size 24 suit that fit. I knew something had to be done. I felt bad about myself. I did not know where to turn. I had tried everything

and was tired of being fat. In addition, my feet hurt, so I could not wear nice heeled shoes. However, there was one thing I had not tried: prayer. I prayed and immediately got the idea to start counting my calories. I searched the Internet for free calorie counters. This search led me to a free diet website (not NutriMirror) with a free calorie counter.

I had started this journey many times before. In fact, seven years prior, I was 279 pounds and lost one hundred pounds with diet pills. I gained all but 10 pounds back. In the seven years I used diet pills, I also used Weight Watchers, and the Dr. Atkins diet. I was trying to get back to 179 pounds. Nothing worked long term.

I started slowly. The first month I concentrated on counting calories. Once I got that under my belt, I worked on an exercise program. My initial goal was to exercise three days a week. It took about two months to be able to do this consistently.

Eventually, I was able to do thirty to forty-five minutes of exercise three days a week.

Along the way I learned more about exercise and how to eat. Although I was staying within my calorie limit, I found that much of the food I was eating was not nutritionally sound. As a result, I was having a hard time getting full. I changed my eating habits slowly. I began eating whole wheat bread instead of white. I increased my fiber intake, eating more fruits and vegetables. This was when I discovered that apples were

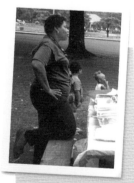

Ola THEN: January '09
269 lbs. / BMI 44.9 / waist 46˝

my best friends. Before, I would get two or three candy bars to curb a sweet attack. To this day, apples are my go-to snack.

In the last three years I have come to realize my mistake. I thought dieting and losing weight was all I had to do. I am a weight gainer. I am an emotional eater. Certain foods affect my appetite and my ability to control it.

As an emotional eater, I will eat instead of dealing with the emotion. I used to think that being an emotional eater meant that I only ate when I was bored, angry, or sad. However, I found that any emotion triggered the overwhelming desire to eat. If I experienced happiness about losing a pound, I would find myself bingeing, because I felt so good. Whatever the emotion, I would overwhelm it with food.

Food sensitivities can be a problem for many. Mine were gluten and artificial sweeteners. These items caused me to experience hunger. Mind you, lowering my calories caused me to be hungry anyway, but I was able to handle it and keep it

under control. However, I found that eating oatmeal, wheat bread, and any other food that had gluten in it was making me extremely hungry all of the time. I found this out by taking a test in a book titled *Ultrametabolism*.

The first day I tried not eating oatmeal or any wheat bread, I found that I was not hungry five minutes after I just finished a meal. In fact, I found that I could go until about two in the afternoon before I had to eat. Other benefits included clearer thinking and more energy.

Weight gain is easy for me. I have accepted this. Every once in a while I indulge. I will have a day when I eat what I want. However, it can take the next six to seven days for my body to pay for this indulgence. I realized that I must, for the rest of my life, count calories. I must eat clean and exercise at least four times a week to keep my weight down and stay healthy. I learned all of this about myself on the other website. However, I still did not understand the science of losing weight and being healthy. Then I was led to NutriMirror.

After going through the site and using its tools, I became aware of what I needed to do to lose and to maintain. I learned the impacts my food and exercise choices have on my calorie balance and my nutritional balance. At the time I was stuck at 175 pounds with a blood pressure reading of 168/85. Once I start using the tools to monitor my calories, nutrition, and exercise, I started losing again. It was through NutriMirror that I learned about net calories. I finally understood that there were calories you expend through your body's routine metabolic activity, regardless of the exercises you perform. I learned that if I overeat one day, it does not mean I have failed. The balance information reporting on the site shows that it is by the longer term trend and not by the day that you determine weight loss and judge success. With NutriMirror, I now have complete control to give my body the fuel it needs for optimal performance. Being green (in balance) is my new goal, not getting skinny.

"What used to be a rarity is now normal and what used to be normal is now a rarity."

—Ron on Biggest Loser

Today I am 163 pounds and my blood pressure is 118/65. Oh, and my feet no longer hurt. I still have thirteen more pounds to lose before I reach my goal. As of June 19, 2009, I will have been on this journey for three years. I still have so much to learn. But I am now living my life like it is golden, a treasure to be protected. What used to be a rarity is now normal—there is no going back.

MY PHYSICAL ACTIVITY

I hate to exercise. I don't care what kind it is; if it is exercise, I hate it. However, I know it is something that I must do. As a result, I have a library of exercise videos. I have a routine that I do, so that I can watch TV and exercise at the same time. For five to six days a week, the routine goes like this:

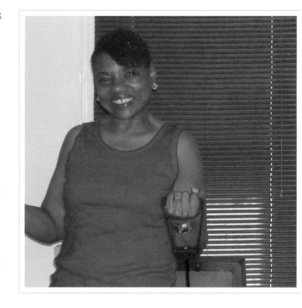

- Five minutes of warm up (One of these: walk up and down the stairs; walk/run in place; jump rope routines, without the jump rope).
- Eight to ten minutes of body strength training (upper or lower, depending on the routine).
- Twenty to thirty minutes of aerobic training: walk/run in place; run up and walk down the stairs; ten minute jump rope routine, twice; or an aerobic video—it depends on my mood.

OLA'S *GREEN* DAY

• Calories Expended: **1,976** • Calories Eaten: **1,283** • Net Calorie Balance: **693**

When I started my new lifestyle three years ago, I cut down my calories, exercised, and lost weight. My food choices were SmartOnes, Weight Watchers dinners, energy bars, and Coke. This was a great improvement over the candy bars and bags of chips I used to eat as snacks. However, I eventually learned that processed food was not the healthiest way to go. It was full of corn syrup, aspartame, chemicals, and empty calories that would contribute to my cravings and an overwhelming desire to binge. I would eat and still be hungry. So I started eating fresh vegetables, fruit, and lean meat and found I could eat so much more food for the calories. And I feel healthier for the change.

MY GREEN DAY NUTRITIONAL FACTS

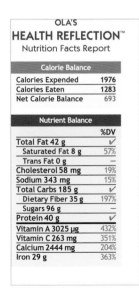

OLA'S
HEALTH REFLECTION™
Nutrition Facts Report

Calorie Balance	
Calories Expended	1976
Calories Eaten	1283
Net Calorie Balance	693

Nutrient Balance		
		%DV
Total Fat 42 g		✔
Saturated Fat 8 g		57%
Trans Fat 0 g		—
Cholesterol 58 mg		19%
Sodium 343 mg		15%
Total Carbs 185 g		✔
Dietary Fiber 35 g		197%
Sugars 96 g		—
Protein 40 g		✔
Vitamin A 3025 µg		432%
Vitamin C 263 mg		351%
Calcium 2444 mg		204%
Iron 29 g		363%

MY BREAKFAST—227 calories

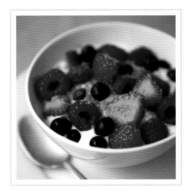

Since I am gluten sensitive my breakfast does not include the normal grains like bread, oatmeal, or many cereals. To get fiber and vitamin C, I eat apples and flax seed. Also, flax seed is a good source of Omega 3 fat and protein. I eat the yogurt with Truvia, along with frozen berries. Sometimes I use it as a dip for my apple.

APPLES, BERRIES, YOGURT, FLAX SEED, AND VITAMINS
• Apple, 72 calories
• 2 calcium 600 + D supplements, 0 calories
• 1/2 cup plain yogurt, nonfat, 55 calories
• 1/2 cup berry blend (frozen blackberries, raspberries, and blueberries), 35 calories
• 2 tbsp. whole ground flax seed, 60 calories
• Women's multivitamin, 5 calories

MY LUNCH–407 calories

Taco Bell was my lunch in the past. One Taco Bell taco with fries and a drink was three quarters of my total daily calorie allowance for the day. Consuming all that fat with no nutrients was like eating seasoned cardboard—what a waste. Now I eat twice as much food for a third of the calories in that lunch. I make fresh tacos with high quality corn tortillas (vitamin B1, B5, phosphorus, and fiber), lettuce, and ground turkey. I round things out with almonds for good fat, a sweet potato, and apple (for more fiber, vitamin A, and vitamin C). Now that's green!

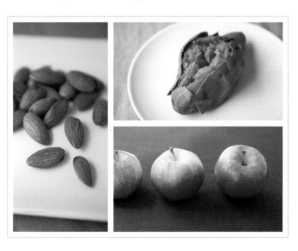

TURKEY TACO, SWEET POTATO, APPLES, AND ALMONDS
- Apple, 72 calories
- 1/2 oz. almonds, roasted, unsalted, 91 calories
- Sweet potato, baked in skin, 139 calories
- 22 g ground turkey, 45 calories
- 1 corn tortilla, 60 calories

MY SNACKS–375 calories

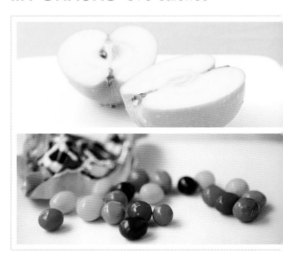

My snacks are eclectic. I eat what I want, as long as it fits my clean lifestyle. Every once in a while I will eat candy in moderation (M&M's, mmmm). The cocoa powder is natural cocoa, mixed with two packets of Truvia. I eat it dry and enjoy the taste. It also provides the iron, antioxidants, and mood booster I need in the mid-afternoons.

I used to be a candy bar addict. I could eat five candy bars a day. That addiction has been replaced with apples. Not a bad trade.

APPLES, CANDY CHEESE, AND ALMONDS
- Apple, 110 calories
- 1/2 oz. peanut M&M's, 72 calories
- Mozzarella cheese, 50 calories
- 15 grams almonds, 103 calories
- 2 tbsp. cocoa powder, unsweetened, 40 calories
- 2 packets Truvia, 0 calories

MY DINNER—274 calories

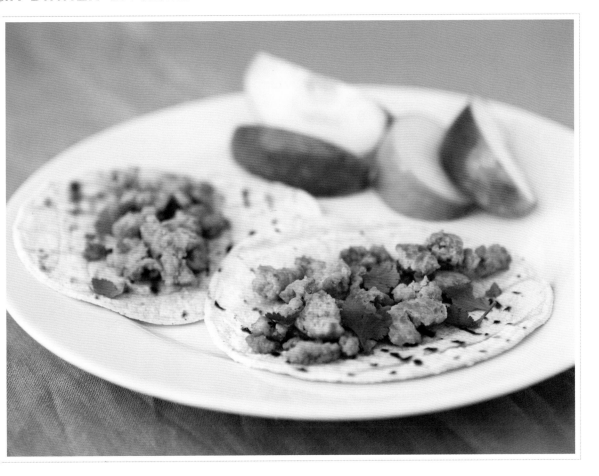

Dinner is a smaller version of lunch. I find that when I don't want to think about what to eat, I just repeat. That way I know that I am still in the zone. Adding lettuce and tomatoes (not enough to count) just keeps things green.

TURKEY TACO AND APPLE
- Apple, 72 calories
- 2 corn tortillas, 120 calories
- 22 g ground turkey, 45 calories

"I MADE THE CONNECTION THAT THE MORE I WORKED OUT THE MORE I COULD EAT."

username: paddy0286 / *first name:* Paddy / *location:* Minneapolis

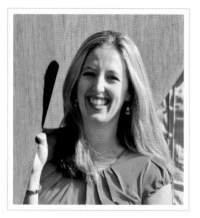

Paddy NOW: October '09 / age: 27
143 lbs. / BMI 21.2 / waist 26.75˝

I am a twenty-seven-year-old recent law school graduate with a very busy lifestyle. My schedule makes it difficult to find time to exercise and I often find myself making quick and easy, though not always healthy, food choices. Consequently I have struggled since college with a weight fluctuation of ten to twenty-five extra pounds.

By the time I graduated from college I had unwittingly packed on twenty-five extra pounds thanks to four years of unhealthy choices at the campus cafeteria. But since I was young, busy, and physically active, the simple transition from dorm food to mostly home-cooked meals and the fact that I began training to run a marathon resulted in losing the twenty-five pounds I had gained without even really trying.

Then I started law school, began working twenty hours a week, and found myself busier than ever. Though my eating habits were not the healthiest, I kept fit by extensive training for more marathons and half-marathons. At the time I considered myself to be a relatively healthy person. I ate whatever I wanted but I still managed to maintain my pre-college weight, give or take a few pounds. If I happened to notice any upward movement on the scale I simply worked out a little longer the next day or limited my food intake for a day or two.

Then, in June 2008, I faced a major setback. I broke a rib! During the six months that it took for my rib to heal I found that I was unable to do any exercise more strenuous than walking. Little by little I began to gain weight again. Without exercise as part of my normal routine I had to rely on my food choices to control my weight, and that presented itself as a whole new challenge.

I had no idea how much I should eat to lose the weight I had gained since my injury. Nor did I know what foods my body actually needed for nutritional balance and optimal health. Sometimes I would start out the day eating very little, but

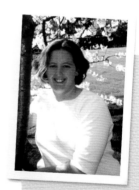

Paddy THEN: March '04
172 lbs. / BMI 25.2 / size 12

by the end of the day I would feel starved. I tried not to eat. Sometimes I would give in and eat too much late in the day. Other times I was able to resist. No matter what I did, my weight gain continued. By September, just three months after my rib injury, I had already gained ten pounds. I felt discouraged, frustrated and demoralized. I knew I needed to find a way to track my calories and somehow figure out what was a reasonable amount for me to eat on a daily basis. I searched the Internet to see if such a tool existed and that's when I stumbled onto NutriMirror.

By January 2009, still frustrated with my weight, I was ready for change. I started using NutriMirror with new resolve and a commitment to take back control of my weight. By this point my rib had healed enough to where I was able to ease back into an exercise program. It felt so good to get back to my old routine. And I loved the way that whenever I logged my exercise for the day, the site automatically allotted more calories to my food log. I made the connection that the more I worked out the more I could eat! This gave me just the motivation I needed to exercise consistently.

NutriMirror gives me the tools to manage my health successfully. I now have the information I need to make positive choices, the flexibility to eat what I enjoy, and the motivation to stick to an exercise plan.

With the renewed dedication that comes from being in control, I began to work on some of my bad eating habits. My greatest challenges were too much sodium and not enough fiber. I decided to be more proactive and, for the first time, I began reading labels in the grocery store. I avoided buying processed foods high in sodium. I replaced my white bread with whole grain bread. Sometimes I even use whole wheat pasta. I never thought I could part with my beloved white bread, but I was beginning to view health and nutrition from a new perspective.

At first I had difficulty recording everything I ate. I would do well throughout the week and I was seeing a lot of green in my food logs, but I seemed to lose control on the weekends. I avoided logging on the days I knew I had made poor choices, but after a few weeks I realized that it was important for me to log both the good and the bad for an honest assessment of how I was doing.

Honesty in logging is an important part of being successful. We need accurate and complete feedback in order to make informed choices. What I don't record only hurts me and keeps me from assessing my needs accurately. I am learning that a healthy diet isn't about "being on a diet." It is not just a phase and something I do to lose weight. Healthy eating is a lifestyle and something I plan to do for the rest of my life. To be successful I have to be able to eat the things I like and find pleasure in choices that I make in order for my healthy lifestyle to be sustainable. To be successful I have to be able to find pleasure in my choices before they will every become sustainable for the long-term. So sometimes I choose to have dessert to avoid feeling deprived.

Now I look at my longer term diet and exercise trend, rather than at individual good days or bad days. I am no longer obsessed about reaching a certain number on the scale. I am more concerned that I look and feel healthy. I don't stress anymore if one day has too many calories or my sodium is too high another day as long as my general pattern is on target and in balance. I am no longer worried that on any particular day I have failed and ruined my "diet" because I am not "on a diet."

I am almost back to my pre-injury weight, though a specific number on the scale no longer matters. I feel great, my BMI is within the normal range, and I comfortably fit into my clothes again. I am still working on toning up my body a little more, particularly in the tummy area. But I am confident that I will continue to see positive changes in my overall health.

MY PHYSICAL ACTIVITY

My main form of exercise is running. I'm not very fast, and I don't particularly like it, but that's what I do. It is the easiest, cheapest way to get exercise. Also, I don't need to belong to a gym or have any special equipment other than a pair of running shoes. Because I don't particularly like running, I sign up for races to keep myself motivated. It's a lot harder to skip a day of training when you know how much pain you will be in when running a half or full marathon if you skip the run. Even when I'm not training for a particular race, I try to run a couple of miles three or four times a week to keep up my general fitness level. As a bonus, I can eat more calories!

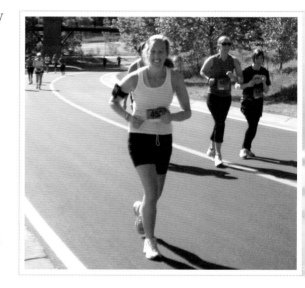

PADDY'S *GREEN* DAY

- Calories Expended: **2,082**
- Calories Eaten: **1,603**
- Net Calorie Balance: 479

Before I joined NutriMirror I thought that I ate pretty healthily. It only took one day to realize that there were some areas in which I was seriously lacking. Generally, I ate the right amount of calories, but I was not getting enough fiber, calcium, or iron. So I started making changes. My first change was to find a cereal that gave me more bang for the buck—or better nutrition for the calories.

The next big change was to add snacks. Simply adding snacks made it easier to control my portion sizes and meals. I also learned that if I ate the right snacks, I didn't have to worry quite so much about making sure I ate the "perfect" dinner.

MY GREEN DAY NUTRITIONAL FACTS

PADDY'S
HEALTH REFLECTION™
Nutrition Facts Report

Calorie Balance	
Calories Expended	2082
Calories Eaten	1603
Net Calorie Balance	479

Nutrient Balance	
	%DV
Total Fat 43 g	✓
Saturated Fat 10 g	56%
Trans Fat 0 g	—
Cholesterol 87 mg	29%
Sodium 1705 mg	74%
Total Carbs 244 g	✓
Dietary Fiber 29 g	129%
Sugars 82 g	—
Protein 73 g	✓
Vitamin A 2033 µg	290%
Vitamin C 119 mg	159%
Calcium 2521 mg	252%
Iron 34 g	189%

MY SNACKS–464 calories

Adding snacks made it possible to control my portion sizes. They help keep my blood sugar at a level where I don't feel the urge to overeat. I also use snacks to selectively target the nutrients I need. I try to include some kind of treat so I don't start feeling deprived. I find that a Tootsie Pop works wonders most days and packs the taste to satisfy my sweet-tooth.

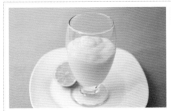 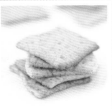

FRUIT, CRACKERS, YOGURT, CHEESE, AND CANDY
- Apple, 104 calories
- 1 1/8 oz. All Bran crackers, 120 calories
- Key lime pie yogurt, light, 100 calories
- 1 Tootsie roll pop, 60 calories
- String cheese, 80 calories

MY BREAKFAST
—322 calories

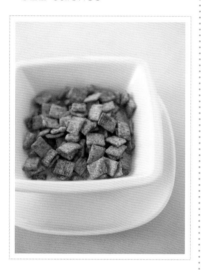

I have always loved breakfast.
I don't feel right without it.
Before Nurtrimirror I didn't
pay attention to how much
sodium was in my cereal. I also
didn't think about what else
was on the side of the box. I
now eat a cereal that is high in
fiber and nutrients. It allows
me to get a jump start for the
day on the things I had the
most trouble with.

CEREAL AND MILK
• 1/2 cup milk, nonfat, 43 calories
• 2 5/8 oz. Total Cinnamon Crunch
  cereal, 279 calories

MY LUNCH—357 calories

My lunch needs to be easy to make and easy to pack up. I decided
that my old lunch of a sandwich and carrots could work if I
tweaked it a little. No more high sodium lunch meat. No more
white bread. So I spent some time at the store figuring out what
best fit both nutritional needs and my taste buds. The answer was
peanut butter and jelly on whole grain bread.

SANDWICH AND CARROTS
• Carrots, baby, fresh: 7 3/4 oz, 77 calories
• PB & J (whole grain bread): 1 serving, 280 calories

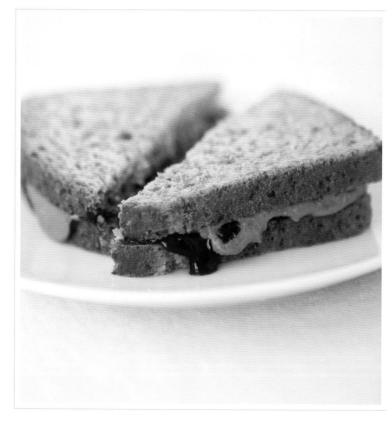

MY DINNER—460 calories

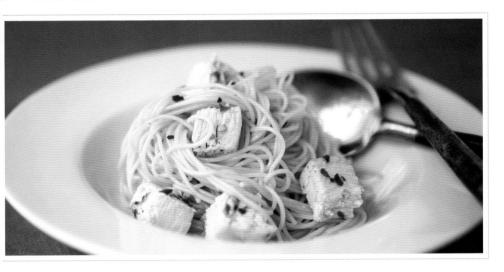

My biggest change for dinner has been portion size. In planning a meal to help me achieve a Green Day, the most important targets are protein and some healthy fats. (I try to take care of the rest of my nutrients before dinner.) I usually have a boneless chicken breast with a side of a starch such as pasta. I eat whole grain pasta if I haven't had enough fiber, but regular pasta if I have. I also eat a few more calories at dinner, but my goal is to keep dinner at or below 500 calories.

CHICKEN AND LEMONADE
- Red pepper chicken with pasta (see recipe), 450 calories
- Crystal Light lemonade, 10 calories

RED PEPPER CHICKEN WITH PASTA

Makes 4 servings

INGREDIENTS
8 oz. angel hair pasta
4 tbsp extra virgin olive oil
16 oz. chicken breast
4 cloves garlic
1 tsp. crushed red pepper flakes, or to taste

PREPARATION
1. Boil water and cook pasta.
2. While water for pasta is heating, add oil, garlic, and red pepper flakes to a sauté pan and cook over medium heat.
3. Add chicken and cook until done.
4. Drain the cooked pasta, add it to the chicken, toss together, and serve.

"AFTER GRADUATION FROM HIGH SCHOOL THE ATHLETICS WERE OVER…THINGS BEGAN TO FALL APART."

username: bearcatrpc / *first name:* Rick / *location:* Rising Sun, IN

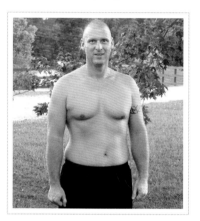

Rick NOW: August '09 / age: 41
240 lbs. / BMI 29.8 / waist 38˝

I grew up and still reside in a very small town in Indiana. Any person who has lived for any amount of time in a small town understands the "everybody knows everybody" mentality that comes with living in these rural burgs.

As a 5´10˝ ten-year-old, I was tagged as fat early in my life by other kids simply because the number on the scale was higher than everyone else's. This tag stuck with me throughout my school years. I was six feet tall when I was thirteen years old. I don't remember the actual weight. I knew I was hefty

but not really fat. I was active in baseball, basketball, cross country, and track in junior high school, so I was at least able to keep myself out of the obese range. As I moved into high school, I grew to 6´3˝ and my weight was in the 220-pound range. It was never a concern then, because I was an athlete who burned lots of calories playing baseball, basketball, and running track.

After graduation from high school the athletics were over and the weight issues began. College brought on the freshmen fifteen (or in my case twenty). After college, I married and began working in a warehouse. I tossed around hundred-pound bags eight hours a day so I was able to maintain my weight at about 240 pounds. Five years later, I was promoted from the warehouse to an office job. That is when things began to fall apart. After a year of office work and getting no exercise, my weight increased to 260 pounds.

I was diagnosed with high blood pressure shortly after that. My physician told me that I "needed to lose weight to keep from going on medication." That is when I realized I had a problem. I have always been a picky eater who only liked meat & taters and sweets, including my biggest vice, peanut butter sandwiches. How can a person lose weight when they don't like any of the typical diet foods like salads, veggies, and fruit? I then began a low fat diet. I was able to get my weight back down to 240 pounds by

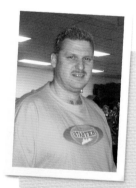

Rick THEN: January '09
310 lbs. / BMI 38.5 / waist 48˝

consuming the same amount of foods that I always had, only low fat versions and cutting out my beloved peanut butter.

Once I reached the 240-pound mark, I was happy with myself and went back to my former eating habits. I ballooned up to 280 pounds. This was the beginning of my series of yo-yo diets. I would go back on the low fat diet and lose weight successfully only to stop and balloon back up. I reached 310 pounds in 2005 and was on high blood pressure medication. I could no longer play on the company softball or basketball teams. My weight was causing my knees to hurt when I tried to run.

In January of 2009, I decided to stop the weight climb. I searched for a tool to help me track my calories and fat on the Internet. I heard people that track their foods were more likely to stay on a diet for a longer period of time. I stumbled across NutriMirror. I learned from this tool that I could lose weight by counting calories. I began to monitor my foods and saw some success in losing weight.

I searched for foods that would help my nutritional values become balanced. One example was sodium. I thought the doctor meant to stop putting salt on things when high blood pressure was diagnosed. I learned, however, that the processed foods I was eating played a major role in my sodium woes. I really had to search for ways to get my sodium level down. I started cooking my lunches instead of eating those frozen "healthy" microwavable dinners.

I also learned my fiber intake was too low. I began eating apples (one of the few fruits that I like) and my fiber started to climb. A side benefit to eating the apple for a snack was that my hunger was satisfied, and then I wasn't as eager for my next meal.

That was when the bell went off in my head. I started eating more small meals during the day. This strategy allowed me to control the amount of food that I ate at main meals. I was able to get all of my nutrients balanced but was still short on calories and the fat that my body needed to keep it

from going into "starvation" mode. (That is where your body thinks that you are starving it, so it holds on to the food you eat and stores it as fat.) I realized that one food that had "healthy fat" and some calories was peanut butter. I was able to still eat my beloved peanut butter (with a fibrous apple) and still maintain my nutritional balance.

I started telling everybody I knew who complained about "needing to go on a diet" that what they really needed to do was to get their food intake balanced. If they did that, they would start to see the results they desired with something they could maintain for life. No more diet-binge-diet-binge living.

I have reached 235 pounds as I write this and continue to lose about a pound a week. I have a goal of 220 pounds and, with the help of my doctor, will evaluate if I need to lose more. Whatever the doctor may say, I will continue to effectively control my body weight and maintain my nutritional balance for the rest of my life. If a picky eater can be successful, any one can do it.

MY PHYSICAL ACTIVITY

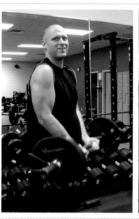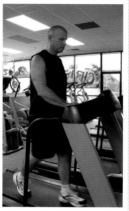

My typical exercise day consists of twenty-five minutes of walking (twenty of which are at 4.3 mph and five at 3.4 mph). My goal is to burn approximately 250 calories during this cardio portion of my workout. The balance of my exercise consists of weight training. I am not talking about hardcore vein-and-muscle-bulging weight training. I just do moderate lifting to help tone certain areas of my body. I burn approximately 120–140 calories with the weight training. All of this physical activity helps me augment my daily food intake with the extra calories I burn off.

RICK'S *GREEN* DAY

- Calories Expended: **3,095**
- Calories Eaten: **2,371**
- Net Calorie Balance: **724**

By logging everything that I put into my mouth and every exercise I perform, I am able to make small adjustments to either my exercise or my meals to help maintain a caloric balance. That ensures that I am on track to meet my weight goal in the time frame I have chosen. I can plan my meals and exercise for the day first thing in the morning. I am then able to tweak things to get my numbers where they belong. If something comes up during the day that alters my original plan, I can always go back and make changes to my plan to get things back in line.

MY GREEN DAY NUTRITIONAL FACTS

RICK'S
HEALTH REFLECTION™
Nutrition Facts Report

Calorie Balance	
Calories Expended	3095
Calories Eaten	2371
Net Calorie Balance	724

Nutrient Balance	
	%DV
Total Fat 74 g	✔
Saturated Fat 16 g	61%
Trans Fat 0 g	—
Cholesterol 146 mg	49%
Sodium 2278 mg	99%
Total Carbs 332 g	✔
Dietary Fiber 49 g	148%
Sugars 164 g	—
Protein 115 g	✔
Vitamin A 1839 µg	204%
Vitamin C 214 mg	238%
Calcium 1326 mg	133%
Iron 18 g	225%

MY BREAKFAST—292 calories

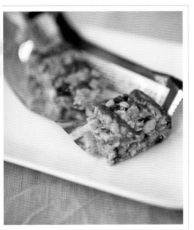

I have never been one who can eat a great deal for breakfast. I always take a vitamin supplement to get my vitamin A into the "green." I also have a fiber bar to help with my daily fiber intake, and a glass of nonfat chocolate milk for calcium. I know that it is often said that you should have a big breakfast but that is not my makeup. Plus it isn't long after that I have my first snack of the day. I still get my caffeine in the form of a diet soda.

FIBER BAR, CHOCOLATE MILK, VITAMIN, AND MORNING SNACK-DIET COKE
• Fiber One Chewy Bar, 140 calories
• Equate men's health supplement, 0 calories
• 1 cup chocolate milk, nonfat, 150 calories
• 24 oz. diet Coke, 2 calories

MY LUNCH—273 calories

My lunches in the past have always consisted of frozen microwavable dinners that were very, very high in sodium. With very little effort I am able to broil some chicken breasts for an entire week's worth of lunches. Throw in some green beans and I have a meal that is better in taste than a frozen dinner and the sodium is almost negligible in comparison. I add another fiber bar for a small dessert and to help get the fiber in line.

CHICKEN, BEANS, AND AFTERNOON SNACK
• 2/3 cup green beans, 23 calories
• 4 oz. chicken breast, 110 calories
• Fiber One Chewy Bar, 140 calories

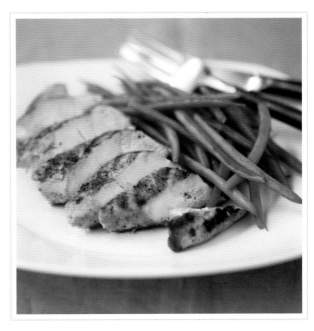

MY SNACKS–1,098 calories

My snacks are the highlight of my day partly because I have learned to look forward to the fruits that make up my Green Day and partly because I know that the next snack is just a couple of hours away. I try to have one of my snacks every two hours between each of my main meals. This helps me get the feeling that I'm not depriving myself in any way.

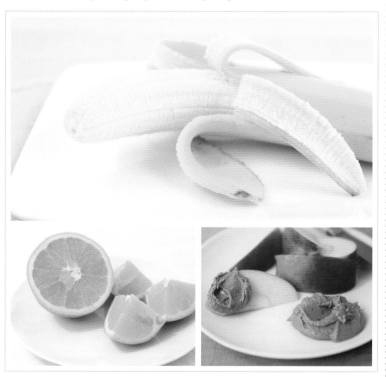

EVERY COUPLE OF HOURS
- Apple, 110 calories
- Banana, 105 calories
- Orange, 86 calories
- 12 oz. Diet Coke, 2 calories
- 3 tbsp. peanut butter, 285 calories

- 2 snack pack puddings, nonfat, 180 calories
- Instant oatmeal, 100 calories
- 2 devil's food cookies, 120 calories
- Whey protein, 110 calories

MY DINNER
—708 calories

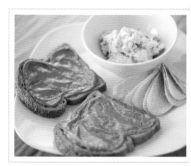

My dinner consists of some canned tuna and fat-free mayo out of a bowl and a couple of slices of bread with peanut butter. Peanut butter used to be my Achilles heal and saboteur of my previous attempts to lose weight. Now I realize that peanut butter is the food that actually helps me get up into the "green" for my daily fat intake.

MY QUICK DINNER
- 1 tbsp. Miracle Whip, nonfat, 13 calories
- 2 slices whole wheat bread, 220 calories
- 2 oz. light tuna, 50 calories
- 1 serving Pringles, 140 calories
- 3 tbsp. peanut butter, 285 calories

username: granny / *first name:* Florence

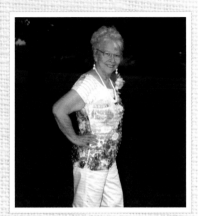

Florence NOW: November '09 / age: 79
132 lbs. / BMI 23.4 / size 10

. . . .

Most of my life (since I was twelve years old) has been spent on diets—first one and then another. I feel like I have been on every diet that ever existed. They all ended the same way. I lost weight only to gain it all back … and then some.

I lost my mother and my baby brother to heart attacks when they were each forty-five. At forty-seven, my father had a stroke. My sister and my other brother had heart attacks and open-heart surgery early in life. Given this history I knew I had the genes for an unhealthy body. From time to time I would attempt to eat healthily, and then revert to the same old routine of off-and-on dieting.

Often I would look into the mirror and say, "You big fat slob." I hated the way I looked. I joined the YMCA and started going to a class called Choose to Lose. The nutritionist stressed to us that we should eat no less than 1,500 calories. However, I just kept with my diet mentality that you had to eat less than 1,000 calories to lose weight.

Then, in February of 2009 at the weight of 162 pounds, I stumbled upon NutriMirror and began logging my food. I quickly saw that I was not satisfying my nutritional needs.

Little by little it began to seep in that I really did need to eat more, but I didn't start doing so until I got down to within five pounds of my goal. Then, my weight loss momentum just stopped cold. I thought, "I'll try doing what everyone is telling me to do and eat more." I did, and lo and behold the weight came off. Now I wish I had done it much sooner. With more calories to eat, the journey would have been so much easier. Now I am at 132 pounds, 8 pounds below my original goal of 140.

My health has improved so much. I remember that my

cholesterol was running about 195. After only a couple of months of healthy living, it had dropped all the way to 122. My triglycerides are 65; HDL 41; LDL 68; cholesterol/HDL ratio 3.0. The doctor is very pleased that I went from being obese to a normal weight and that my health benchmarks are much improved.

I believe this healthy living is something that will add active years to my life. At seventy-nine years young, I can tell you it is never too late to improve your health and your life.

. . . .

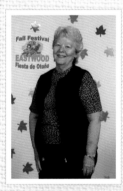

Florence THEN: April '09
. . . .
184 lbs. / BMI 32.6 / size 16

"HEALTHY EATING DOES NOT MEAN SACRIFICING FLAVOR."

username: PuraVida / *first name:* Pamela / *location:* Oceanside, CA

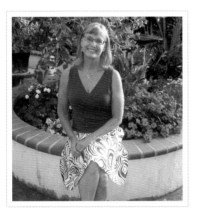

Pamela NOW: October '09 / age: 56
124 lbs. / BMI 21.2 / waist 29″

I have always loved cooking, but a few years ago I began taking my kitchen creations to a new level. I adopted a new hobby of gourmet cooking, complete with food and wine pairings. Retired from teaching high school Spanish, I had plenty of time to dedicate to my new form of artistic expression. As one can imagine, my body began slowly "growing" accustomed to my new lifestyle of eating too much and too many rich foods.

In January 2009, after a medical physical exam, my doctor suggested that I start taking a medication to help lower my cholesterol. I was only 55 years old but at 5′4″ I weighed 165 pounds. In addition to having high cholesterol, I had a number of other health problems, including the beginning of atherosclerosis. My mother experienced extremely debilitating side effects from taking cholesterol-lowering medication. I did not want to take that type of drug. I promised my doctor that I would eat better and exercise instead. He agreed to give me six to eight months to lower my cholesterol on my own without medication. He ordered new tests for the end of that time period. I was ready to make some serious life transformations.

Just two months prior, my husband had brought home a NutriMirror brochure that was still sitting on my desk. He described NutriMirror as a tool I might like because I enjoy playing games and I am very competitive. However I was neither interested nor ready to make any changes. After the doctor visit, I went straight to my computer and brought up the NutriMirror website. My husband was right about the food journal appealing to the game lover in me. The challenge was on and I resolved to be a winner. I was and still am determined to live a long and healthy life. So began my journey. Five months from my start date, I had dropped thirty-five pounds. I lost lots of inches from all parts my body and decreased my total body fat from 42 percent to 29 percent.

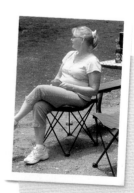

Pamela THEN: January '09
165 lbs. / BMI 28.3 / waist 41.5″

After seven months of mostly balanced (green) days with NutriMirror, I have lost forty-one pounds and lowered my cholesterol by seventy-five points.

When I began using this amazing tool, it clearly showed me how my poor food choices had led to my unhealthy state. As I began reading labels and weighing my food, I was surprised that what I considered "one portion" was in fact two or three portions according to the package labels. Right away I saw that my sodium was out of control when I ate packaged foods or ate at fast-food restaurants. Now I often plan my meals and snacks for the day first thing in the morning, entering everything into NutriMirror to make sure I meet all of my nutritional requirements. I balance the calories between carbohydrates, healthy fats, and proteins. I love being able to see what choices contribute to a "green" day and what choices do not.

For me, this site has also given rise to a much more active lifestyle. The natural side effect of healthy eating is feeling better and having more energy. Seeing the impact that my daily exercise has on the number of recommended daily calories I need to reach my goal weight is quite motivating.

When I first began exercising, I was hard pressed to get through five minutes on the elliptical machine. Two minutes on the stair climber really got my heart racing. Little by little I have been able to increase my activity level and I feel great. I might even join my twenty-five-year-old daughter in running a 5K. My husband thinks it is great that I no longer need his encouragement to get to the gym. For the first time in my life I actually look forward to exercise, whether it is going to the gym, kayaking, playing tennis, or going for a run.

Here is the fun part. I have combined my newly acquired love for healthy eating with my passion for gourmet cuisine. I consider myself a "healthy gourmet" and I sacrifice absolutely nothing in terms of taste and visual appeal. I have been able to create new menu items from wholesome ingredients that are as pleasing to the palate as any of the rich food creations I used to make. I still love food and wine pairing but I have learned to prepare food in a manner that celebrates the textures, flavors and nutrients of wholesome elements and combine them into nutritious, satisfying, and mouthwatering meals.

MY PHYSICAL ACTIVITY

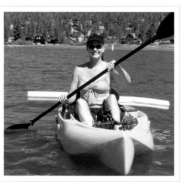

For the first time in my life I actually look forward to exercise! I've started various workout programs in the past, but this is the first time I have actually stuck with one. Initially, I think I was motivated by the fact that NutriMirror showed me how I could eat additional calories and still lose weight if I exercised. Now I exercise because I really like it. I enjoy a variety of activities at my gym: elliptical, stair climber, treadmill on maximum incline, balance exercises, weight training, and racquetball. Outside of the gym I play tennis, ride my bike, and run four to eight miles a week. For Valentine's Day I treated my husband and myself to a Wii, complete with Wii Sports, Wii Fit, and EA Active.

PAMELA'S *GREEN* DAY 1

- Calories Expended: **2,129**
- Calories Eaten: **1,273**
- Net Calorie Balance: **856**

My goal for each day is to meet as many of the essential nutrients as possible through my food choices alone, although I do take daily vitamin and mineral supplements. I focus on food selections that pack the most nutritional value per calorie, combining them into healthy meals that celebrate the natural goodness of whole foods. It is important for me to achieve a healthy daily balance between complex carbohydrates, proteins and healthy fats. NutriMirror has made it easy for me to see whether or not I am on target.

On this particular Green Day, with my breakfast less than 300 calories, lunch under 400 calories, and dinner under 500 calories, I could easily add a glass of wine and still be completely green!

PAMELA'S NUTRITION FACTS, GREEN DAY 1

PAMELA'S
HEALTH REFLECTION™
Nutrition Facts Report

Calorie Balance	
Calories Expended	2129
Calories Eaten	1273
Net Calorie Balance	856

Nutrient Balance	
	%DV
Total Fat 40 g	✔
Saturated Fat 9 g	64%
Trans Fat 0 g	—
Cholesterol 73 mg	24%
Sodium 1614 mg	70%
Total Carbs 164 g	✔
Dietary Fiber 40 g	224%
Sugars 75 g	—
Protein 68 g	✔
Vitamin A 2808 µg	400%
Vitamin C 347 mg	463%
Calcium 1212 mg	101%
Iron 14 mg	175%

MY BREAKFAST—282 calories

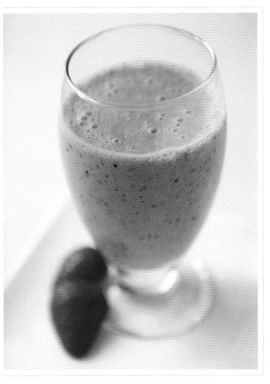

I used to skip breakfast and then eat too much the rest of the day. Now I love to jump-start my day with a smoothie. To get a nice creamy texture I always include a banana or six ounces of plain yogurt. Most of the time I use whatever fresh fruits are in season such as cantaloupe, strawberries, blueberries, pineapple, kiwi, peaches, nectarines, and apples. Often, especially in the winter, I use frozen fruit, including strawberries, mixed berries, and peaches. Some days I even add spinach and beets for extra fiber and iron.

FRUIT SMOOTHIE
25 blueberries, 19 calories
2 cups frozen strawberries, 101 calories
1 1/4 oz. Body Wise chocolate/vanilla, 81 calories
Plain yogurt, nonfat, 81 calories
1 cup water, 0 calories

MY SNACKS—159 calories

I tend to reach for whatever is convenient for my snacks so I make sure to keep lots of fresh fruits and vegetables on hand. I love roasted and grilled vegetables (hot or cold) so I like to prepare lots of them in advance so they are available whenever I need a snack. Now I find grapes, almonds, raw carrots, apples, and roasted vegetables to be so much more satisfying than my old favorites of candy, cookies, and chips!

FRUIT AND VEGGIES
• 25 grapes, 86 calories
• Tangerine, 45 calories
• 8 baby carrots, 28 calories

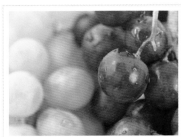

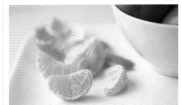

MY LUNCH–369 calories

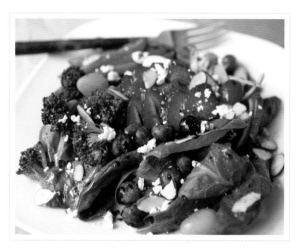

One of my favorite lunches is what I call my "Power Foods Salad." The term "power foods" comes from The Sonoma Diet by Dr. Connie Guttersen, where she identifies ten foods containing essential nutrients in low-calorie packages. Power foods include spinach, broccoli, bell peppers (all colors), strawberries, blueberries, grapes, almonds, olive oil, and whole grains. Although olive oil and almonds are not that low in calories, they contain healthy fats necessary for good health. This salad, served with whole grain bread, contains eight of the ten power foods. Not only is this salad visually appealing, it is a delicious blend of sweet and savory!

SALAD AND BREAD
- 1 piece whole wheat bread, 70 calories
- 1 serving Power Foods Salad (see recipe), 299 calories

SPINACH SALAD
(AKA POWER FOODS SALAD)

Makes two servings.

INGREDIENTS
4 cups baby spinach
12 grape tomatoes
3 large fresh strawberries, sliced
25 fresh blueberries
1 small sweet red pepper
3 broccoli florets, finely chopped
1/4 cup sliced raw almonds (unsalted)
1 oz. feta cheese, crumbled
6 basil leaves, cut into long, thin strips
1 oz. purple onions, sliced
1 tbsp. balsamic vinegar
1 tbsp. extra virgin olive oil

PREPARATION
Combine the first ten ingredients in a large bowl. Toss with the balsamic vinegar and olive oil.

NOTES
In this recipe, the only ingredients that are not power foods are the onions, basil, feta cheese, and balsamic vinegar. The two power foods not in this recipe are grapes and whole grains.

MY DINNER—463 calories

Healthy eating does not mean sacrificing flavor! I love gourmet cooking, especially cooking with wine. In the past this always meant cooking with butter and other foods high in saturated fat and simple carbohydrates. I have learned to be even more creative, using wholesome and healthy ingredients while avoiding those foods that originally led to my weight gain. This grilled salmon with strawberry Pinot noir reduction and strawberry mango salsa (277 calories) is an example of how pleasurable nutritious food can be.

Until a few months ago I had never heard of quinoa and now it is one of my favorite whole grains. It can be served hot or cold, as in this simple quinoa salad. I have even found pasta made from quinoa.

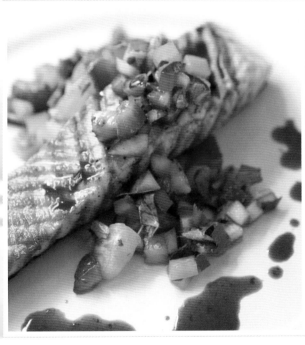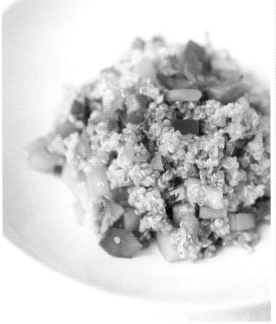

SALMON, VEGETABLES, QUINOA, AND FRUIT SALSA (RECIPES ON PAGES 216-217)

- 2 spears asparagus, 7 calories
- 3 oz. Brussel sprouts, 33 calories
- 1/4 tsp. salt
- 3/4 cup French haricort vert (green beans), 20 calories

- Strawberry mango salsa (see recipe), 35 calories
- Strawberry pinot noir reduction, 72 calories
- 2/3 serving quinoa salad (see recipe), 126 calories
- 4 oz. Salmon (see recipe) 170 calories

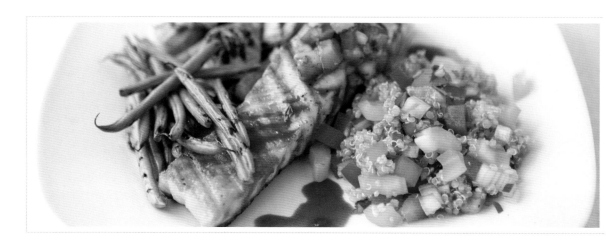

QUINOA SALAD

Makes six 3/4-cup servings.

INGREDIENTS
1 cup quinoa
3/4 cup chopped celery
1/2 cup chopped fresh cilantro
3 tbsp. diced purple onion
3 tbsp. diced sweet red or yellow pepper
3 tbsp. extra virgin olive oil
3 tbsp. balsamic vinegar
1/4 tsp. kosher salt

PREPARATION

1. Prepare quinoa according to package directions. Let cool before assembling salad.

2. Add celery, cilantro, onion, pepper, and salt to quinoa.

3. Mix with balsamic vinegar and olive oil.

NOTE
In my logged foods for this day, I only ate 1/2 cup of the salad rather than a full 3/4-cup serving.

STRAWBERRY MANGO SALSA

Makes six to eight servings.

INGREDIENTS
4–8 strawberries
1/2 mango
4 diced sweet red or yellow peppers
3 tbsp. diced purple onion
4 kumquats, skin on, seeds removed
1/2 tangerine
1/4 cup chopped cilantro
Juice from 1/2 lime

PREPARATION
1. Finely dice strawberries, mango, kumquats, and tangerine. Mix together in a small bowl.
2. Add the diced onion, sweet peppers, and cilantro.
3. Add the lime juice and mix.

NOTE
For easy entertaining, you can prepare this recipe up to one day ahead of time.

STRAWBERRY PINOT NOIR REDUCTION

My original recipe. Makes four servings of one tablespoon each.

INGREDIENTS
4-8 strawberries
3 tbsp. shallot, diced
1 tbsp. balsamic vinegar
1 cup Pinot noir
4 sprigs thyme, fresh (optional)
1 leaf sage, fresh (optional)
1 large basil, leaf (optional)

PREPARATION
1. Purée strawberries in food processor or blender.

2. Heat 1/2 cup strawberry purée in heavy skillet and sauté diced shallot on medium heat in the purée, stirring constantly, about 3 minutes.

3. Add the pinot noir, scraping the sides of skillet.

4. Add herbs.

5. Simmer uncovered until reduced to 1/2 cup, stirring frequently, about 10 minutes.

6. Strain and return liquid to skillet.

7. Add balsamic vinegar and continue simmering until liquid has reduced to 1/4 cup, about 8 minutes.

NOTE
For easy entertaining, double this recipe and make the reduction up to a day ahead of time. Keep refrigerated until ready to use. Reheat on top of the stove in a small saucepan.

GRILLED SALMON WITH STRAWBERRY PINOT NOIR REDUCTION AND STRAWBERRY MANGO SALSA

My original recipe. Makes four servings of four ounces each.

INGREDIENTS
16 oz. Atlantic Salmon, skinless, cut into 4 steaks
Dash of Kosher salt
1 tsp. olive oil
Strawberry Pinot Noir Reduction (see recipe)
Strawberry Mango Salsa (see recipe)

PREPARATION
1. Prepare strawberry mango salsa.
2. Lightly brush salmon steaks with olive oil and sprinkle with a dash of kosher salt.
3. Let sit at room temperature for about 15 minutes before grilling.
4. Meanwhile, prepare the strawberry Pinot noir reduction.
5. When the strawberry Pinot noir reduction has been strained and returned to the skillet for its last 8 minutes of simmering, begin to grill the salmon for 3-4 minutes per side.

TO SERVE
1. Drizzle about 2 tsp. of the strawberry Pinot noir reduction on each plate.
2. Place each salmon piece on top of the reduction.
3. Drizzle 1 tsp. of the reduction on top of the salmon.
4. Top each piece of salmon with 1/4 cup strawberry mango salsa.

PAMELA'S NUTRITION FACTS, GREEN DAY 2

PAMELA'S
HEALTH REFLECTION™
Nutrition Facts Report

Calorie Balance	
Calories Expended	1906
Calories Eaten	1676
Net Calorie Balance	230

Nutrient Balance	
	%DV
Total Fat 40 g	✔
Saturated Fat 10 g	54%
Trans Fat 0 g	—
Cholesterol 194 mg	65%
Sodium 2264 mg	98%
Total Carbs 205 g	✔
Dietary Fiber 43 g	184%
Sugars 78 g	—
Protein 90 g	✔
Vitamin A 5694 µg	813%
Vitamin C 324 mg	432%
Calcium 1210 mg	101%
Iron 17 mg	213%

MY BREAKFAST—395 calories

This smoothie is one of my favorite breakfasts because it gives me more than 100% of my vitamin A and C requirements, 72% of my daily fiber, 39% of my daily calcium and 51% of my daily iron! And it tastes delicious! I don't even notice the spinach because of the apple and berries.

SMOOTHIE (394 CALORIES)
- Apple, 72 calories
- 4″ banana, 61 calories
- 1 cup frozen blueberries, 79 calories
- 7 frozen strawberries, 26 calories
- 2 cups baby spinach, 20 calories
- 1/2 oz. beet, 7 calories
- 1 1/4 oz. vanilla protein powder, 130 calories

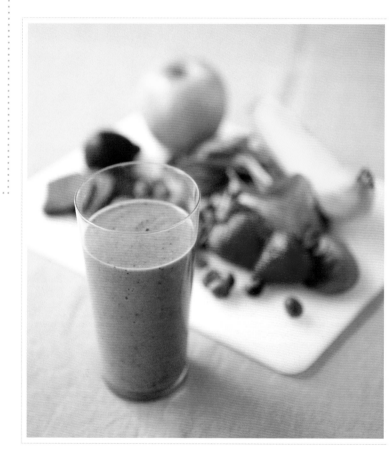

MY LUNCH—308 calories

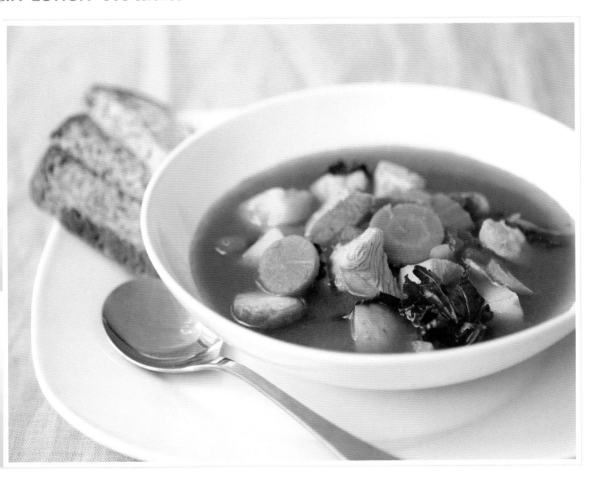

HOMEMADE CHICKEN VEGETABLE SOUP WITH BREAD

- 1/4 chicken breast, 50 calories
- 3/4 tsp. chicken stock, 4 calories
- 1/2 carrot, 7 calories
- 1/2 potato, 64 calories
- 1/4 cup sweet corn, 40 calories
- 1 oz. sugar snap peas, 13 calories
- 1/4 cup green beans, 23 calories

- 1 Brussel sprout, 8 calories
- 1 oz. tomato, 7 calories
- 1/4 cup spinach, fresh, 2 calories
- Dash kosher salt, 0 calories
- Dash pepper, 0 calories
- 1 slice whole grain bread, 90 calories

MY SNACKS—274 calories

- 1 orange, 86 calories
- Mozzarella cheese stick, 80 calories
- 2 1/4 oz. baby carrots, 22 calories
- 1/2 oz. almonds, dry roasted, unsalted, 86 calories

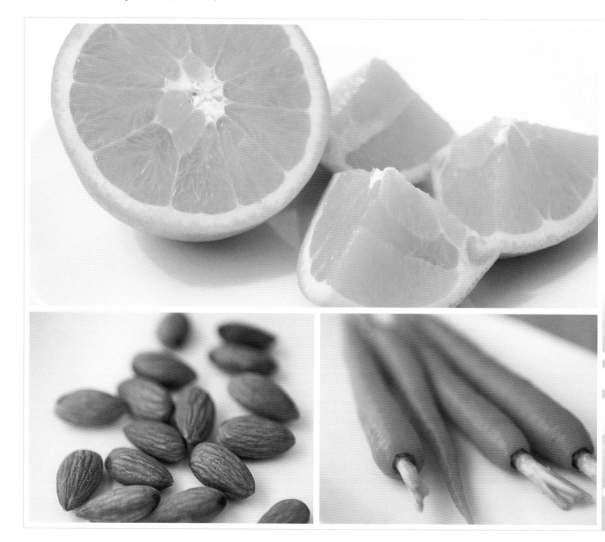

MY DINNER—699 calories

Friends were coming for dinner this particular evening and, with a little preplanning, it was easy to stay "green." Our guests were treated to a healthy and nutritious meal, but they were more impressed with the celebration of unique flavors and the perfect wine pairing!

GREEN SALAD
- 3 oz. mixed baby greens, 15 calories
- Grape tomato, 18 calories
- 2 tbsp. sweet red pepper, 5 calories
- 1/4 small red onion, 7 calories
- 1/2 oz. gorgonzola cheese, 50 calories
- 1 tsp. extra virgin olive oil, 40 calories
- 1/3 tbsp. balsamic vinegar, 3 calories
- Sweet basil garnish

GRILLED SHRIMP WITH SPICE RUB
- 5-6 large shrimp, 70 calories
- 1 tsp. extra virgin olive oil, 40 calories
- Fennel spice rub (chili powder, cinnamon, dried coriander, fennel seed, black pepper, red pepper flakes, kosher salt), 9 calories

COUSCOUS WITH SUNDRIED TOMATOES AND LENTILS
- 1/2 cup cooked couscous, 85 calories
- 1/4 cup lentils, cooked, 60 calories
- 1/4 cup sun-dried tomato halves (not oil-packed), 18 calories
- Dash kosher salt
- Dash cumin seeds
- Pepper to taste

THE REST
- 1 3/4 oz. grilled asparagus, 20 calories
- 4 oz. white wine (sauvignon blanc), 96 calories
- 5 oz. red wine (syrah), 123 calories

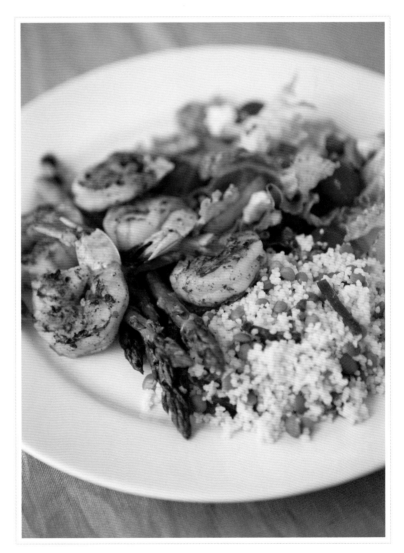

PAMELA'S NUTRITION FACTS, GREEN DAY 3

PAMELA'S
HEALTH REFLECTION™
Nutrition Facts Report

Calorie Balance	
Calories Expended	1878
Calories Eaten	1486
Net Calorie Balance	392

Nutrient Balance		%DV
Total Fat 45 g		✔
Saturated Fat 7 g		42%
Trans Fat 0 g		—
Cholesterol 5 mg		2%
Sodium 1547 mg		67%
Total Carbs 211 g		✔
Dietary Fiber 38 g		183%
Sugars 77 g		—
Protein 36 g		✔
Vitamin A 2038 µg		291%
Vitamin C 158 mg		211%
Calcium 1406 mg		117%
Iron 15 mg		188%

MY BREAKFAST
—278 calories

STEEL CUT OATMEAL WITH BERRIES
AND WALNUTS
- 1/4 cup steel cut oats, 120 calories
- 10 blueberries, 8 calories
- 3 strawberries, 17 calories
- 1/8 cup raisins, 65 calories
- 4 tsp. walnuts, 67 calories
- 1/8 tsp. cinnamon, 1 calorie

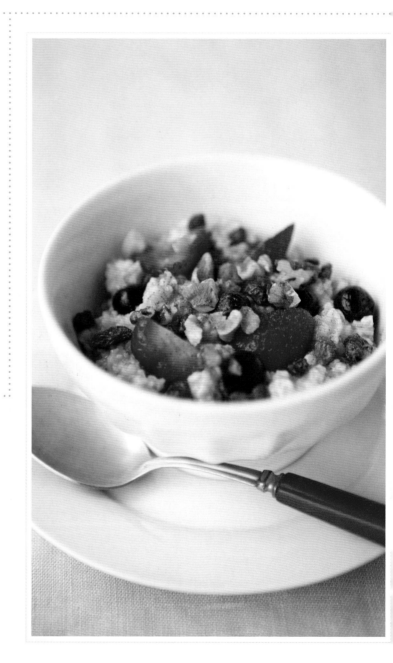

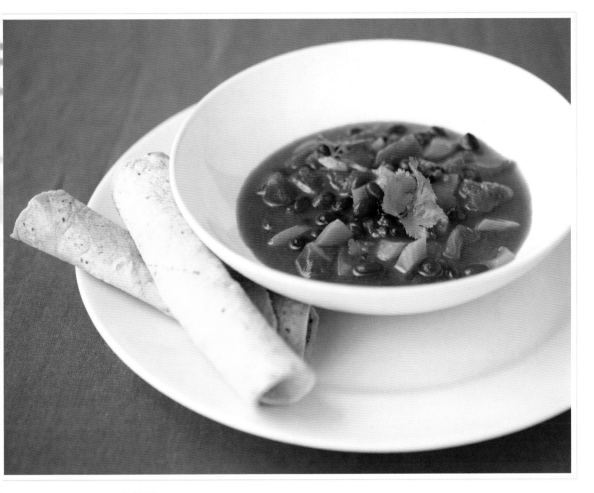

BLACK BEAN AND TOMATO SOUP

Makes five 237-calorie servings.

3 1/2 cups black beans, 770 calories

3 1/2 cups diced tomatoes, 87 calories

3/4 cup carrots, 36 calories

1 tsp. vegetable broth, low sodium, 5 calories

- 1 tsp. red pepper flakes, 6 calories
- 1/2 cup cilantro, 2 calories
- 1/3 cup onion, 31 calories
- 2 tsp. garlic, 9 calories
- 2 tbsp. olive oil, 240 calories

SERVED WITH
- 2 corn tortillas, 104 calories

MY SNACKS–254 calories

- 25 grapes, 86 calories
- 1 apple, 72 calories
- 2 1/4 oz. carrots, 22 calories
- 1/2 oz. pumpkin seeds, roasted, unsalted, 74 calories
- Calcium supplement

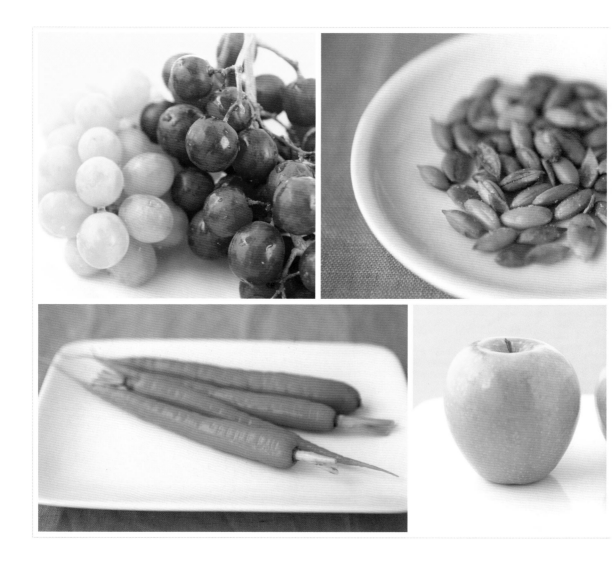

MY DINNER—613 calories

WALNUT PEAR SALAD
- 1 1/2 oz. mixed baby greens, 8 calories
- 1/4 pear, 24 calories
- Gorgonzola or bleu cheese, 25 calories
- 1 tbsp. red onion, 4 calories
- 1/4 oz. walnuts, chopped, 47 calories
- 1 tsp. extra virgin olive oil, 40 calories
- 1 tsp. balsamic vinegar, 3 calories

VEGETARIAN TOMATO SAUCE WITH PURÉED BROCCOLI
Makes six 117-calorie servings.
- 1.5 tbsp. extra virgin olive oil
- 3 tbsp. sweet red, yellow, or green peppers
- 3 cloves garlic
- 3 tbsp. onion
- Kosher salt, to taste
- 45 oz. tomatoes
- 11 1/2 oz. cooked broccoli, puréed
- 3 tsp. oregano
- 10 leaves basil
- 1/2 tbsp. rosemary
- 4 oz. red wine

SERVE OVER
- 3 oz. polenta, 75 calories

GRILLED WHOLE GRAIN BREAD
- 1 oz. whole grain bread, 80 calories
- 1 tsp. extra virgin olive oil, 40 calories
- Kosher salt to taste

AND FINALLY
- 6 oz. red wine, 150 calories

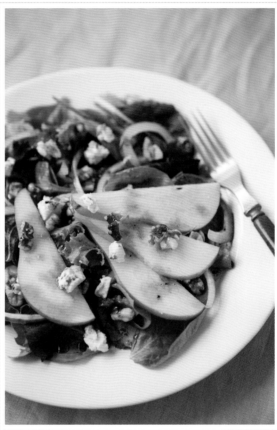

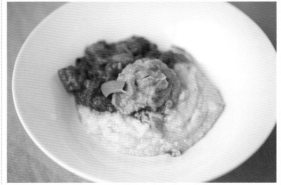

PAMELA'S NUTRITION FACTS, GREEN DAY 4

PAMELA'S
HEALTH REFLECTION™
Nutrition Facts Report

Calorie Balance	
Calories Expended	1898
Calories Eaten	1527
Net Calorie Balance	371

Nutrient Balance	%DV
Total Fat 48 g	✔
Saturated Fat 10 g	59v%
Trans Fat 0 g	—
Cholesterol 107 mg	36%
Sodium 2002 mg	87%
Total Carbs 194 g	✔
Dietary Fiber 47 g	220%
Sugars 86 g	—
Protein 85 g	✔
Vitamin A 3636 µg	519%
Vitamin C 153 mg	204%
Calcium 1248 mg	104%
Iron 18 mg	225%

MY BREAKFAST
—239 calories

CHOCOLATE SMOOTHIE
- 1 tsp. cinnamon, 6 calories
- Banana, 61 calories
- 1/2 cup canned pumpkin, 42 calories
- 1.2 oz. chocolate protein powder, 130 calories

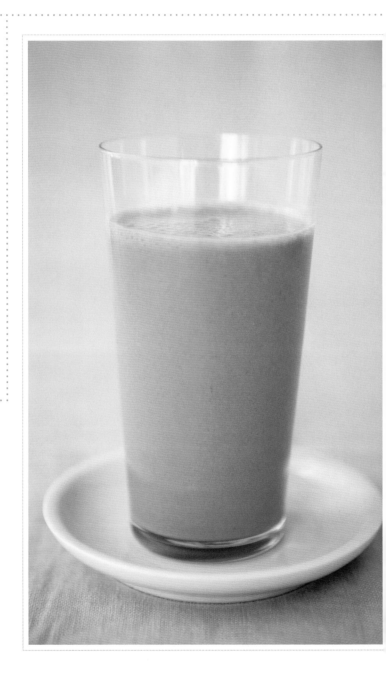

MY LUNCH—265 calories

LENTIL SOUP

- 2/3 cup vegetable or chicken stock, 7 calories
- 1/4 cup lentils, 70 calories
- 1 oz. sweet red, yellow, or green peppers, 8 calories
- 3/4 oz. carrot, 9 calories
- 3/4 oz. onion, 10 calories
- 1/3 cup Yukon gold potato, 32 calories
- 1 oz. tomatoes, 5 calories

- 2 oz. spinach, 13 calories
- 1 tsp. extra virgin olive oil, 40 calories
- 1 1/8 tsp. parsley, 1 calorie
- Kosher salt to taste
- Black pepper to taste
- Fresh herbs (thyme, marjoram) to taste

SERVE WITH

- 2 whole grain crackers, 70 calories

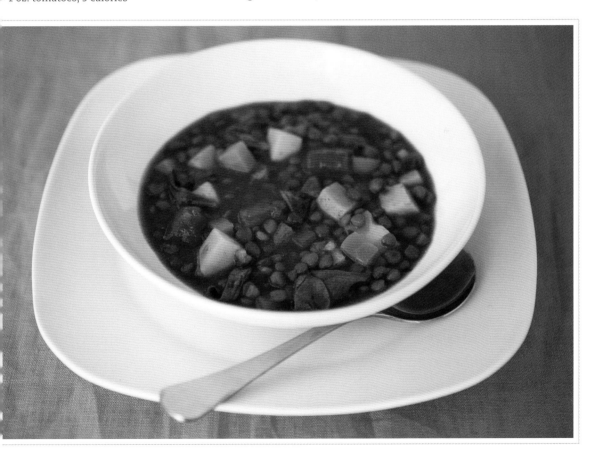

MY SNACKS—464 calories

- 1 apple, 72 calories
- 20 grapes, 69 calories
- Mozzarella cheese stick, 108 calories
- 2 1/4 oz. carrots, 22 calories
- 1/4 cup raisins, 108 calories
- 1/2 oz. almonds, dry roasted, unsalted, 85 calories

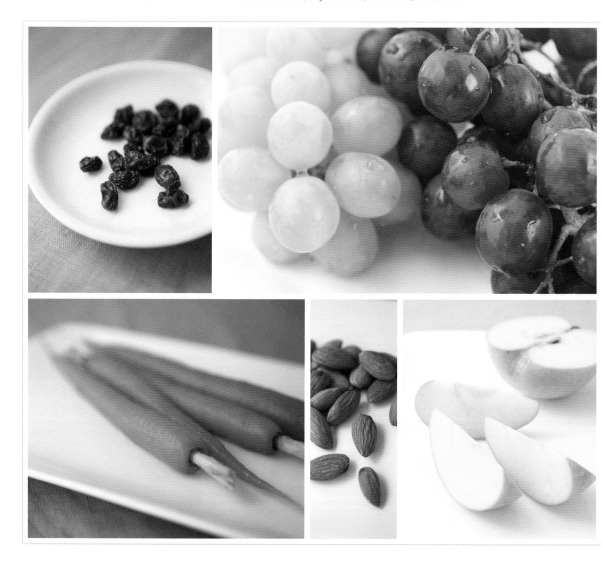

MY DINNER—559 calories

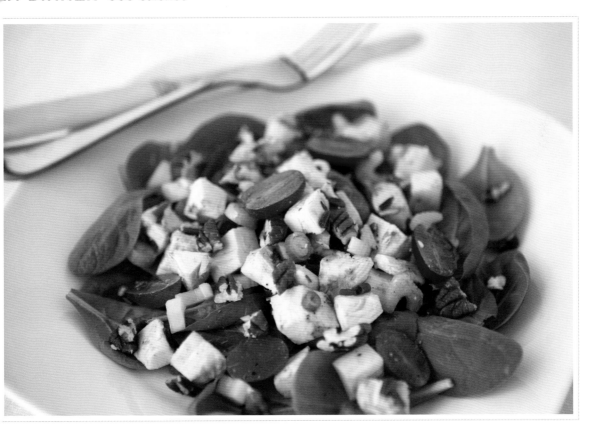

TURKEY-TARRAGON SALAD OVER CHOPPED SPINACH

Makes six 292-calorie servings.

- 24 oz. roasted turkey breast
- 2 cups grapes (or substitute dried cranberries or dried cherries)
- 1 cup chopped celery
- 3/4 cup diced onion

- 6 cups fresh spinach
- 4 tbsp. fresh tarragon leaves
- 2 tbsp. white balsamic vinegar
- 1/4 cup extra virgin olive oil
- 1 tbsp. fresh lemon juice

OPTIONAL GARNISHES

- 1/4 oz. chopped pecans, 49 calories
- 1 1/8 oz. avocado, 48 calories

ACCOMPANIED BY

- 1 slice whole grain bread, 70 calories
- 5 oz. white wine, 100 calories

PAMELA'S NUTRITION FACTS, GREEN DAY 5

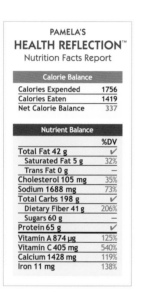

PAMELA'S
HEALTH REFLECTION™
Nutrition Facts Report

Calorie Balance	
Calories Expended	1756
Calories Eaten	1419
Net Calorie Balance	337

Nutrient Balance		%DV
Total Fat 42 g		✔
Saturated Fat 5 g		32%
Trans Fat 0 g		—
Cholesterol 105 mg		35%
Sodium 1688 mg		73%
Total Carbs 198 g		✔
Dietary Fiber 41 g		206%
Sugars 60 g		—
Protein 65 g		✔
Vitamin A 874 µg		125%
Vitamin C 405 mg		540%
Calcium 1428 mg		119%
Iron 11 mg		138%

MY BREAKFAST
—207 calories

GALLO PINTO

Makes six 161-calorie servings.

- 6 cups whole grain rice
- 1 1/2 cup black or small red beans
- 3 tbsp. sweet red or yellow (or both) peppers, 9 calories
- 3 tbsp. cooked onion
- 1/2 cup cilantro
- 1/8 tsp salt
- 1 tbsp. extra virgin olive oil

ALSO

- 1 wedge cantaloupe, 19 calories
- 2 oz. fresh pineapple, 27 calories

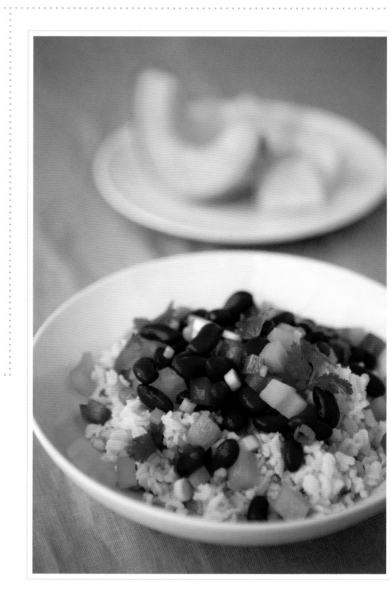

MY LUNCH—532 calories

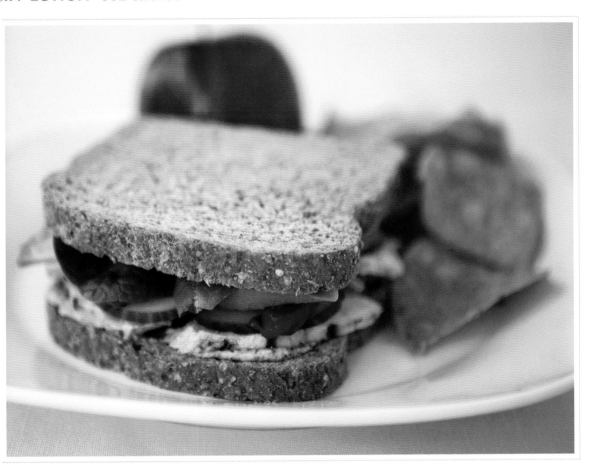

CHICKEN BREAST SANDWICH
- 2 slices whole grain bread, 140 calories
- 3 pieces thinly sliced chicken breast, 70 calories
- 1/4 avocado, 80 calories
- 1/8 cup cucumber slices, 2 calories
- 0.84 oz. sweet red peppers, 16 calories
- 1/8 cup spinach, 1 calorie
- 1 tbsp. mustard, 11 calories

PLUS
- 10 multigrain tortilla chips, 140 calories
- 1 apple, 72 calories

MY SNACKS—151 calories

- 20 grapes, 69 calories
- 4 strawberries, 23 calories
- 2 1/4 oz. carrots, 22 calories
- 1/4 oz. pumpkin seeds, roasted, unsalted, 37 calories

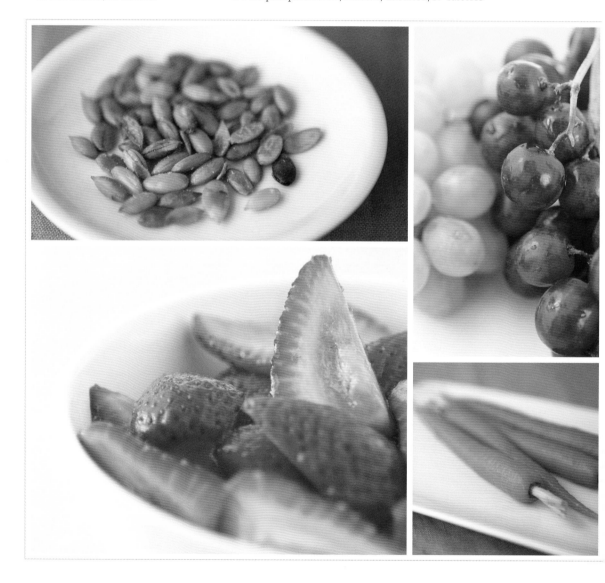

MY DINNER—529 calories

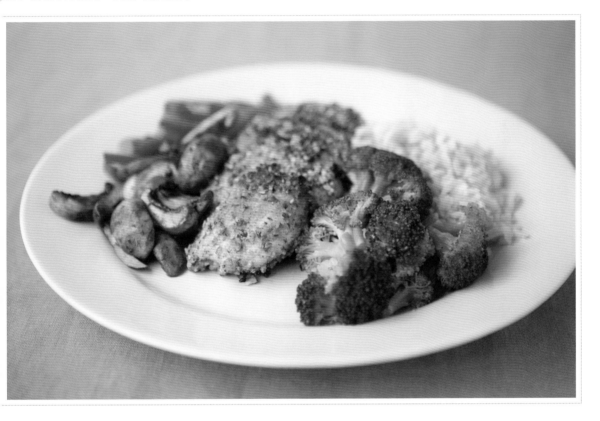

ALMOND CRUSTED CHICKEN BREAST
Makes four 172-calorie servings.
- 1 lb. chicken breast, boneless, skinless
- 1 tbsp. extra virgin olive oil
- 1 oz. almonds, roasted, unsalted, ground
- Dash kosher salt
- Dash black pepper
- Herbal seasoning

ROASTED BROCCOLI WITH BABY PORTOBELLO MUSHROOMS
Makes four 130-calorie servings.
- 17 oz. broccoli
- 5 oz. baby portobello mushrooms
- 3 oz. onion
- 3 3/4 oz. sweet red or yellow peppers
- 2 tbsp. extra virgin olive oil
- 1/4 tsp. kosher salt
- Dash black pepper

SERVED WITH
- 1/2 cup whole grain rice, 102 calories
- 5 oz. red wine, 125 calories

"I HAD ASSUMED I WAS IN GOOD SHAPE. WRONG!"

username: SheilaM / *first name:* Sheila / *location:* Oceanside, CA

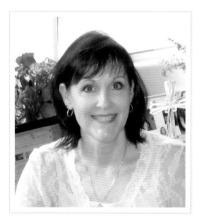

Sheila NOW: October '09 / age: 56
131.2 lbs. / BMI 19.9 / waist 31˝

How did I get here? When I was first approached about being a contributor to the *Balanced Days, Balanced Lives* book project I was a bit hesitant. Who, me? I have never really had a weight issue, maybe ten to fifteen pounds now and then but never anything like the difficult journey some of the other members were taking. But because I had been logging my food intake in one way or another for so many years, it had become habit. So I agreed. Here is my journey and how I use the NutriMirror tool in my life.

I used to do the fad diet thing every now and then and was always successful when I needed to be. One fad diet in particular really made me stop and think. Many years ago my step-daughter wanted to lose weight. She brought home a diet plan she was going to try so I decided I'd do it with her. I forget what it was called but we were instructed to eat hardboiled eggs one day, then spinach on another day, and bananas on another, and so on for two weeks. At the end of the two weeks we had lost some weight, were happy with our progress, and went on our way. That's where the trouble began for me. I couldn't stop losing weight. Each day I would wake to continued weight loss no matter what I ate. I am 5´8˝ and I was down to a little more than 100 pounds. I went to my GP who recommended I supplement my diet with Sego (now that will date me) three times a day and eat whatever I wanted. I still had no weight gain. Then I became pregnant with my first

child and finally began to regain the weight I had lost. The only answer the doctor had was that this diet had completely messed with the electrolytes in my system and was creating havoc. When I became pregnant my system seemed to right itself. So for me that was the end of fad diets. It was very scary. I am a control freak and anything I do that is not under my control I don't like.

It wasn't until after my first grandchild was born that again I wasn't happy with my weight (again nothing major). I tried

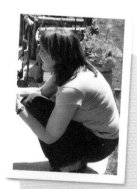

Sheila THEN: November '05
143 lbs. / BMI 21.7 / waist 32˝

a program that had me count points. It sounded like a game and was sort of fun. I was successful on this program and lost the few pounds I wanted to lose. The program was expensive, though, and the costs were going up. It was about that time that Jim Ray, NutriMirror's founder, was having personal health issues. He was in development of an Internet tool with his son, Michael, to help him find an efficient way to monitor calories and certain nutrients. He was looking for testers to get feedback and asked for volunteers in the office. I had already done a lot of leg-work and some research to help in the early development stages. And now that it was ready for testing, I started using it. It was really exciting to use something that I had actually had a hand in creating.

From the very first moment I used the program I realized that all the time I had been with the point-counting program, I had been missing a huge part of why I *should* be logging. I had been under the impression that all my choices were healthy, providing my body with exactly what it needed.

My family history is filled with heart and high blood pressure problems. So I had assumed that by keeping my weight under control by exercising regularly and by counting points, I was in good shape. Wrong!

When I began logging with NutriMirror, the very first thing I saw was the amount of sodium I had been consuming. Nothing too major, but I was still high (in the "red") every day. I was also deficient in fiber and calcium. If I had just looked at it as a daily thing, I could have told myself those imbalances of five to ten percent were no big thing. However, over the course of several weeks, months, and years I was probably headed for disaster. With this site I could see exactly where I was going and what dietary changes I needed to make.

Now that I am able to see my intakes I am "in the green" almost every day. As a result my mind and body feel so much better. Although I don't use NutriMirror for weight loss issues, it is a comfort for me to know that as long as I control my calorie balance, I control my weight. NutriMirror has become an invaluable part of my daily life and will be for the long haul. I look at it as my life plan. I can actually look at each day or week and know I am doing something good for myself and my family. Too many family members have passed way too early due to lifestyle issues that hopefully I can avoid by staying "green" (in balance).

Looking back, I am simply amazed by what we have created. I know now that all the work we did in those early days has led to something very special and very important. I see it and hear it all day long through the people that gather in the Journal Room. They have become like family to me and I feel great pride in the role I get to play assisting and serving these wonderful people.

MY PHYSICAL ACTIVITY

My exercise … hmmmmm. I don't have a regular daily routine for exercise. I love being outside so I am constantly doing something like walking the dog, gardening, swimming, or walking to the park with the grandkids. Indoors, of course, the inevitable house work keeps me active. I know that others might not consider all of this to be physical activity, but it works for me.

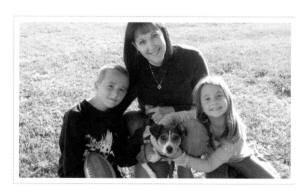

Active in the park with grandkids.

SHEILA'S *GREEN* DAY

- Calories Expended: **1,563**
- Calories Eaten: **1,322**
- Net Calorie Balance: 241

This has been a journey of personal discovery for me—more about healthy eating and snacking habits than weight loss. Sure, everyone wants to lose that extra ten to fifteen pounds but for me it was about the health issues that plague my family—high blood pressure and heart disease being the main ones. I never grasped the impact that my careless snacking and soda habit had on my nutritional balance. After a few weeks of logging I quickly saw that the extra-large diet coke at lunch during the week and the chips after work were driving my sodium levels completely off the charts. With a few simple tweaks I found that iced tea was much better and more satisfying and I've found much healthier snacks options!

MY GREEN DAY NUTRITIONAL FACTS

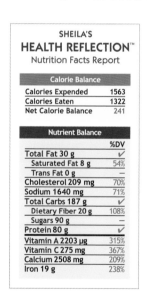

SHEILA'S HEALTH REFLECTION™
Nutrition Facts Report

Calorie Balance	
Calories Expended	1563
Calories Eaten	1322
Net Calorie Balance	241

Nutrient Balance	
	%DV
Total Fat 30 g	✔
Saturated Fat 8 g	54%
Trans Fat 0 g	—
Cholesterol 209 mg	70%
Sodium 1640 mg	71%
Total Carbs 187 g	✔
Dietary Fiber 20 g	108%
Sugars 90 g	—
Protein 80 g	✔
Vitamin A 2203 µg	315%
Vitamin C 275 mg	367%
Calcium 2508 mg	209%
Iron 19 g	238%

MY BREAKFAST—234 calories

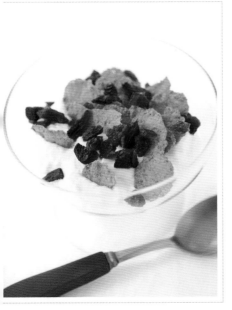

You'll notice throughout my day that I'm a grab-and-run eater. I do plan meals most evenings but for work I need it to be quick and easy. I used to grab a Zone bar and eat half when I first got to work and half late morning. When I began using NutiMirror and watching the sodium monster I noticed there was way too much in each bar. I also struggled getting my fiber into the green. By switching to Total, yogurt, and craisins my 234-calorie breakfast got my day off to off to a great green start. And my sodium score was much improved.

CEREAL, YOGURT, AND FRUIT
- 1 oz. cranberries, dried, sweetened, 87 calories
- 1/2 cup Total cereal, 67 calories
- 1/2 cup yogurt, nonfat, 80 calories

MY LUNCH—235 calories

On this day, I ate leftovers from the night before. I typically bring leftovers from home or something simple that I can pop into the microwave—add a salad and presto! I make up a large salad Sunday evening for lunches during the week, or I grab a side salad at McDonald's. I found the "spritz" type dressings are a wonderful invention. They give the salad that little extra pizzazz without all those calories. I always add a calcium supplement.

SHRIMP PRIMAVERA, SALAD,
ICED TEA, AND VITAMINS
- 5 oz. shrimp primavera with sauce, 185 calories
- 3 outer leaves romaine lettuce, 14 calories
- 1 tbsp. onion, chopped, 4 calories
- 1 radish, 1 calorie
- 1 tbsp. sweet red pepper, 2 calories
- 3 baby carrots, 11 calories
- 42 oz. unsweetened iced tea
- 12 sprays honey-mustard dressing, 18 calories
- Calcium supplement (with vitamins D & K), 0 calories

MY SNACKS–440 calories

I am a snacker—especially when I'm at home. So I try to find things that will satisfy me in small amounts. After realizing that my snacking habits were leading to my sodium issues, I found healthy alternatives that would stop the cravings yet be a healthier. Also measuring/ weighing my snacks (and meal portions) became a must. I found that a handful of tortilla chips are not one serving. So a scale in the kitchen has become a fixture.

FRUIT, CHEESE, CHIPS, GRAHAM CRACKERS, AND VITAMINS
- 1 orange, 72 calories
- 1.5 oz. Swiss cheese, light, 72 calories
- 1 oz. dried blueberries, 92 calories
- 1 honey graham cracker, 55 calories
- 1 oz. mini white tortilla rounds, 140 calories
- Proanthenols 100 supplement, 0 calories
- Mature multivitamin, 0 calories
- Calcium supplement (with vitamins D & K), 0 calories
- 1 oz. fish oil, 10 calories

MY DINNER–413 calories

This was my first homemade roast chicken. My husband was always asking me to purchase whole chickens but I didn't want to mess with them. If the chicken wasn't already boned, skinned and cut up, I really didn't want to bother. But when I finally did, I bought one of those great little roasters and OMG it turned out so yummy and juicy that I was shocked. Needless to say we now buy whole chickens. Along with a baked potato and a steamed veggie this was a quick and easy dinner for a work night.

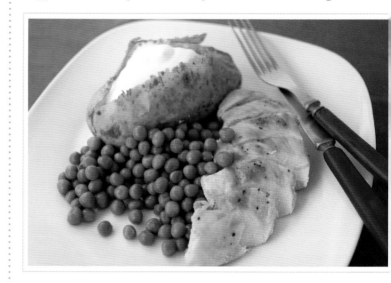

CHICKEN, POTATO, LIGHT SOUR CREAM, AND PEAS
- 5 oz. roasted chicken breast, meat only, 234 calories
- 3 oz. baked potato with skin, 79 calories
- 2 tbsp. sour cream, light, 40 calories
- 1/2 cup peas, 60 calories

username: jessica / *first name:* Jessica

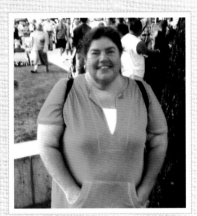

Jessica NOW: November '09 / age: 51
213 lbs. / BMI 41.9

. . . .

I have been fat forty-five of my fifty-one years. I can't say I have tried every diet but I've had my share of them. I've done diet pills, Weight Watchers, nutrition classes, and more. And I exercised whenever I went on "serious" diets, always losing 25 pounds or more. I would soon tire of dieting, finding excuses to quit. With the increased rate of obesity in our country, I felt more comfortable as a fat person and decided to just live my life and eat whatever. Thankfully, I quite liked healthy foods, but it was just prepared in bad ways and I ate too much of it. I ate out as often as I ate at home. If I hadn't had a job requiring me to be on my feet and lifting all day I would have gotten even larger than I did. The pain started from being on my feet eight hours a day. When my husband and I went places that required a lot of walking, I usually had to sit a lot of it out.

Then I turned fifty and something had to change. My hours were cut back, which meant that the granddaddy of all excuses—not enough time to do anything about it—was gone. I Googled something or other and found the NutriMirror site. To this day, I swear it was an answer to a prayer.

There is no food plan or "system." This is good, because once I am told I cannot eat this or that, I want it all the time. Here, all I had to do was make well informed food choices and NutriMirror would show me exactly where, and how much, I was out of balance. Once I started making better food decisions and feeding my body what it needed to function properly, it responded. I don't crave empty calorie foods in large amounts any more and, believe it or not, I'm rarely hungry. When I do want more to eat, I earn it by moving my body more.

I have started walking and slightly modified the types and amounts of food I eat. I still go out to eat and really do not feel like I am depriving myself. I have learned to read labels on everything. I have high blood pressure so my number one nemesis is sodium. In four months, I have lowered the daily sodium in my food choices from 4,313 mgs to 2,149 mg. I can plan a balanced day in relatively little time. Although I've lost thirty-seven pounds, I am still a work in progress. I am certain my ideal weight will come in time. I now have a mindset for life long success and I am in control—something I never was before.

. . . .

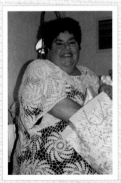

Jessica THEN: May '09
. . . .
249.8 lbs. / BMI 49

MY MOTHER: "SOMETIMES WHEN YOU'RE READY FOR A THING, YOU'LL FIND IT." THE TRICK IS TO BE READY.

username: SteppinUp / *first name:* Steph / *location:* Witchia, KS

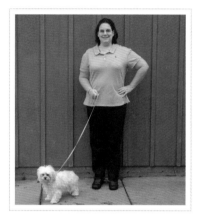

Steph NOW: October '09 / age: 41
210 lbs. / BMI 35 / waist 41.75˝

I cannot begin to talk about my relationship with food and eating without mentioning my mother and grandmother. However, make no mistake about this, in no way do I set any of the blame for my excess weight upon their shoulders. I choose what I place within my body, they don't. What they gave me was a love for food, cooking, and trying new things. As I began to think about the many foods that I adore, it brought back many fond memories of these great ladies. Mother is a fantastic

cook, and grandmother was a professional chef for a great many years. I never knew what new thing would be served for dinner, or what stranger might be invited to dine with us.

Somewhere along the way, I took this love of food straight from my lips to my hips. I packed on the pounds. I could spout off a half-dozen excuses, but it all comes down to one word: choice. I chose to eat in an unhealthy manner and my body responded in kind.

For years, I took prescription acid blockers, popped antacids, and even took a trip to the ER when I woke up one morning with blood all over my pillow due to severe reflux. That was when I found out that eating a brownie and popping Ibuprofen just before bed was not a good idea.

Years went by and I continued to put garbage into my body and my body continued telling me to stop. I had to look for a way to figure out exactly what was causing the problem.

I found Nutrimirror and quickly learned that I was giving my body a lot of calories, fat, and sodium and not a whole lot of anything good. I now thank God for acid reflux, because it helped to teach me a lesson that I needed to learn! I am not completely reflux-free, but I am now able to tell when it is food-related and when it is just an ordinary stress event. I have more pain-free days than not. I'm not popping pills every day, and I feel great!!

I am a mother of three, and I realize that I am passing

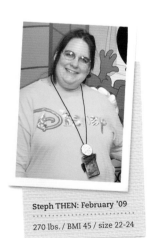

Steph THEN: February '09

270 lbs. / BMI 45 / size 22-24

on my nutritional legacy to my children. I adore that my parents gave me a love for trying new things, and I now prepare newer, healthier versions of old favorite recipes: meat loaf, tacos, chili, pasta alfredo, scampi—the list goes on and on. I have found that my children usually like these recipes. Not all have been a hit, but most have. My kids are learning good nutritional habits right along with my husband and me. They understand that we are getting healthier every day, and thinner too! I'd be lying if I said that they don't sometimes say that they miss some of the high-fat, high-sodium, low nutritional value treats that used to be in the pantry. However, we all have discovered healthier alternatives that we now love. Instead of pizza and potato chips, we snack on fruit, veggies, and healthier versions of those calorie-laden crutches we used to trip over. Instead of a bag of greasy chips, we'll eat just a few lower fat, lower sodium chips that the kids insist taste just as good as their greasy cousins.

My daughter and I like to share a few baby carrots after dinner, just for a snack. It's our thing. We have made determining wise food choices a way of life. True, they don't relish spending what must seem like an eternity (to them) at the grocery store while Mom compares food labels making sure that she gets the most nutritional bang for the buck, but it always puts a smile on their face when a fruit leather or other fun, healthy treat makes its way into the cart.

Little by little, choice by choice, day by day, we are bringing new habits and new attitudes about food into our lives. We have found that we enjoy and taste our foods more instead of horsing down greater quantities of nutritionally empty calories. Special events don't cause us trouble, or send us back to our former nutritional wasteland. We eat, make merry, and log it all. Each day is a new day to make new nutritional choices, and we love ours.

I often tell my children great stories about their grandmother and great-grandmother. I truly wish that my grandmother had lived long enough for them to have met and known her. I know that they would have adored one another. She lived a good life, but succumbed to heart disease, diabetes, and cancer. There may never be a single thing in the world that tastes better than her Sunday Fried Chicken, but I will still think of her every time that I serve my healthier oven-baked version. With some good fortune, maybe my great-grandkids will get the chance to know their great grandmother. I owe it all to God, acid reflux, and the information I get from using NutriMirror. This awesome combination keeps me in control of all the choices that determine my health. My mother once said something to me that I will never forget: "Sometimes when you're ready for a thing, you find it." The trick is to be ready.

MY PHYSICAL ACTIVITY

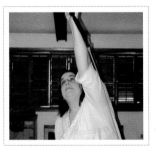 I have never been one to exercise with any regularity, and in many ways I'm still not. However, my terminal couch potato ways are changing. I may take the dog for a walk, splash around in the pool with the kids, or even do some stretching and toning while watching my favorite television show. I take the stairs instead of the elevator. These are small steps to be sure, but a great improvement. Gone are the days of going out to eat a high-calorie meal and coming back home to a nap. Ultimately, I'd like to start taking some dance classes, as that is something that I once enjoyed. I just haven't summoned the courage yet to join all those toned and trimmed bodies. As the pounds keep ticking away, though, I can see that goal coming much closer!

STEPH'S *GREEN* DAY

- Calories Expended: **2,284**
- Calories Eaten: **1,466**
- Net Calorie Balance: 818

For me the beauty of constructing a Green Day is the understanding that it's all about the nutrition. It's not about a bunch of guidelines to follow, or a menu that I have to stick to. I can't do that and succeed in making myself healthy. I've learned to balance my choices (how I love that word) so I eat what I like while at the same time giving my body the nutrients it needs. The ability to have this kind of control has been such a blessing.

I began this journey with the mindset that I wanted to get healthy, not thin. The weight loss is a fantastic side-effect of getting healthy. Using the NutriMirror tools has helped me to see the reality of what it is that I am putting into my body. But it doesn't deliver a result. The choices and responsibilities are all mine.

MY GREEN DAY NUTRITIONAL FACTS

STEPH'S
HEALTH REFLECTION™
Nutrition Facts Report

Calorie Balance	
Calories Expended	2284
Calories Eaten	1466
Net Calorie Balance	818

Nutrient Balance	
	%DV
Total Fat 35 g	✔
Saturated Fat 6 g	37%
Trans Fat 0 g	—
Cholesterol 179 mg	60%
Sodium 1495 mg	65%
Total Carbs 193 g	✔
Dietary Fiber 30 g	146%
Sugars 88 g	—
Protein 106 g	✔
Vitamin A 3114 µg	445%
Vitamin C 133 mg	177%
Calcium 1332 mg	133%
Iron 25 g	139%

MY BREAKFAST
–271 calories

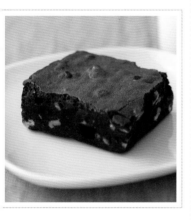

Breakfast was the meal that I either skipped altogether, or got out of a fast-food wrapper. Now, it is a huge part of making my day come out green. I have learned that getting enough fiber and lowering sodium are key to making everything else balance. Also, starting out the day correctly strengthens my resolve to make better decisions throughout the day.

CEREAL, COFFEE, AND BROWNIE
- Decaf coffee, 8 oz., 0 calories
- 1 packet sugar, 11 calories
- 1 serving Simple Harvest multigrain cereal (vanilla, almond, and honey), 160 calories
- 1 chocolate Vita Brownie, 100 calories

MY SNACKS–186 calories

Hey, I can have my jelly beans and eat them too! Carrots may not seem like a snack to a lot of people, but for me they are… and so much more. My daughter and I regularly share a snack of carrots; we "toast" our carrot sticks together and munch in unison. How cool is it to round off your Green Day (and boost your calcium level as well) with a fudge bar?

FRUIT, CARROTS, JELLY BELLYS, AND SKINNY COW
- 1 apple, 71 calories
- 7 baby carrots, 25 calories
- 10 Jelly Belly candies, 40 calories
- 1 mini Skinny Cow fudge bar, 50 calories

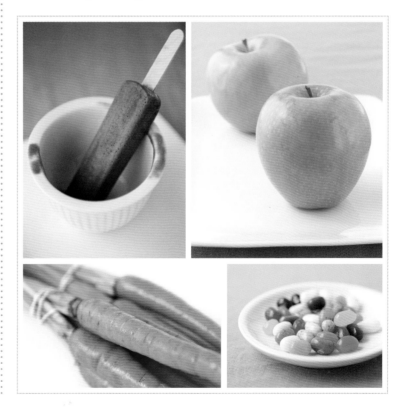

MY LUNCH–318 calories

I often ate fast-food or other high-calorie, nutrient-poor food for lunch. Now, I am a big fan of the protein-topped salad. I switch it up and choose different proteins and experiment with different flavors in their preparation. When I go out to eat, I ask for the dressing on the side so that I can control the amount.

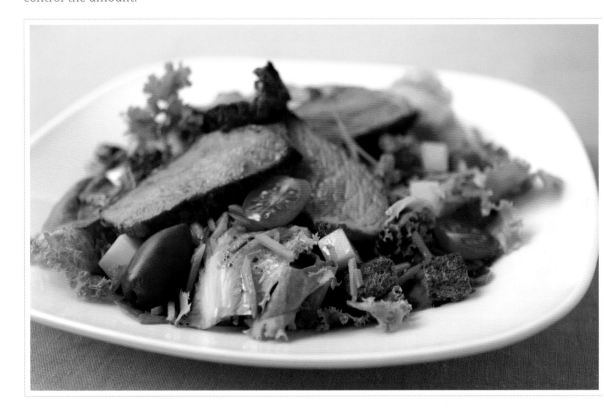

SIRLOIN SALAD AND TEA

- 1 cups green leaf lettuce, 10 calories
- 1 cup fresh spinach, 7 calories
- 2 baby carrots, 7 calories
- 3 oz. top sirloin, 155 calories
- 5 cups tea, 13 calories
- 1 tbsp. croutons, 8 calories
- 5 large olives, 31 calories
- 4 tsp. balsamic Italian dressing, 73 calories
- 1/2 tbsp. mild cheddar cheese, 10 calories
- 1/2 oz. tomatoes, 4 calories

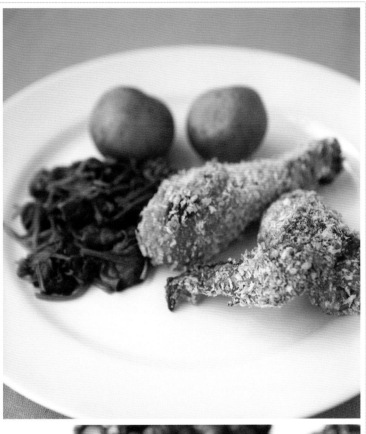

MY DINNER—691 calories

Fried Chicken is a classic, but it's high in calories and saturated fats. Since I could never make it as well as my Grandmother, it made sense to reinvent it and still love it! I wish she were still here to try some. I think she would have had a lot of fun with the panko. No matter what, she'd always swear that she "dipped her toe in the salt on that one!" Well, I didn't here. So that I don't break tradition, let's just pretend that I did!

CHICKEN, VEGATABLES, FRUIT, AND MILK
- 4 oz. panko oven-fried chicken, 345 calories
- 3 oz. red potatoes, baked, 76 calories
- 1 cup spinach, cooked, 41 calories
- 1 cup blackberries, 62 calories
- 2 cups milk, nonfat, 167 calories

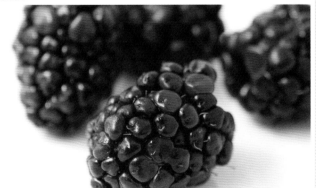

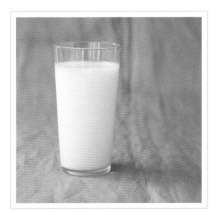

"IF I DID NOT CHANGE MY HABITS AND FAST, I WAS HEADED FOR A TWENTY-POUND WEIGHT GAIN IN A MATTER OF MONTHS."

username: susano / *first name:* Susan / *location:* North Carolina

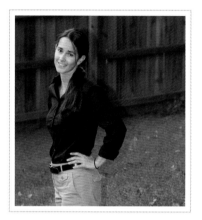

Susan NOW: November '09 / age: 40
110 lbs. / BMI 19.5 / waist 26.5˝

I am what most would call "one of the lucky ones" as I have lived my life never having to think about what I ate. I never gained weight, even without exercise. Aside from a few gains along the way—some added weight in my freshman year of college, twelve pounds when I quit smoking after close to twenty years, and a thirty-pound gain while pregnant—I have pretty much weighed the same since high school. Admittedly, it had been a great ride—I have always loved food and I truly enjoyed indulging myself—sometimes to the point of being so stuffed

I could barely move. (I used to find this amusing but more recently, not so much.)

The negative side to my great metabolic luck was that it also enabled me to form some very bad habits. When I think of how little exercise I have done in my life it makes me cringe. For years I have eaten more fats and salts than anything else— the bulk of my consumption taking place after dinner and sometimes into the wee hours. After my daughter was born I stopped cooking for the most part. She turned out to be a very picky eater and it just wasn't worth my time or energy to fix meals that only I would be eating.

Whenever I got the chance to eat at someone else's home and have a "real home-cooked meal" I would especially stuff myself Perhaps it was that I didn't know when I would eat like that again that made me feel like I had better get as much as possible! Yikes. I also tended to eat out of boredom, or when I came home from a trip to the

grocery store I would have to sample just about everything I had gotten there at once. I also ate very fast; this has always been my habit but it only got worse when motherhood arrived, perhaps because I am almost always in a hurry and eating had to fit in quickly between other things.

As all great rides must come to an end, I found myself being (rudely, if I say so myself!) kicked off the "lucky metabolism" train a couple years ago. I stood there in a

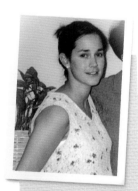

Pregnant, and the beginning of a big lifestyle change

cloud of dust as the train rolled away, scratching my head and wondering what I had done to be treated that way. Since I turned thirty-eight I have arrived at each new season with last season's clothes embarrassingly tight and uncomfortable. In my thirty-ninth year I developed a little "gut," which definitely got my attention. For years I have been aware of the lack of muscle tone in my thighs and rear, but since I couldn't see them (wink!) they were easy to ignore – and not such an issue since I was still skinny. Previously I could see my stomach, and it had always been flat and tight. I had been lucky to get away with a thirty-pound pregnancy gain without any signs of it left on my belly. However the sudden appearance of a gut was unsettling because I was fully aware of the implications. And yet, I continued to eat nachos as soon as my daughter went to bed—and popcorn with butter and salt, and whatever else came to mind.

This year I turned forty, and when it got cool enough to wear jeans I was dismayed (but shouldn't have been surprised) to find that none of them fit. In fact, the ones that were baggy last season were too tight! I had to go out and buy all new jeans—a whole size up. I tried on my spring clothes and was aghast at how they fit. This was a rude awakening because not only did I not want to go out and buy a new spring wardrobe—I couldn't afford to. There was no way I was going to extend my debt to pay for clothes just because of my irresponsible eating habits. Plus, that little gut was now big enough that it hung over my pants a little bit and I could feel it jiggle when I walked—oh no! It hit me like a ton of bricks how fast I was gaining and that if I did not change my habits and FAST, I was headed for a twenty-pound weight gain in a matter of months.

I am a single mother and it is important that I be an example of healthy and balanced living for my daughter—in every aspect of life. Raising a daughter in this culture that worships celebrity, especially the skeletal variety, is daunting. I am determined that my girl have a healthy relationship with her body. This begins with me.

The idea that the right foods (the whole foods that nature provides) can do more to prevent disease than any medication, has long been a firmly-held belief of mine.

Over the years I have read much about the benefits of certain foods and have had the long-term goal of ridding myself of reflux acid through diet and exercise to get off the toxic medications that I currently take. Many times I have started a food journal to keep track of what I was eating and how I felt. I could go through it and see if specific foods triggered flare-ups or alternatively improved my well-being. I'm not very organized or consistent, and procrastination is a finely honed skill of mine, so this never lasted more than a few days before I would forget where I put the notebook and just decided to forget it all together. Despite all the research I did on nutrition, I never kept the specific information in my head for long.

In March of 2009 I was Googling "weight loss and nutrition" and came across the NutriMirror site. I signed up just to see what it was all about and was instantly hooked. Even though I already had a pretty healthy diet, I could suddenly see exactly how much I was eating with regard to calories. No wonder I was so full and gaining weight so fast! Being able to see immediately how what I ate affected my calorie allowance was incredibly motivating. I was able to lose those few pounds quickly and keep them off. What is even more exciting to me is that I can keep track of the nutrients I get. If I'm low in vitamin A I eat a carrot and see the numbers go

up instantly. WOW. And as I log my food daily I can jot down how I am feeling on that day, so now I have a health and food journal to refer to at a moment's notice and I always know where it is. This is invaluable to my goal of treating my autoimmune disease through diet! I can see the trends and address them easily.

My love of eating has in no way been hindered by all of this. The truth is I can now eat even more, but without the consequences. Being able to see the nutritional information on my foods enables me to make smarter choices about what I can eat. Instead of a piece of pizza that uses up almost half of my daily calorie allowance, I can eat

loads of fruits and vegetables and beans—things I more fully enjoy anyway. No more empty calories for me! Eating this way frees me up to have more variety in my day, and variety is something I value. Life is for living! I have never believed in self-deprivation of any sort. Eating good food has always brought me joy and I will not relinquish that. I don't have to.

NutriMirror has also illuminated my current most pressing need: exercise. I am finally motivated to work out. And I can see through the measured feedback how much room that thirty-minute walk gives me for that extra treat I may be wanting.

MY PHYSICAL ACTIVITY

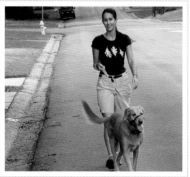

Excercise has always been my biggest challenge. I did not work out at all and it has been difficult to find time in my busy day. Hiking in the mountains is how I would most like to exercise. Since I don't have that mountain access on a daily basis, I take walks in the neighborhood or around town. I have also started to really enjoy working out with my Wii. Although I am still going slowly I have already noticed an increase in strength and this is a big motivator for me. I have even started to look forward to exercising.

SUSAN'S *GREEN* DAY

- Calories Expended: **1,494**
- Calories Eaten: **1,278**
- Net Calorie Balance: **216**

I have learned to make smarter food choices that allow me to indulge in my love of food and cooking. I love soup, and the act of taking a variety of ingredients—vegetables, beans, and spices—and tossing them into a pot together is a joyful experience for me. It's becoming a regular routine for me to put up a pot of soup to eat all week. Some goes into the freezer in single servings so I have meals ready to go in a pinch, which is important for me since I am generally rushed.

MY GREEN DAY NUTRITIONAL FACTS

SUSAN'S **HEALTH REFLECTION™** Nutrition Facts Report	
Calorie Balance	
Calories Expended	1494
Calories Eaten	1278
Net Calorie Balance	216

Nutrient Balance	
	%DV
Total Fat 29 g	✔
Saturated Fat 9 g	63%
Trans Fat 0 g	—
Cholesterol 30 mg	10%
Sodium 1114 mg	48%
Total Carbs 209 g	✔
Dietary Fiber 38 g	212%
Sugars 69 g	—
Protein 62 g	✔
Vitamin A 1734 µg	248%
Vitamin C 271 mg	361%
Calcium 1264 mg	126%
Iron 39 g	217%

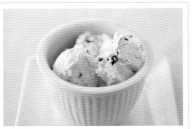

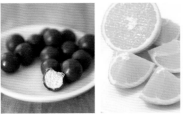

MY SNACKS–450 calories

I really do love that soup. I had two bowls as snacks on this day. Now I make it a point to take things like this to work with me so I don't get hungry and eat empty junk calories that will leave me drained. I also like to have apples and oranges on hand—self-packaged, time-saving snacks that taste great and fill me up without a lot of calories. I was even able to treat myself with a little ice cream and some candy while keeping green!

MY SOUP, FRUIT, CANDY, AND ICE CREAM
- 1 orange, 62 calories
- 2 Whoppers malted milk balls, 20 calories
- 1/2 cup mint chip ice cream, 160 calories
- 1 tbsp. nutritional yeast, 30 calories
- 2 servings vegetable soup (see recipe), 178 calories

MY LUNCH–414 calories

I made a big pot of this soup over the weekend and it was delicious! It is so colorful and full of flavor and nutrition that on some days I eat it for lunch and dinner. Sometimes I add nutritional yeast—it adds flavor as well as protein and lots of other micronutrients. I get a big kick out of knowing how nutrient-dense and calorie-friendly it is, and my neighbor likes it so much she keeps asking me to make more.

MY SOUP, BREAD, AND YEAST
- 1 serving multigrain bread with touch of honey, 180 calories
- 2 tbsp. nutritional yeast, 60 calories
- 1 serving vegetable soup (see recipe), 174 calories

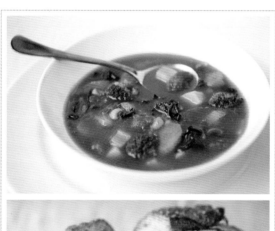

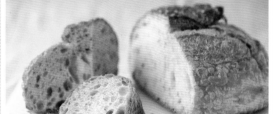

THIS WEEK'S SOUP

Makes approximately twenty-one 1-cup servings.

INGREDIENTS
1 tbsp. olive oil
2 1/2 cups chopped yellow onions
1 cup chopped celery
4 cups carrots, chopped wide
15 cloves garlic
1 32-oz. can diced tomatoes (unsalted)
2 tsp. turmeric
1 tsp. garam masala
1/2 tsp. black pepper
1 tsp. salt
1 tsp. curry powder
1 tsp. SPIKE vegit seasoning
6 1/2 oz. chopped mushrooms
2 15-oz. cans black eyed peas (unsalted)
1 15-oz. can adzuki beans (unsalted)
6 cups chopped kale
1 1/2 cups chopped spinach
1 cup sweet potatoes, chopped wide
1 1/2 cups Yukon gold potatoes, with skin, chopped wide
3 1/2 cups broccoli florets
10+ cups water

PREPARATION
1. Heat olive oil in a large pot. Add onions and celery, cooking until soft and great smelling. Add carrots, garlic, and a cup or two of water. Let this cook a bit to get a good, flavorful base.

2. Add tomatoes with juice, turmeric, garam masala, pepper, salt, curry powder, and vegit seasoning.

3. Slowly, one at a time, add the mushrooms, black eyed peas, adzuki beans, kale, and spinach. Add water as needed to keep ingredients covered. Save the potatoes and broccoli for near the end so they don't overcook.

MY BREAKFAST—119 calories

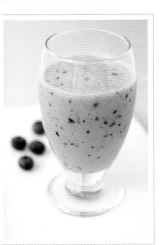

I have always been a smoothie fan and am even more so now that I have a little one to feed. My daughter is a healthy eater, but she's very picky and hates to try new things. However, she'll eat just about any smoothie I make for her. Not only are they packed with nutrition, but also they are easy to mix up quickly and can be eaten on the ly, which is perfect for our hectic mornings.

SMOOTHIE, COFFEE, AND VITAMINS
• 8 oz. coffee, 2 calories
• 1/2 cup vanilla soy milk, 50 calories
• Iron supplement, 0 calories
• Folic acid supplement, 0 calories

ERB SMOOTHIE

Makes one serving.

INGREDIENTS
1/4 extra small banana
1/8 cup blueberries
1 small wedge cantaloupe
1 oz. pineapple juice
4 frozen strawberries
2 oz. orange juice

PREPARATION
Mix in a blender and serve.

• Calcium 600 + D, 0 calories
• 1/2 serving ERB smoothie (see recipe), 67 calories

MY DINNER—295 calories

This dinner is one of my daughter's favorites. I made tofu like this back when my daughter was tiny and it is the only way she will eat it. Paired with some brown rice and steamed broccoli drizzled with lemon juice, it's a great meal and one we have often. What is new about this meal is that before I became so mindful of how much I eat, I'd have eaten the equivalent of three times this amount and been painfully full afterwards. It's very empowering now to be to be able to control those impulses.

VEGETABLE, BROWN RICE, AND TOFU
• 1/2 tsp. lemon juice, 1 calorie
• 1 cup chopped broccoli, cooked, 55 calories
• 1/2 cup brown rice, 108 calories
• Tofu, 131 calories

"I WILL CONTINUE TO ACHIEVE A GREEN BALANCE AND ENJOY MY FOOD AND LIFE."

username: SylviaAnn / *first name:* Sylvia / *location:* Henderson, NV

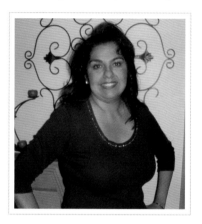

Sylvia NOW: September '09 / age: 44
175 lbs. / BMI 24.5 / waist 32.75˝

I am the wife of a very loving and supportive husband. He is very active in the community and that also keeps me busy. We have two wonderful teenagers. Our kids are active in school with karate, football, cheerleading, and dance. This means a lot of bleacher-sitting for me. I work a forty-hour week and have been with my employer for twenty-one years. I sit at a desk most of the time; very little walking is involved.

My father passed away when I was seventeen. I have four siblings. My mother says that I am more like a mother hen than a sister or daughter. Three of the four siblings have lived with me at one time or another. And the one who has not is now my next door neighbor. My brothers say that I am the Hispanic version of Martha Stewart because of my creative nature. I make gift baskets, decorate cakes, make my own cake fillings, try new recipes and I am always trying to organize one thing or another. I have worked and earned money since I was old enough to baby-sit. I look forward to living a long, healthy life. I look forward to being a grandmother and a great-grandmother.

As a young person I was always very thin. People called me skinny. The word skinny makes me angry to this day. I used to hear comments like, "you must eat like bird," "where does the food go?" and "you are so skinny, don't you eat?" Being overweight was never an issue for me until I hit my forties.

At age forty I reached 180 pounds. I accepted this weight gain, believing that, as we get older, we just gain weight naturally. Slowly over the next four years my weight continued to climb. By the time I hit 190 pounds, my size 14 was too snug and made my muffin-top very evident. I bought loose blouses. I eventually graduated to size 16 to make the muffin-top go away. My knees hurt and I was tired at the end of day.

I went to the doctor and she ran tests that came back normal.

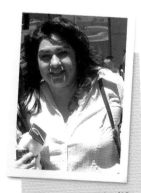

Sylvia THEN: November '08
203.8 lbs. / BMI 28.9 / waist 42.5˝

She gave me the drill about eating balanced meals and eating appropriate calories. She told me to incorporate exercises into my daily routine. Possibly I was eating more fast-food than I realized. It was certainly easier to grab fast-food than actually prepare a meal. Before I knew it, I was repeating the same pattern in my size 16 as I had in my size 14.

I tried one of the programs that delivered food to your front door. What was I thinking? Out of desperation I was willing to do anything to lose weight. Within the first week, I realized that I could not buy this food for a lifetime. Furthermore, the meals were not that great. I wanted to enjoy my food. I briefly tried counting points, yet another program that I quickly realized was not my style. I did't want to eat points. I wanted to eat food!

In October of 2008 I realized that my weight was out of control; I was now 203.8 pounds. I refused to go into a size 18 but I had already purchased three size 18 blouses.

I began to search the Internet and found NutriMirror. NutriMirror made it simple; there are two colors, red and green. I could work with those colors. I knew healthy eating promoted healthy weight. I just needed a tool that could guide me in the right direction.

I accepted the fact that exercise is also important to increase your metabolism. Beginning my journey to achieve a healthy weight, I did not see myself as a vigorous exercise person. My exercise of choice is walking; I set my goal at a minimum of fifteen minutes and a maximum of sixty minutes a day.

In six months I managed to lose twenty pounds, I reduced my waist measurement from 42 inches to 33 inches, and my hips from 48 inches to 42.5 inches. In addition to losing weight, I noticed the migraine headaches had started to go away. (I had previously averaged three to four migraines a month that had to be treated with prescription medicine.) Currently I have one migraine a month and I can treat it with

an over-the-counter medicine. I will continue to achieve a green balance and enjoy my food and life. I am currently back to size 14, and in no time at all I will be in a size 12.

MY PHYSICAL ACTIVITY

My exercise of choice is walking. I walk an average of five days a week, for a minimum of thirty minutes and a max of one hour per session. My energy level has increased over time allowing me to walk at a 3.8 mph pace and at times I can increase my pace to 4.0 mph. Walking is simple and it allows me to just use that time for thinking things through.

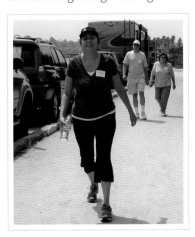

SYLVIA'S *GREEN* DAY

- Calories Expended: **1,923**
- Calories Eaten: **1,482**
- Net Calorie Balance: 441

I love the immediate feedback I get that measures the choices I've made, telling me if I am in balance or out of balance. I have such control and am not depriving myself of my favorite foods. I've learned how to incorporate my favorites by balancing and meeting the nutritional needs of my body. I re-discovered many foods that I had eaten as a child, along with new foods introduced to me via the NutriMirror community. This is a Green Day that typifies my new healthy eating lifestyle.

MY GREEN DAY NUTRITIONAL FACTS

SYLVIA'S
HEALTH REFLECTION™
Nutrition Facts Report

Calorie Balance	
Calories Expended	1923
Calories Eaten	1482
Net Calorie Balance	441

Nutrient Balance	
	%DV
Total Fat 48 g	✔
Saturated Fat 8 g	49%
Trans Fat 0 g	—
Cholesterol 55 mg	18%
Sodium 1731 mg	75%
Total Carbs 199 g	✔
Dietary Fiber 22 g	106%
Sugars 102 g	—
Protein 81 g	✔
Vitamin A 2830 µg	404%
Vitamin C 162 mg	216%
Calcium 1906 mg	191%
Iron 26 mg	144%

MY SNACKS–374 calories

I really look forward to my snacks each day. Snacking between meals prevents my overeating at main meals. I especially enjoy my evening snack because it is typically a treat such as ice cream.

YOGURT, FRUIT, NUTS, AND ICE CREAM
- 1 orange, 45 calories
- 10 almonds, 69 calories
- Greek yogurt, 120 calories
- Vanilla ice cream sandwich, 140 calories

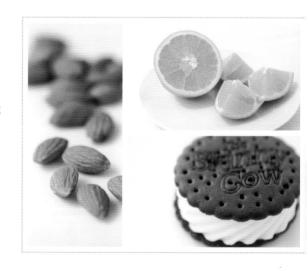

MY BREAKFAST—350 calories

I wake up fifteen minutes earlier now to eat breakfast. I love steel-cut oatmeal and I eat it just about every morning. I change my flavorings often; I add canned pumpkin, blueberries, peanut butter, raisins, or strawberries. My breakfast is never boring.

OATMEAL, MILK, SEASONINGS, COFFEE, AND VITAMINS
- Oatmeal, 150 calories
- 1 tbsp. canned pumpkin, 5 calories
- 1 tbsp. brown sugar, 45 calories
- 1/2 cup milk, nonfat, 43 calories
- 6 oz. coffee, 2 calories
- 3 tbsp. Coffee-mate, 105 calories
- One-A-Day supplement, 0 calories
- Calcium + D supplement, 0 calories

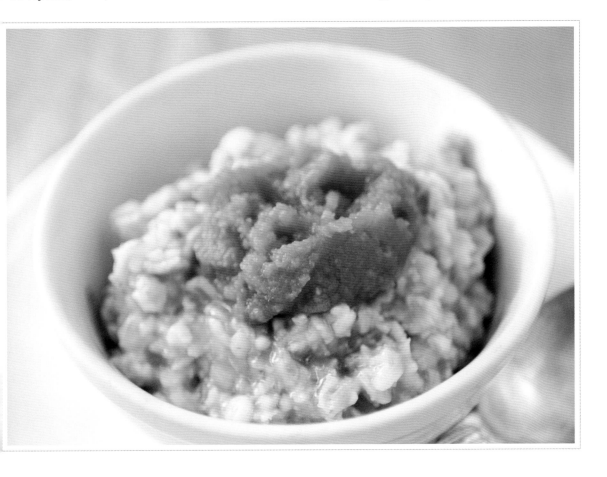

MY LUNCH–345 calories

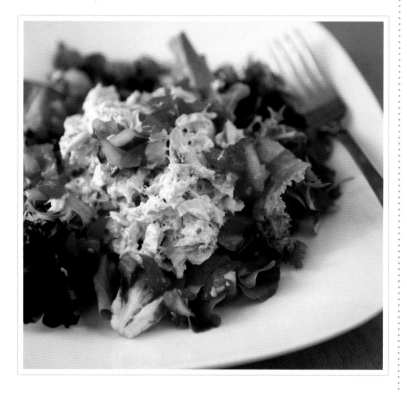

I love salads. I'm happy as long as I have on hand a mix of baby greens, romaine or spinach, any protein such as canned salmon, tuna, chicken, shrimp, or leftover cooked chicken, pork, or steak. I buy a package of vegetable medley which contains broccoli, cauliflower, and carrots. One bag can make three salads. I love to use salsa as a substitute for dressings

SALAD WITH PROTEIN AND DRESSING, AND YOGURT
- 1 tbsp. mayonnaise, 90 calories
- 3 tbsp. fire roasted vegetable salsa, 15 calories
- 5 oz. Greek yogurt, 120 calories
- 1 serving pink salmon, 90 calories
- 6 oz. European salad mix, 30 calories

MY DINNER
—413 calories

When my family is running in different directions, sometimes something as simple as a peanut butter and jelly sandwich is perfect for dinner.

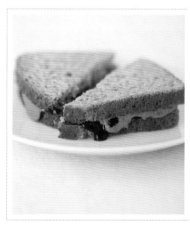

PB&J WITH MILK
- 2 tbsp. peanut butter, 180 calories
- 2 slices whole wheat bread, 140 calories
- 1 tbsp. grape jelly, 50 calories
- 1/2 cup milk, nonfat, 43 calories

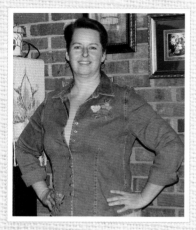

Dawn NOW: November '09 / age: 42
188.8 lbs. / BMI 29.6 / waist 34.5˝

For the past twenty years or so, my weight had slowly crept up. I always told myself I'd change tomorrow, but tomorrow never came. I was obese and unhealthy. I watched what I ate but had no compass for what was balanced. Without the information I needed, I acted as if my choices didn't affect my health—that a fast-food meal was okay because I was in a hurry or I deserved a treat. I yo-yo exercised, starting strong for six to twelve weeks and then slacking off when I started seeing change. I was completely disconnected from the reality of my eating habits and what I was doing to my health and my happiness. My weight-losing efforts were half-hearted and the results didn't last. I needed to change my thinking.

Then, one day last spring, something inside just clicked and I decided I wasn't going to live like that anymore. I had to find a way to make what I looked like on the outside match who I truly am on the inside and so I decided to find a food log online. I did, and I have never looked back!

Using the feedback provided helps makes me knowledgeable and guides my choices. I am in control. I just log my food and exercise and instantly learn which of my choices need refining. I got sodium under control and learned to plan my meals, both at home and away. I decided not to try to make any weight loss speed records, but work toward the recommended one pound per week.

After losing ten pounds, I finally started to believe my progress wasn't a fluke. I realize I am in control of my choices and I can make good choices for my health. I don't turn to food to fix my emotional lows and I don't deny myself the foods I really like. But I do plan for my treats.

And I have learned that when I make poor food or exercise choices, it is not the end of the world. Because I am in control I have no need to feel guilt over bad choices. I just log them, learn, and move on. Conscious choice is empowering. I fully believe that I am developing habits that will be sustainable for the rest of my life.

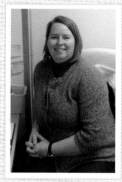

Dawn THEN: April '09

220 lbs. / BMI 34.5 / waist 40˝

"HAVE YOU ALWAYS BEEN A BIG MAN?"

username: tomgerrity / *first name:* Tom / *location:* Haslet, TX

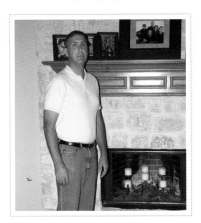

Tom NOW: October '09 / age: 46
205 lbs. / BMI 25 / waist 33˝

I was on the cross country and track teams in high school. I could eat anything and not gain weight. I continued to run throughout college and even into the first several years of marriage. When I graduated college, I weighed 168 pounds. I was a 6´4˝ beanpole. When I met my wife, I was over 200 pounds, but definitely not overweight. I remember looking at a picture of myself from high school. I realized that my face had filled out and I looked different. I actually looked healthier than I did in high school and college. That same healthy image is what I thought others always saw.

Over the past twenty years, my weight had slowly risen to 245 pounds. My weight steadily grew to new all-time highs. Periodically, I would begin an exercise regimen, make an effort to watch my calories, or simply increase my daily water consumption and quickly lose ten pounds. Within weeks, however, the pounds would always be back with five or more friends. This pattern continued for the better part of four years.

In October of 2008, an employee at my restaurant asked me a question that made me rethink everything. After a full day of climbing a ladder, installing cameras, one of my younger employees asked me if I'd always been a "big man." I was shocked. I replied, "It depends on what you mean by a "big man." He went on to point out that he was 6´4˝ and that I seemed about the same height. He said that no matter what he tried, he could not put on weight. I told him to get married, have a couple of kids, and sign a mortgage ... the weight would come.

To make matters worse, I was preparing my laptop to access the security cameras remotely and caught a glimpse of myself on camera. I immediately thought of the line from the television show, *Friends*, where Monica states that the camera adds ten pounds and Chandler asks, "How many cameras did they have on you?" Coincidentally, I had installed eight cameras that weekend.

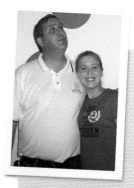

Tom THEN: October '08
265 lbs. / BMI 32.3 / waist 38˝

The conversation with my employee continued to bother me. The Monday after I returned home from installing the cameras, I mentioned to a friend at work that I could tell he had lost weight. He told me about a website he was using to log his foods and exercise. That same day, I signed up on NutriMirror and entered my height and weight. The data came through. At 265 pounds, I was obese for my height (or more than a foot under-tall for my weight.) On October 29 I set my goal weight, logged my first day, and began the learning process.

A funny thing happened on my way to achieving my goal: I learned a lot about what makes me tick. I found that the NutriMirror website really appealed to the geek in me. It quickly became very important to me that I achieve at least the weight loss projected for me on the site based on my net calorie surplus. Making sure that I recorded exercise conservatively and calorie intake aggressively became almost an obsession.

From the beginning, each night, I would prepare the foods to take to work the next day. My co-workers all know my "Jethro Bodine" lunch pail—an ice chest that could hold a twelve-pack of soda. Immediately after transferring all of the snacks and lunch into the company fridge, I log all the foods for the workday. In doing so, I like to believe I've created a contract with myself. To date, I have eaten every food I've pre-logged. When workday foods are planned in advance, reaching my balance goals seems much easier.

The typical day starts off with a light breakfast after my workout, a snack at ten o'clock, lunch at noon, and another snack at two o'clock. Every "feeding" is light, but the frequency keeps me from feeling hungry during the day. One other key to feeling full has been drinking two liters of water before noon every day.

Exercise is as important to me as making good food choices. My workout regimen is a mix of cardio and circuit training. Each of the first four days starts with twelve minutes on the elliptical followed by seven minutes running hard and a five-minute cool down. Throughout the hard run, I try to maintain a pace of more than 240 strides per minute. During the cool down, I keep a pace of 220 strides per minute. My target calorie burn is 190 for the twelve-minute warm-up.

I follow the elliptical with a varied circuit workout: day one—chest and triceps; day two—back and biceps; day three—shoulders and abs; and day four—legs. To reward myself for working out, I finish each day swimming ten laps in less than fifteen minutes. If I get to the gym for a fifth day, it is a pure cardio day that starts with thirty-five minutes on the cross-country elliptical and finishes up with my ten-lap reward. Each new week, I start with day one regardless of the number of days I made it to the gym the previous week.

Planning and recording both exercise and caloric intake has been critical to my success. My current weight is 205 pounds—a loss of 60 pounds.

MY PHYSICAL ACTIVITY

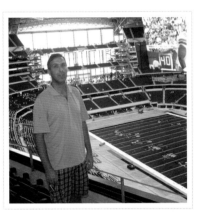

My daily exercise routine takes less than forty-five minutes to complete. I start with twelve minutes on the elliptical machine, followed by fifteen to twenty minutes of circuit training and finish with fifteen minutes of lap swimming. For the first 7 minutes of the elliptical workout I maintain a pace of 240+ strides per minute. During the five-minute warm down I maintain a pace of 220+ strides per minute with a goal of burning 190 calories in twelve minutes. Each day, the circuit varies based on working different areas of the body: chest & triceps, back & biceps, shoulders & abs, and legs. Swimming laps is both my warm down and my reward. I try to complete ten laps in less than fifteen minutes.

TOM'S *GREEN* DAY

- Calories Expended: **2,895**
- Calories Eaten: **1,920**
- Net Calorie Balance: 975

Success for me seems to depend on planning. Each night, assembling the meals and snacks for the next day makes it easy to pack my lunch pail and head to the gym. After working out, I log both my exercise and all of the prepared foods for the workday. Throughout the day, my mind still wanders to food as it always has. The difference is that my focus is on the healthier meals and snacks that I know await me in the fridge. When the next "feeding time" hits, I am thinking about nothing other than the next logged fare. The workday food menu is structured to provide high nutritional value while taking in less than half of the calorie allowance for the Green Day goal.

MY GREEN DAY NUTRITIONAL FACTS

TOM'S
HEALTH REFLECTION™
Nutrition Facts Report

Calorie Balance	
Calories Expended	2895
Calories Eaten	1920
Net Calorie Balance	975

Nutrient Balance	
	%DV
Total Fat 43 g	✔
Saturated Fat 17 g	80%
Trans Fat 0 g	—
Cholesterol 96 mg	32%
Sodium 2272 mg	99%
Total Carbs 288 g	✔
Dietary Fiber 42 g	156%
Sugars 132 g	—
Protein 102 g	✔
Vitamin A 3411 µg	379%
Vitamin C 1509 mg	1677%
Calcium 1836 mg	184%
Iron 11 mg	138%

MY BREAKFAST
–304 calories

Fresh fruit and coffee are the mainstays of breakfast for me. I created a standard K-cup recipe to make logging easy. I start with a banana after my workout. At ten in the morning, I eat a cup of fresh pineapple or grapefruit. Fresh pineapple is my favorite, and the grapefruit is both delicious and convenient.

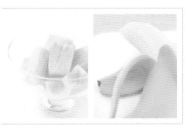

FRUIT, CEREAL, AND VITAMINS
- 1 cup pineapple, 74 calories
- 1 banana, 105 calories
- K-cup (coffee with creamer and sweetener), 95 calories
- Vitamin C supplement, 0 calories
- Flax seed oil supplement, 30 calories
- One-A-Day men's multivitamin, 0 calories

MY SNACKS–448 calories

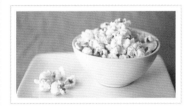

Fruit, veggies, and nonfat yogurt make up my afternoon snacks. To make it to dinner, I often whip up a batch of my homemade kettle corn recipe. I discovered kettle corn a few weeks before beginning my journey to health. Creating a low sodium alternative to the prepackaged options became almost an obsession.

FRUIT, VEGETABLES, WALNUTS, AND DESSERT
- 1 cup pineapple, 74 calories
- 30 oz. Diet Rite cola, 0 calories
- 6 oz. lemon chiffon yogurt, nonfat, 80 calories
- 2 servings Tom's zucchini in tomato sauce, 128 calories
- 2 tsp. walnuts, 33 calories
- 1 serving kettle corn (see recipe), 133 calories

LOW SODIUM KETTLE KORN

Makes approximately 3 1/2 cups.

INGREDIENTS
3 tbsp. popping corn
3 sprays I Can't Believe It's Not Butter
1/4 tsp. Splenda brownsugar blend
1/2 tsp. Great Value Altern no calorie sweetener

PREPARATION
1. Measure popcorn into microwaveable bowl.
2. Spray kernels with I Can't Believe It's Not Butter.
3. Spread the brownsugar blend and Altern over the kernels.
4. Microwave on high for three minutes.

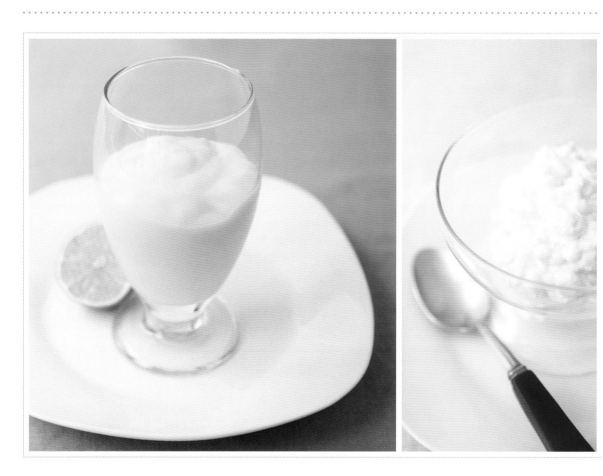

MY LUNCH–482 calories

The ability to eat the same basic lunch four days a week is a trait that I consider to be important to my personal success. I really enjoy cottage cheese and fruit. In addition, I frequently add a side of vegetables. The zucchini in tomato sauce is a favorite of mine. For dessert, I have one of my favorite Weight Watchers yogurts.

COTTAGE CHEESE, YOGURT, FRUIT, VEGGIES, AND DIET RITE
- 1 key lime pie yogurt, nonfat, 100 calories
- 1 cup cottage cheese, low fat, 180 calories
- 3 cup diced pineapple, 74 calories
- 24 oz. Diet Rite soda, 0 calories
- 2 cups Tom's zucchini in tomato sauce, 128 calories

MY DINNER—686 calories

Growing up, lasagna was a family favorite. As an adult, creating a healthier version that held true to the flavors I remember has been a personal goal. This dish uses a small amount of sausage to flavor the zucchini and veggie mixture that serves as the meat layer in the traditional version. I tend to make a very large batch and eat it several days in a row.

LASAGNA, SALAD, AND DIET RITE

- 2 servings meat-flavored lasagna, 655 calories
- 1/4 zucchini, 5 calories
- 1/4 tomato, 5 calories
- 1/4 cup lettuce, 9 calories
- 1 tbsp. light balsamic vinaigrette, 12 calories
- 24 oz. Diet Rite soda, 0 calories

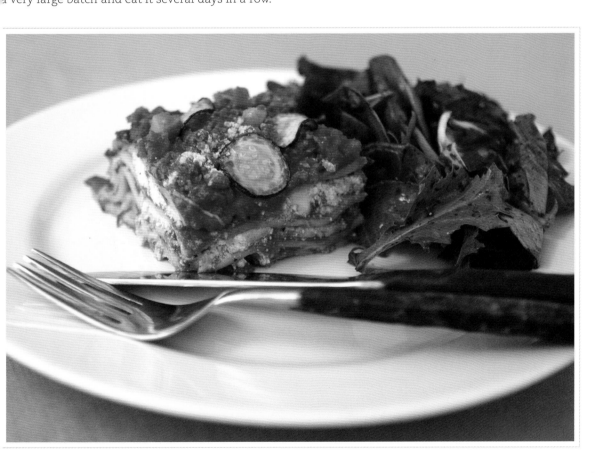

"I AM IN MY FIFTIES ... ENOUGH IS ENOUGH."

username: cactusman / *first name:* Tony / *location:* Escondido, CA

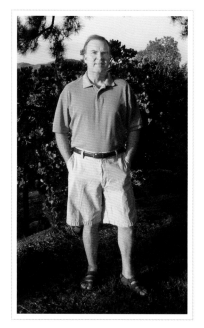

Tony NOW: October '09 / age: 58
182 lbs. / BMI 25.5 / waist 37˝

Healthy eating is something I have paid little attention to for most of my life. I was a bit of a "porker" from my early-to-mid-teen years, but I have a very good reason for that.

I grew up in the south and was fortunate enough to experience my mom's and grandmother's great southern cooking during those early years. For breakfast, there were homemade biscuits with sausage gravy, and on special occasions there were those biscuits with chocolate gravy and bacon or sausage with a large bowl of scrambled eggs. For supper, we had traditional meat, potatoes, and vegetables. Dessert was either a delicious pie or cake of some sort. Those were the days. I can still picture all those wonderful times.

Back then, words like "diet" or "overweight" were not used as much as they are now. In those days if a diet or weight loss program was mentioned, people would just say, "Oh you are not fat."

When I reached my teen years, I gained an interest in sports and the weight came off. I was able to maintain a healthy weight on a fairly consistent basis through my twenties and early thirties. The weight problem began during my late thirties. I was not thinking about or paying much attention to the foods I ate. The weight just sort of crept up on me. Over the past fifteen years, I have gone from 180 pounds to 235 pounds.

Because of this excess weight I take medication for high cholesterol and high blood pressure. My mother has had three triple bypass surgeries over the last ten years. I was very concerned that this may be where I was headed. A typical day for me didn't include breakfast. I ate a ham and cheese sandwich with mayonnaise on white bread for lunch. Snacks would be donuts, cookies, potato chips,

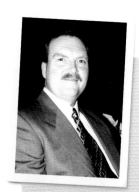

Tony THEN: April '09
225 lbs. / BMI 31.5 / waist 44˝

and diet colas. Dinner would be Mexican take-out or a homemade, high fat, high calorie meal. I would have ice cream for dessert. I wondered why I had high cholesterol.

I sat at a desk all day. I would come home after a day's work and watch television until it was time to go to bed. I would fall asleep on the couch. I had trouble sleeping at night because of the excess weight.

Over the years I tried many diets. I would set weight-loss goals because of a vacation, trip, or a special event. It was always just a quick fix so I could look good. I would always lose the weight while on the diet. However, when I stopped following the meal plan or stopped buying the packaged food, I would put the weight back on and more. I never thought about long term. I never thought about keeping it off for my health.

Then, one day my wife told me about NutriMirror. I checked out the site and began using the food log. I have learned to look at the calories and fat/

cholesterol levels in all the food before deciding if I really want to put it in my body. I really get excited when I have a complete "green" chart at the end of the day. Every day I look forward to being green.

I am in my fifties and have decided enough is enough. My goal is to get my weight down, eat healthy every day, exercise six days a week, and enjoy the life I have been given.

When I look back at all the bad eating habits I had and then look at my NutriMirror food logs, I'm in total amazement at how much my food choices have changed. I am enjoying lots of food and my choices are healthy. I can still have the foods I love, but I have made changes to how often I have them or I change the portion size so that it still gives me a "green" day. I have lost forty-three pounds and two belts sizes. I notice a definite difference in my energy level.

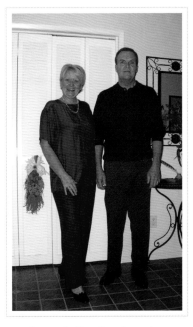

Couples are finding that the path to lasting change and improved health is easier to travel together than alone. Tony and his wife Carla (page 74) are united in their pursuit of more active lifestyles and wiser food choices.

MY PHYSICAL ACTIVITY

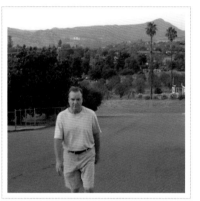

Playing basketball has always been my favorite form of exercise. I had put on so much weight in recent years that it had kept me from being able to play a good game. I was having trouble keeping up with the other guys, getting winded often. Since losing about forty pounds, I am back in the game. I play one day a week now and also try to walk four days a week at a brisk pace. These two forms of exercise have helped me to maintain my weight loss and will help me to lose the additional ten pounds to reach my goal weight. I keep track of my exercise by using the NutriMirror exercise log. On the day that I play basketball I am rewarded with an additional 517 calories that I can consume. That makes for a treat, like a chocolate bar or a bowl of ice cream—without guilt!

TONY'S *GREEN* DAY

- Calories Expended: **2,162**
- Calories Eaten: **1,739**
- Net Calorie Balance: 423

One thing that I have discovered about myself is that I really like to eat, and often. I keep foods that I can snack on throughout my workday. I find that I like to eat about every two hours. In the past I would have skipped breakfast altogether, had a high calorie lunch and dinner, and then continued to eat late into the evening, sometimes ending right before going to bed. Now I spread my calories out so that I am not eating such large meals. This strategy has also kept me from snacking late into the evening. I still eat a snack at night, but not as much as before.

MY GREEN DAY NUTRITIONAL FACTS

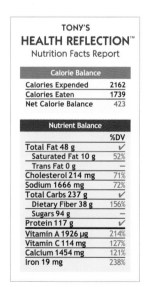

TONY'S
HEALTH REFLECTION™
Nutrition Facts Report

Calorie Balance	
Calories Expended	2162
Calories Eaten	1739
Net Calorie Balance	423

Nutrient Balance	
	%DV
Total Fat 48 g	✔
Saturated Fat 10 g	52%
Trans Fat 0 g	—
Cholesterol 214 mg	71%
Sodium 1666 mg	72%
Total Carbs 237 g	✔
Dietary Fiber 38 g	156%
Sugars 94 g	—
Protein 117 g	✔
Vitamin A 1926 µg	214%
Vitamin C 114 mg	127%
Calcium 1454 mg	121%
Iron 19 mg	238%

MY BREAKFAST—284 calories

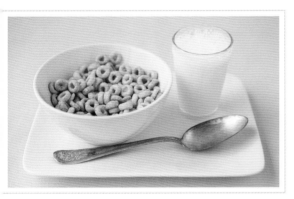

I have always loved breakfast, but rarely took the time for it. And when I did it was not made up of healthy choices. Most of the time my breakfasts were in restaurants and included the usual—eggs, ham, fried potatoes and pancakes. Now I make an effort to eat breakfast at home. On this day I had cereal with low fat milk and coffee. This is all I need to start my day and it keeps me going strong until my a mid-morning snack.

CEREAL WITH MILK, COFFEE, AND JUICE
- 1 cup Cheerios, 100 calories
- 12 oz. coffee, decaf, 0 calories
- 12 oz coffee, 4 calories
- 1 1/2 cup milk, low fat, 180 calories
- Calcium + D supplement, 0 calories

MY SNACKS—506 calories

I create a snack pack each day to take to work. By using the NutriMirror custom menu tool, I can enter all of these items into my food log in just one click. The snacks that I take to work are the things that have kept me from eating way too much for lunch and have helped me avoid the candy machines or the inevitable boxes of donuts and pastries that people bring to the office. I always try to have a mid-morning snack, sometimes two. Then after lunch I have another. The snacks, which I took with me on this day were a fairly large peach, two granola bars, and some bite-sized pita crackers. I cut the peach in half so that I could enjoy it twice. My evening snack that I call my *watching TV snack,* was a vanilla ice cream sandwich.

GRANOLA BAR, CRACKERS, AND ICE CREAM
- 9 bite-sized pita crackers, 120 calories
- Crunchy granola bar, 180 calories
- 1 peach, 66 calories
- 1 vanilla ice cream sandwich, 140 calories

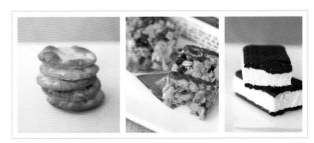

MY LUNCH–538 calories

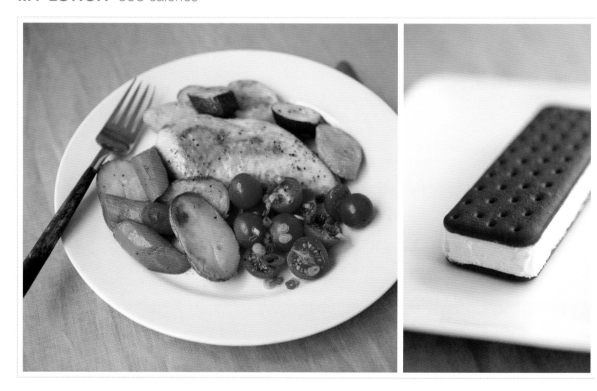

I like to have a fairly good-size lunch. On this day I had roast chicken, steamed red potatoes with a pat of butter, summer squash, and sliced tomato. For dessert I had a low-fat ice cream sandwich. In the past my choices would have been something from a fast-food restaurant like a high-sodium ham sandwich on white bread with lots of mayonnaise and probably some cheese and a bag of potato chips. The lunches I have now satisfy me more than the fast-foods I use to have. I have lowered my sodium levels considerably

CHICKEN, VEGETABLES, AND ICE CREAM
- 4.6 oz. roasted chicken breast, 215 calories
- 1/2 cup carrot slices, 24 calories
- 1.2 oz. spring onions, 11 calories
- 2 1/2 oz. red potatoes, 63 calories
- 1/2 cup summer squash, 18 calories
- 1 tsp. butter, 34 calories
- 6.6 oz. red ripe tomatoes, 33 calories
- 1 vanilla ice cream sandwich, 140 calories

MY DINNER—411 calories

Why head to a fast-food restaurant for a wrap (what I used to do) when you can create a better-tasting version at home and also control the sodium, fat, and calories? I made my wrap with a multigrain flatbread, lean roasted chicken breast, fresh spinach, avocado slices, onions, diced tomato, and a Greek olive oil dressing. I also have some cucumber and carrot slices on the side. By taking charge and making this myself I have controlled the amount of dressing and the quality of ingredients that go into this awesome (and delicious) meal.

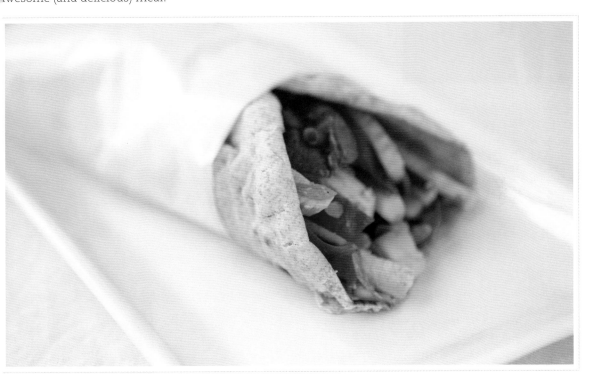

CHICKEN WRAP WITH VEGETABLES
- 2 1/2 oz. roasted chicken breast, 116 calories
- 1 piece multigrain flatbread, 100 calories
- 2 oz. avocado, 91 calories
- 1 oz. carrots, 12 calories
- 1/2 oz. cucumber, 8 calories
- 1 small spring onion, 2 calories
- 1.8 oz. spinach, 12 calories
- 4 oz. red ripe tomatoes, 20 calories
- 1 tbsp. Greek dressing (with olive oil), 50 calories

"AS AN EMERGENCY ROOM NURSE FOR TWENTY YEARS, I KNOW THE CONSEQUENCES OF OBESITY."

username: cocorhum / *first name:* Valerie / *location:* Central, AL

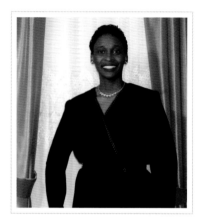

Valerie NOW: August '09 / age: 44
198.4 lbs. / BMI 31 / waist 35.5˝

In 2000, my marriage of only nine years ended in divorce. My daughter was six and my son was ten months old. While I've always been slightly heavy, I had maintained my weight at a bearable 160-170 pounds. I then let myself go and paid a dear price.

What was the price? Well, two years later I found myself at a whopping 235 pounds, the heaviest I had ever been. I had elevated blood pressure to boot. Seventy-five pounds above my ideal weight, feeling poorly, appearing like a beached whale and ashamed, I joined a well-known weight loss group. I started exercising and in a year was back to a fit 160 pounds. I felt great and in charge of my life. It was so easy to lose the weight, but maintaining the loss wasn't. Within four years I weighed 224 pounds.

Based on personal experience and direct observation of others, I knew that without immediate action I would keep gaining weight and end up with multiple health concerns. As an emergency room nurse for twenty years I know the consequences of obesity. It stares at me daily in the faces of patients who battle preventable illnesses brought on by poor eating habits and sedentary lifestyles.

It is a sad business seeing someone just thirty-five years old lose their leg due to the effects of uncontrolled diabetes. It's distressing to tell a wife and mother that she is now a widow and single parent at forty because all attempts to resuscitate her young three-hundred-pound husband after a heart attack were unsuccessful. And it's wretched to observe obese patients with sleep apnea unable to lie flat in a bed, having to wear oxygen and a mask at night just to stay alive. Unfortunately, these situations are becoming more common in our country with every new day that passes.

These events and many others like them also wear on the minds and the spirits of caregivers. I saw myself

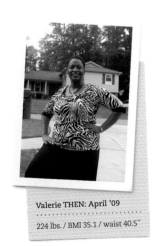

Valerie THEN: April '09
224 lbs. / BMI 35.1 / waist 40.5˝

becoming one of these patients and it was an earth-shattering wake-up call. To top it off, a recent study shows that 54% of nurses are overweight.* Sadly, I am one of them, but not for long. After many years of unhealthy yo-yo dieting I have taken complete responsibility for myself and am finally in control and on the path to healthy living.

Alabama, where I have lived all of my life, was ranked third in the 2008 United States Adult Obesity Rankings with 31% obese and 36% overweight. Collectively, 67% of adult Alabamians are fat. Ironically, nine of the top states for obesity are in the south (Michigan ranks tenth). Even states that are historically ranked as "thin" have had marked increases in obesity. It is becoming epidemic. Without intervention, the healthcare delivery system will be swamped with chronically sick patients. More frightening is the thought that there may not be many nurses to provide care

since they too are so at risk of becoming patients themselves.

With childhood obesity also on the rise, all healthcare providers must step up and become positive role models to help combat this epidemic. Bedside, nurses have the greatest of impacts on patients and their families. So we nurses must make a stronger commitment to becoming healthy healthcare workers. We must take our positive examples to a position at the front of the stage.

Upon graduating nursing school, all nurses take the Florence Nightingale Pledge that reads *"I solemnly pledge myself before God and in the presence of this assembly, to pass my life in purity and to practice my profession faithfully. I will abstain from whatever is deleterious and mischievous, and will not take or knowingly administer any harmful drug. I will do all in my power to maintain and elevate the standard of my profession, and will hold in confidence all personal matters committed to my keeping and*

all family affairs coming to my knowledge in the practice of my calling. With loyalty will I endeavor to aid the physician in his work, and devote myself to the welfare of those committed to my care."

As a young nurse I thought drugs and alcohol were the behaviors considered most harmful or injurious. It has taken me twenty years to fully realize that behaviors leading to obesity are also deleterious acts. My poor eating habits and sedentary lifestyle were a direct contradiction to what I had pledged and a disservice to my profession. I have a responsibility to live in healthy balance so that my example might positively impact patients, their families, and others whom I encounter daily.

How do I convince a patient that exercise and eating properly is good if I am waddling up to their bed short of breath, and wearing a size twenty plus? How do I tell the diabetic patient that they need to control portion size and count carbs?

Overweight and obesity in nurses, advanced practice nurses, and nurse educators: Journal of the American Academy of Nurse Practitioners, United States. Author/s: Miller, Sally K ; Alpert, Patricia T; Cross, Chad L, 2008-May; vol. 20 (issue 5): pp 259-65

My quest for a healthy lifestyle is not just for myself but also to be a better role model for my children. With personal health, I can freely educate patients and their families without embarrassment or hypocrisy. I can talk with them about the ill effects of obesity and share with them ways to achieve and maintain healthy living.

And one of the ways to personal health I will share with them is NutriMirror. It has been a fun, interactive tool that assists me every day in achieving optimal health. My daily commitment is *"GOING for GREEN."* Exercising and meeting my caloric/nutrient requirements is moving me closer to awesome health and life benefits. For once in this long, somewhat discouraging battle against obesity, I no longer consider myself on a diet. DIE-ting is dead.

Healthy living through lifetime weight control and nutritional balance is now my goal.

MY PHYSICAL ACTIVITY

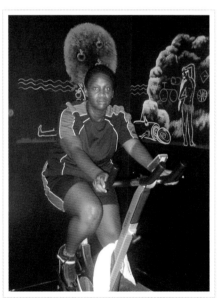

I like hardcore, sweat-pouring exercise! It may not be for everyone, but it works for me and I feel energized and refreshed when it's over. My favorite programs are Boot Camp and Spin Cycle as both burn many calories in a short forty-five minute session. And I can manage forty-five minutes even when time is limited. Since I'm a morning person, my workout begins at 5:30 A.M., Monday through Friday. Exercising early almost always assures there are no interruptions. Last minute obstacles don't seem to pop up before the sun rises. Interestingly, the most important thing I've learned about exercise and its relationship to weight loss is that I MUST consume at least 75% of the calories I burn through exercise to maintain my weight loss and not get stuck in the plateau rut. Yes, the body must have adequate fuel to burn fat, so EAT. But make sure you're making good food choices with those calories by *Going for GREEN!*

VALERIE'S *GREEN* DAY

- Calories Expended: **2,039** • Calories Eaten: **1,741** • Net Calorie Balance: **298**

Before getting the measured feedback I receive through logging with NutriMiror, I thought overall I was eating healthy. Surprisingly, I discovered that many of the low calorie/low fat foods I consumed were heavily laden in sodium and deficient in iron, calcium, and fiber. Being female, I definitely need adequate calcium to prevent bone loss.

A great untruth is that healthy food cannot taste good. Well I beg to differ; I eat many great-tasting foods with minimum or no added flavor-enhancing ingredients. My logs have a variety of foods in them as I like to try new things. Logging my daily meals takes only about ten to fifteen minutes and with the instant feedback given I am always in control of my weight and nutrition.

MY GREEN DAY NUTRITIONAL FACTS

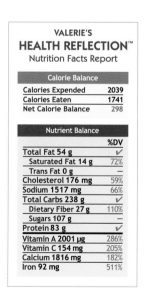

VALERIE'S
HEALTH REFLECTION™
Nutrition Facts Report

Calorie Balance	
Calories Expended	2039
Calories Eaten	1741
Net Calorie Balance	298

Nutrient Balance		
		%DV
Total Fat 54 g		✔
Saturated Fat 14 g		72%
Trans Fat 0 g		—
Cholesterol 176 mg		59%
Sodium 1517 mg		66%
Total Carbs 238 g		✔
Dietary Fiber 27 g		110%
Sugars 107 g		—
Protein 83 g		✔
Vitamin A 2001 µg		286%
Vitamin C 154 mg		205%
Calcium 1816 mg		182%
Iron 92 mg		511%

MY BREAKFAST—369 calories

This is the easiest meal and a must for me. If missed, it will not be a good day. I mainly eat at home, but because I exercise before going to work and may be pushed for time, breakfast must be quick, nutritional, and portable. I typically eat some type of fiber-filled hot or cold cereal with low fat or soy milk. Then I'll have some fruit at work to complete my breakfast. On mornings when I'm hungrier I'll eat turkey sausage or low fat bacon with double fiber bread, which is more filling than the cereal. Coffee is my morning comfort drink and I enjoy every sip! I also add my multivitamin and calcium supplement here. I don't take iron (unless I need to) until the end of the day.

OATMEAL. FRUIT, AND COFFEE

- 12 oz. coffee, 7 calories
- 2 packets sugar, 22 calories
- 1 cup soy milk, 100 calories
- 1 packet oatmeal with flax, 140 calories
- 2/5 cup sliced peaches, 40 calories
- Vitamin supplement, 0 calories
- Calcium chew, 20 calories
- 4 tsp. creamer, 40 calories

MY LUNCH–716 calories

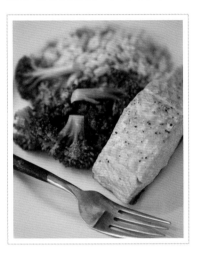

I usually prepare lunch at home so that I have control over ingredients and cooking methods. This meal took very little time to prepare. I've been baking, broiling, and steaming foods for quite sometime now, so my palate is acclimated to the taste and consistency of foods cooked these ways. The boxed rice meals are convenient and quick, but the sodium is high, so I make sure I monitor this closely when I do use them.

SALMON, RICE, AND BROCCOLI
• 3/4 cup chopped broccoli, 41 calories
• 6.5 oz. salmon, 425 calories
• 2 oz. brown and wild rice with herbs and seasonings, 250 calories

MY SNACKS–421 calories

I use snacks to add more fiber-rich foods since I struggle to meet this daily requirement. I also eat fruit, other dairy products, and a sweet treat if desired. I take an iron supplement if I'm still low.

FRUIT, GRANOLA, CANDY, FIBER BAR, AND YOGURT
• 3/4 cup fruit cocktail, 82 calories
• 1/3 oz. almond granola, 39 calories
• 1 oz. Twizzlers candy, 100 calories
• 1 Fiber One Chewy Bar, 140 calories
• 6 oz. vanilla yogurt, 60 calories
• Iron supplement, 0 calories

MY DINNER–235 calories

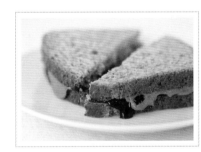

Now this is not a typical dinner for me but I wanted a PB&J on this day. I LOVE peanut butter. I choose not to eat a low fat version or other substitute as I enjoy the smooth taste of regular JIF. I no longer overeat to satisfy a craving. Instead, I eat more slowly and savor every bite.

PB&J
• 1 tbsp. grape jelly, 50 calories
• 1 tbsp. peanut butter, 95 calories
• 1 serving double-fiber wheat bread, 90 calories

username: karynd / *first name:* Karyn

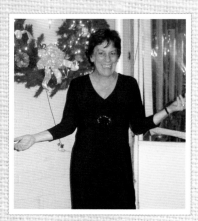

Karyn NOW: November '09 / age: 56
147.2 lbs. / BMI 25.1 / waist 32.5˝

· ·

My weight was normal in my early twenties, but by the time I hit forty-five I was obese at 210 pounds. I lost 10 pounds just in the course of living, but for eight years I weighed 200 pounds. For the last couple of those years, I felt horrible every morning when I woke up. At fifty-six, I felt old, fat and bloated, like my life was pretty much over. I wanted to lose weight and eat healthy, but had no idea how to do that. I knew that if someone would only tell me what to eat to be healthy, I would do it. But I needed someone to tell me every meal to eat, every bite. I really didn't know how.

On July 4, 2009, I went online, searched on "calorie counter," and found NutriMirror. It was a calorie counter, but also had a nutritional feedback component that told me exactly what I needed to know!

From day one I have been motivated by the information feedback and the journal posts of the other members. By assessing the feedback, I began changing my diet. I began to eat more fresh fruits and vegetables, and smaller meals about six times a day. I was feeling full and satisfied all the time. By the end of my first week I felt great when I woke up, and enthused about the day ahead. At first, because I was so full all the time, I could not eat the allotted number of weight loss calories. But after a while I started craving the nutritious foods.

About five weeks into self-monitoring, I ate all my calories plus some! With exercise added to my life, I had earned those additional calories. I started walking with my dog, going bowling, parking far away from the entrance to work, and adding whatever activities I could. Once I get to the point where I'm able to eat all my calories including those I burn through exercise, I will step up the intensity or time of my exercise sessions to earn even more calories. Although I have no doubt that I will reach my goal weight, my focus has changed from weight loss to loving my new diet and lifestyle. I will continue logging for the rest of my life. I have found the person who could tell me how to eat healthy and that person is me. With the measured feedback I get from NutriMirror, I will successfully manage calorie and nutritional balance for the rest of my life.

· ·

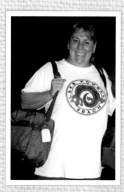

Karyn THEN: July '09
· ·
195 lbs. / BMI 33.3 / waist 43˝

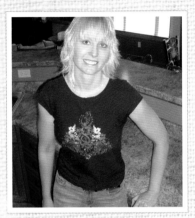

Dena NOW: November '09
146 lbs. / BMI 20.6 / size 8

. . . .

Mike and I were married in August of 1996 and settled into the typical American lifestyle—work all day and eat an evening meal in front of the television where we remained until bedtime, only to get up the next day and begin the cycle again. Of course we also enjoyed going out to eat, and usually had two or three restaurant meals per week.

After five years of marriage, we had our daughter, and a little over two years later, our son. From the beginning, I wanted to feed my kids healthy foods. I wanted them to enjoy fruits and vegetables and all the good-for-you nutritional choices. The problem was that we didn't seem to care as much about what we ate ourselves. I always knew we

didn't eat the healthiest, but I rationalized it with thoughts that it could be worse. After all, we didn't keep junk food in the house and we usually had a vegetable with our evening meal. That's pretty good, right? It must not have been, because between 1996 and 2007, Mike and I each gained about fifty pounds.

Early in 2008 because of a few health concerns, Mike decided to get healthier. He quit drinking soft drinks, quit eating super-sized value meals, and he started exercising. Soon after I also quit drinking soft drinks, and I started walking daily. We began preparing healthier meals at home for our whole family. Mike's excess weight fell off fast. By summer he was down to his goal weight (which he has been maintaining ever since). My weight loss was slow and steady, so far about forty-nine pounds in a year and a half. At first it was discouraging how much slower I was losing. However, I am so glad I stuck with it. Not only did I get there, but I started feeling healthier and more energetic almost right away by simply eating better and doing some exercise.

When I started using NutriMirror, I thought I really wouldn't learn much. Was I ever surprised! I learned that I was consistently consuming too much sodium and not enough iron or fiber! Wow! Who knew? It was also great to learn so much about the foods I was eating. I love that members are encouraged to live a healthy lifestyle more than they are to lose weight. It is not a quick fix or a fad diet. It is a lifelong tool for living a healthy life. With just a few minutes of logging each day, I can see what my food choices are doing for my health.

For me, one of the nicest things I've gained is peace of mind.

. . . .

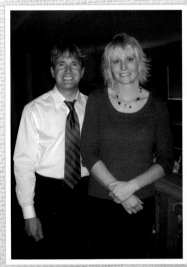

Mike & Dena now.

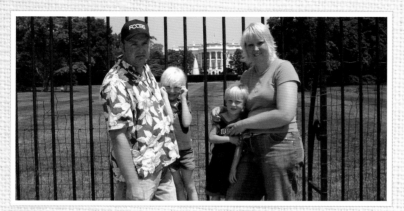

Mike THEN: June '09

212 lbs. / BMI 30.4

Dena THEN: June '09

195 lbs. / BMI 27.3 / size 16/18

Before, if I ate something not-so-good for me I would beat myself up over it for the entire day. I would even think, "well the day is shot; I might as well eat what I want." Now I know that one food choice or one day, once in a while, will not throw off my balance. I can look at my average over the last two weeks and see that there is no damage done. Or, I can assess exactly what choices I need to refine to remain in balance. That is a good, empowering feeling.

Mike started logging after I did, but since he had already reached his goal weight, he uses it for maintenance and to make sure he is nutritionally balanced. He keeps a close eye on his ratios of proteins,

fats and carbs since he is in a weight training program. Even though Mike and I apply the tool somewhat differently, we are together in practicing effective weight control and nutritional balance.

Living healthy is something we will do for the rest of our lives because it is now a lifestyle that brings us great joy each day. We are not depriving ourselves of anything. We enjoy our healthy food choices; we stay full and satisfied, and we still have our treats now and again. I love that I feel better at thirty-one than I did at twenty-one!

I like that our kids are learning what foods make them strong and healthy. They understand

that the main purpose of food is to fuel their bodies and they are learning about balance. I hope they will grow up to have a healthy relationship with food.

It is great that Mike and I have more energy to do things with the kids, and it feels good to have a more active lifestyle. I haven't missed our nightly TV watching ritual of the past! The weight loss is just a side benefit. The happiness we feel in our family and our health are the greatest benefits of all!

. . . .

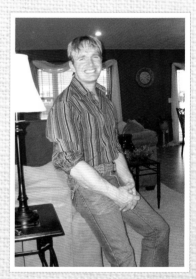

Mike NOW: November '09

174 lbs. / BMI 24.9

"KEEP YOUR SODIUM INTAKE TO ONE TEASPOON A DAY!" THE BIRTH OF NUTRIMIRROR®

username: Jim_Ray / *first name:* Jim *location:* Fallbrook, CA

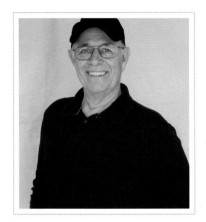

Jim NOW: May '09 / age: 68
198 lbs. / BMI 27.9 / waist 35˝

In 1973, at the age of thirty-three, I lived for weeks on nothing but liquid protein, water, and supplements. That was my first experience at dieting. I lost the weight I needed to lose; told every weight-challenged person I knew "try the liquid protein diet, it really works"; looked admiringly into the mirror while wearing my fatter-pants, considered the "before" and the "after" of me; and vowed to myself, and to everyone else that would listen, "never again." Now, let's fast forward to 2004,

thirty-one years later. The deep looks into the mirror to admire all of my "afters," the evangelizing of "it works,"and the vows of "never again" had, through repetition, become worn-out clichés, meaningless "diet-chatter."

The scale was telling me I weighed 255 pounds (86 more than my 1973 "never again" weight). And the doctor was telling me that my blood pressure reading was 210/110, that my choices had led to hypertension. Although these were not his exact words, the message got through—"get it right this time, or you're going to die ... much sooner than you want!" He advised, "You must move more and eat less. Limit yourself to 1,500 calories a day until you reach a healthy weight; and keep your sodium intake to about one teaspoon a day."

I immediately purchased, for the umpteenth time in my life, one of those calorie counting books. I pondered those

"successful" diet plans and guidance systems I had tried over thirty plus years. Which plan should I follow ... for life this time?

Did I want the high-protein-low-carb Atkins thing again? Or another shot at the low-fat-higher-carb Pritikin plan? Did I want to begin my transformation with yet another "fat-farm" stay? How about I do the Hospital Community Outreach Wellness Plan one more time? Should I have another date with Jenny Craig? Or maybe NutriSystem

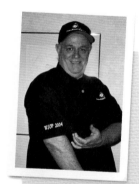

Jim THEN: July '04
255 lbs. / BMI 36.5 / waist 44˝

would be better? I really did love the Mediterranean diet—so balanced, so healthy, and so tastefully satisfying. I refreshed memories of that diet book plus the Zone, South Beach, and the many other best-sellers I had followed during their moments of fame.

Or perhaps a gym membership renewal with yet another kick-ass boot camp style personal trainer would do the trick. Or how about beginning with the favorite of all my past "successful" plans—the "kick start" vacation? Let's just throw on a backpack and walk from San Diego to Morro Bay again; or maybe I should repeat the bike trip from Puget Sound down the coast to San Diego … that was a great trip and I lost so much weight. There were at least a half-dozen of these "kick start" vacations I could immediately recall to reflect upon and consider.

Perhaps Body Wise or some of the other supplement companies I've used over the years could be part of the solution. Whatever my choice, I would need to make sure I consider my nutritional needs and use supplements to offset the harm modernity has done to my food supply, right? But in which nutrients am I deficient? And what measure of each does my body require? And what is that going to cost me?

Maybe if I followed the USDA Food Pyramid … or is the Harvard Medical School version the wiser choice?

But before I decide on anything, maybe another visit to the iridologist—or the guy that clipped and analyzed my hair to give me my vitamin and mineral reading, or the group that put me on a five-day prune juice fast and intestinal cleanse—would be in order.

One thing the doctor said I needed to do, however, presented a problem none of my past experiences or options could do for me. That need kept reverberating. My hypertension, in part, was caused by too much sodium in my diet: "Keep your sodium level to about one teaspoon a day."

How was I going to do that? I began by searching the Internet.

Those searches led to the development of NutriMirror® (www.NutriMirror.com) by my artist, scientist, and life-saving son, Michael.

And the rest is now, as they say, "history!"

Since the earliest stages of Michael's work on NutriMirror, I have consistently been in control of my nutritional balance (including sodium) and my calorie balance. I lost fifty-five pounds within the first year and have maintained my weight ever since.

Moreover, something new and unexpected has happened. Somewhere along the way, I stopped feeling deprived. I have come to find pleasure in this journey and the choices that are keeping me in balance.

I do not say about NutriMirror, "IT WORKS." I am the only "IT" that "WORKS" … or doesn't work.

I recognize that NutriMirror is just a tool. Like a mirror, or a shovel, it does exactly what it is supposed to do, every time. It lets me see the measured impacts of my actions and it guides my choices so that I have a better chance of living in balance.

Although I will never again say about my condition "never again", or ever see myself as a finished work (an "*after*") I can say, without reservation, that I am, finally, enjoying the things that make me healthy; more than I enjoyed the things that made me unhealthy.

And, because of the joy, I am more confident about this journey than I have ever been.

MY PHYSICAL ACTIVITY

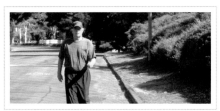

My "boot camp" mentality about exercise is long gone. Now, my exercise of choice is simply walking briskly. On most days I walk at a 4 mph pace for about thirty-five minutes. Occasionally, like on this Green Day, I'll pop with a more strenuous ninety-minute walk at the same 4 mph pace. This regimen helps keep my weight in check and is something I can easily manage for the long haul.

JIM'S *GREEN* DAY

- Calories Expended: **2,344**
- Calories Eaten: **2,165**
- Net Calorie Balance: 179

I had been on a pace that would have led to an additional forty-two pounds of body weight in twelve months. But slowly, over time, I made small, informed modifications to the food choices that had been giving me too many calories and not enough nutrients.

The key to my long term success has been that somewhere along the way I discovered that there is great pleasure in eating healthy—more than in the instant gratification I was getting from foods that had made me fat and sick.

MY GREEN DAY NUTRITIONAL FACTS

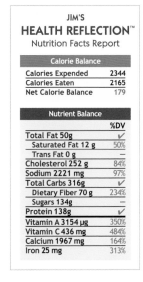

JIM'S
HEALTH REFLECTION™
Nutrition Facts Report

Calorie Balance	
Calories Expended	2344
Calories Eaten	2165
Net Calorie Balance	179

Nutrient Balance	
	%DV
Total Fat 50g	✔
Saturated Fat 12 g	50%
Trans Fat 0 g	—
Cholesterol 252 g	84%
Sodium 2221 mg	97%
Total Carbs 316g	✔
Dietary Fiber 70 g	234%
Sugars 134g	—
Protein 138g	✔
Vitamin A 3154 µg	350%
Vitamin C 436 mg	484%
Calcium 1967 mg	164%
Iron 25 mg	313%

MY BREAKFAST–454 calories

When I saw the damage my old standard breakfast was causing, I knew I had to modify that meal. I replaced fried eggs with Egg Beater omelets (I still have eggs with yolks at least once a week). I replaced the fat, sodium-rich breakfast meats and fried potatoes with healthier, lower calorie choices like the ones you see in this picture—shrimp, fruits, salsa, whole grain, low-sodium bread with avocado (instead of white bread and butter). It seems I am eating as much as before—perhaps even more! And the pleasure factor is higher.

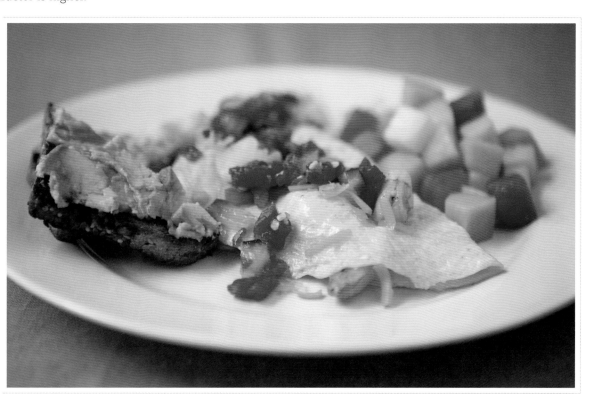

SHRIMP OMELET
- 1/2 cup Egg Beaters, 60 calories
- 2 tbsp. salsa, 10 calories
- 1 oz. shrimp, 28 calories
- 1 oz. sweet green peppers, 8 calories

- 2 cu. inches cheddar cheese, low fat, 59 calories
- 1 piece sprouted grain Ezekiel bread, 80 calories
- 2 oz. avocado, 91 calories
- 2 cups assorted fruit, 118 calories

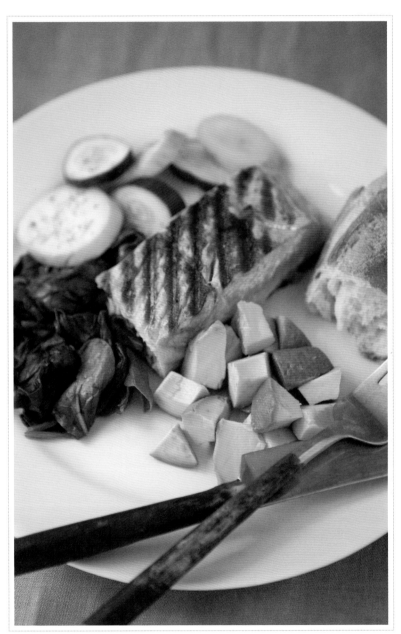

MY LUNCH
—620 calories

This meal took little in the way of preparation and cooking. In the old days I might have had a pizza delivered, or ducked out for a quick trip to a fast-food restaurant for a meal that was probably loaded with lots of sodium, saturated fat, and calories but almost nothing of nutritional value. Today, I find little pleasure in those toxic selections. They simply do not compare to this delightful and healthy meal of salmon, fresh steamed spinach, summer squash, rustic bread, and avocado.

SALMON WITH STEAMED VEGETABLES
- 4 4/5 oz. grilled salmon, 316 calories
- 1 cup steamed spinach, 41 calories
- 2 1/4 oz. steamed summer squash, 13 calories
- 2 1/5 oz. sourdough baguette, 150 calories
- 2 1/5 oz. avocado, 100 calories

MY SNACKS–438 calories

Because I have learned to eat calorie-light, nutrient-dense snacks frequently throughout the day, I am able to better control the portion sizes of what I eat at main meals. I never eat out of hunger anymore. And I always make sure to plan some kind of treat with my discretionary calories that I include in my snacks. I never feel deprived. By themselves, these snack selections (plus a calcium supplement) put most of my scores into "green" territory.

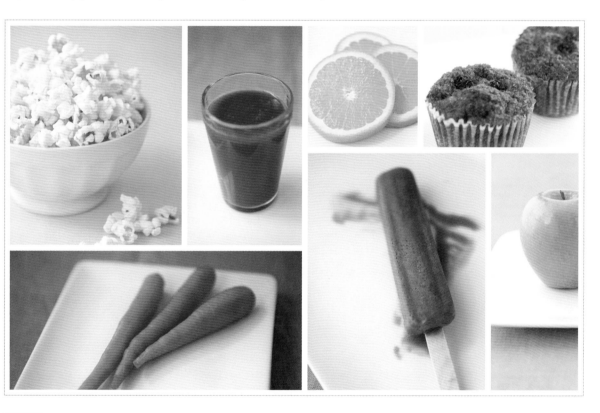

SNACKS

- Apple slices, 72 calories
- 1 cup orange sections, 85 calories
- 3 1/2 oz. carrots, 41 calories
- Calcium + D supplement, 0 calories

- Popcorn, 90 calories
- Blueberry Fiber Cake Bar, 80 calories
- 5 1/2 oz. V8 Juice, 30 calories
- 1 Fudgsicle, 40 calories

MY DINNER–653 calories.

What, at one time, might have been a 2,400-calorie meal with little or no nutritional value, now looks something like this. I have learned to find great pleasure in grains like couscous (something I never had before my sixty-fifth birthday); large amounts of vegetables like fresh asparagus; skinless roasted chicken breast flavored with onion slices and tomato; and finally, to top it all off, angel food cake with assorted in-season berries and light Cool Whip™.

COUSCOUS AND ROASTED CHICKEN BREAST
- 1/2 breast roasted chicken, meat only, 142 calories
- 1/2 cup couscous (cooked with low sodium chicken broth), 154 calories
- 3 oz. red ripe tomatoes, 15 calories
- Grilled, sliced onions, 12 calories
- 8 spears asparagus, 26 calories

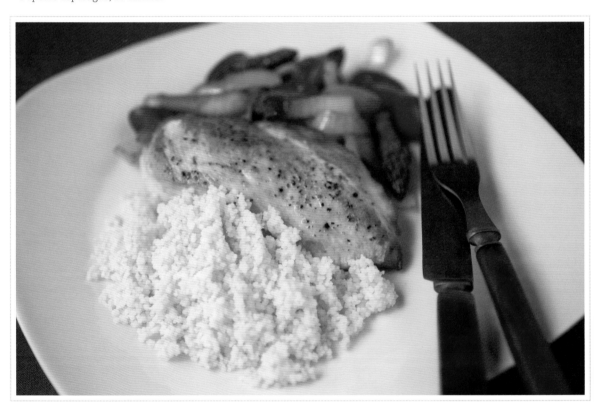

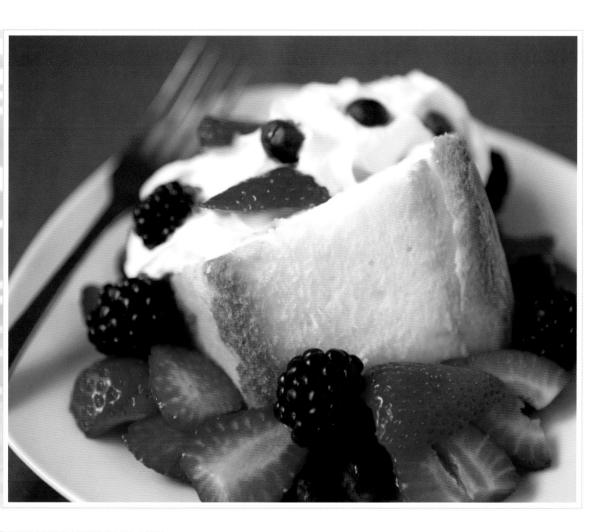

MIXED BERRY ANGEL FOOD CAKE
- 2 oz. angel food cake, 160 calories
- 1 cup fresh strawberries, 53 calories
- 1/2 cup fresh blackberries, 31 calories
- 2 1/2 oz. fresh blueberries, 40 calories
- 2 tbsp. Cool Whip™, light, 20 calories

AFTERWORD

Here are some closing thoughts from Jim Ray about the *Balanced Days, Balanced Lives* project and the NutriMirror experience. Also included is a sampling of affirmations from others who are also changing their behaviors to live healthier lives. These shared experiences provide hope for what Jim sees as a rapidly growing *person-to-person, one body at a time* movement that may help reverse the trend of obesity and chronic disease in our modern world.

Closing Thoughts

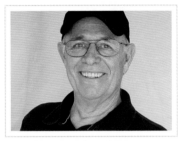

Balanced Days, Balanced Lives Co-Creator and NutriMirror® Co-Founder

My family (my sister Judy Johnston, my wife Pam, and our son Michael) did not set out with any thought to give the world a free, life-changing Internet website. And I certainly didn't know that approaching my seventieth year of life I would be a part of *Balanced Days, Balanced Lives*—a book project that is the launch point of a quiet mission to help reverse our national obesity and chronic disease trends.

My doctor told me in 2004 that because of life-threatening hypertension I needed to make some lasting changes. He told me I needed to lose weight by limiting my daily calories to 1,500, and to keep my sodium intake to no more than one teaspoon a day. I had no idea then that it would lead to the creation of NutriMirror and this book. I only knew that I wanted to live more than I wanted to die.

At the time, I reflected seriously upon thirty-plus years of failure at one diet program or the other. What had I learned? How was I going to manage my calorie balances to achieve and to maintain a healthy body weight? And, how was I ever going to measure a teaspoon of salt (and all the other key nutrients) in my diet? How was I going to get it right this time—and forever? All my questions were answered within months—and beyond my most fervent hopes—when my son, Michael, produced the first working model for what would, eventually, become the NutriMirror.com website.

For more than three years, Michael continued to refine the features of NutriMirror until I was able to log and assess the impacts of all my choices in less than five minutes each day—making it practical for my daily, lifelong use. I have logged every bite of food I've eaten and every step of exercise I've performed for more than six years. I own the behaviors that determine my continuing good health.

In February of 2008, our family decided to release NutriMirror to the public at large—free to any Internet connected adult user. Then, in January of 2009, we opened a public journal room. Here, members could share their journeys to health and provide support to one another. It was only then that the wider impacts of what Michael had created were fully known to us. Not a day goes by without members sharing their personal stories of transformation and expressing their gratitude to us—sometimes in very emotional and moving terms. My personal experience, it seems, was being replicated by ever growing numbers of people throughout the Internet world.

Helping to heal a nation—person-to-person, one body at a time

Each day, members ask us what they might do to repay the free gift of NutriMirror that they have received. Our answer is always the same: *Pay the favor of a free NutriMirror forward by reaching out to others who may be influenced by your good example.* And maybe, together, we can help reverse the prevalent trend of obesity and chronic disease in our nation.

This book helps our members and others extend their outreach. It connects the values of the Eight Guiding Truths at the heart of the NutriMirror experience to others within each of our personal spheres of influence: health care professionals to patients; business owners to employees; non-profit organizations to members; wives to husbands; parents to children; friends to friends; personal trainers to clients; coaches and athletic trainers to athletes; governments to citizens; stores and services to patrons.

I believe that success breeds success. When enough of our nation's people have taken ownership of their behaviors and discover the sustainable pleasure that is so possible in the choices that produce calorie balance and nutritional balance, we will begin to see a reversal of obesity and chronic disease trends. This is the only way it will happen: person to person, one body at a time.

We see NutriMirror as an antidote to the commercal diet industry, and we therefore will never accept advertising on our site for products and services not compatible with the vision and mission at the heart of our *Eight Guiding Truths*. The free NutriMirror website exists because of sales generated by *Balanced Days, Balanced Lives* and other Health Reflection™ publications. We thank you—as do the thousands of members who are making lasting change in their lives—for your purchases and your suppport.

To those readers who may decide to join the NuriMirror.com family, I welcome you with this simple admonition and instruction: Live Green!

Affirmations

Here are some of the affirmations we have received from among thousands of unsolicited member comments that illuminate the NutriMirror experience. We call them affirmations because they affirm the *Eight Guiding Truths* that are at the heart of NutriMirror and this pursuit of better health that we all share—whether or not we ever use the Internet to monitor our food and exercise choices.

"This is not a diet. Diets suck. They make you fat. This ingenious absolutely free site is a tool that helps you learn what you need to know about food and about yourself so that you can make the important decisions that will save your life. I found this site in August of 2008 and have lost 105 pounds ... slow and smart. I have no reason to think those pounds will be back, since I didn't lose them using a gimmick or depriving myself. Sure, I feel wonderful now that I'm lighter, but I felt great immediately upon taking control of my eating. My life had changed by week two. The changes were taking place in my understanding of nutrition and therefore I was able to renovate my relationship with food. If you're tired of the diet industry making money off your poor health and then making it even worse, check out NutriMirror. It's the real deal."

. . . .

"I've been a member of NutriMirror since July 2009. I have lost sixty-five pounds, more than my original goal! I have been maintaining my weight loss since 1/1/10. Before NutriMirror, I had no idea what eating healthy even meant. Now I have the tool I need to make sure I am in balance ... The site is pure genius and I could not be happier for the miracle that brought NutriMirror into my life!"

. . . .

"I joined in Sept 2009 after decades of dieting. I have learned that the key to a healthy weight lies in meeting your bodies nutritional needs, and NutriMirror is just the tool to make that happen. Thanks to this site and its many users, I am finally learning to cook healthy, nutritious meals that my whole family enjoys. I have lost twenty-two pounds so far and feel better than I have in years."

"This site is the best of the best. Never, ever, ever have I succeeded with getting healthy (especially getting to a healthy weight) as I have with this site. I'm in better shape now, at sixty, than I've been since I was thirty. Unbelievably accurate, insightful, supportive, encouraging, and free! Love it!"

"I absolutely love the power and insight that NutriMirror gives me. I know I can take control of my diet and lose weight if I need to; I also have confidence that I can maintain the loss long-term. I believe the user community of NutriMirror is at least fifty percent responsible for my success … NutriMirror ROCKS!"

"I have tried many different ways to lose weight and this is the only one that I feel good about. I know I am balanced, I know that I am getting enough to eat, and I know I am healthy. I dont recommend any other but NutriMirror. I am very happy to be part of NutriMirror family and I will be for life."

"I joined NutriMirror on July 27, 2009. My doctor told me I had to lose sixty pounds. I have lost forty-three pounds without feeling like I am dieting. With NutriMirror it is not really dieting that you are doing. You are getting an education. Before NutriMirror I knew I was eating badly, I just didn't know how badly! Because of NutriMirror, I have lost more weight than ever on any diet, and I can honestly say that I can visualize myself going all the way down to my goal weight of 135ish. Never on any diet did I feel like I could be successful enough to ride it all the way out to goal weight. But because I am not deprived and can eat whatever I want, I can stick with this. NutriMirror has changed my life. I can't sing its praises loudly enough."

"NutriMirror is an amazing site. It is not about dieting, it is about eating in a healthy, satisfying way. The most important feature, in my opinion, is the amazingly positive and supportive people who use the site. I highly recommend you give this site a try!"

. . . .

"I think NutriMirror is mislabeled as a "diet." It is a tool for restructuring your life by bringing your healthy habits to the forefront and helping you avoid your weaker habits. … I've tried other programs before, and like this better than any of the others. It's something that I can use to keep calorie counts, nutrition information and a whole-picture look at my health in one place, all easily accessible. These guys have started a quiet revolution in weight management through sane, controlled eating with the goal on healthy choices to establish a lifelong pattern of new behavior. Just what the doctor ordered!"

. . . .

"NutriMirror is absolutely amazing. I found the site in March of 2009 because I had started to put on a little weight after years of being able to eat whatever I wanted. I was hooked immediately. Those extra few pounds fell off within weeks, and I have been able to keep them off. NutriMirror is not a diet or any kind of "out there" fad that makes you deprive yourself of anything. It is simply a tool that allows you to see exactly what you eat—which foods give you the nutrition you need and which ones don't. It is a tool for self-empowerment that puts your health under your total control and helps you to be able to live well in a balanced way so that you can still eat the foods you love. The journal room is filled with supportive and loving people who are eager to see one another thrive and there is a wealth of information being shared. It's an amazing place, run by amazing people who genuinely care for the members, and when you have people like that in charge—people who sincerely want to see others reach their full potential—there is nothing that can't be done."

"I have lost fifty-five pounds, however this has been far more than a weight loss journey. The number on the scale has become less important than physical and mental changes that have taken place in my life. With the help of NutriMirror and its members, I have become more aware of what I put in my body to fuel it … NutriMirror not only helps you lose weight, it changes lives."

. . . .

"I'm not interested in someone else's diet plan that restricts me in any way—what I want is the knowledge of how to fix the foods I already love in ways that balance my nutrition and health. This is what NutriMirror does for me. Too many people are looking for an easy fix to weight loss and health issues via a pill or a special menu that will do this or that … but that just keeps you dependent on external factors and sets you up for failure. NutriMirror is amazing and I plan to always be a part of it."

. . . .

"This is truly the one place I recommend for those who are seriously wanting to change their lifestyle … When you embark on this journey of proper nutrition, the extra pounds go away … I've lost thirty-one pounds so far just by understanding the right way to eat … Thanks to NutriMirror, I now believe that a slow approach to weight loss is so much better than an instantly gratifying extreme calorie deprival program that is short on loss and short on return … Nutrimirror is for the those who want the lifelong process."

. . . .

"I love NutriMirror! This awesome site has changed the way I relate to food forever, which means I will maintain my weight and give my body all the nutrients it needs, and I will be healthy and live to a ripe old age. Gone are the days of gaining/losing/gaining again. I can still have those days of eating a little too much, say, of the brownies my son "made" me bake, because I am totally conscious of what else has gone in my mouth for that day."

"As a NutriMirror user and healthy adult who has finally conquered the obesity struggle, I believe it would be hard to find any community anywhere that shows the success rates that NutriMirror does among regular users. Instead of stressing eating less and losing weight, the tool encourages balanced eating and improved health. The community support is second-to-none. The results of this winning combination are a whole bunch of happy, healthy, steadily shrinking (in a good way) people. I am down ninety pounds and while the momentum was all mine, the use of the tool is what made it all possible."

· ·

"A million thanks to this website and all those responsible for it! I have tried almost every diet published and was never to be successful in the long term. The NutriMirror system has finally provided me a tool to properly focus on what I am putting in my body, track my progress and make necessary adjustments to my behavior. I was 168 lbs in my early thirties and finally I have a vision of obtaining a healthy weight. You very well may have saved my life! Thank you."

· ·

"I've been using NutriMirror for just over a year now. I lost twenty-plus pounds, but more importantly, I've maintained that loss now for over six months. And the best part is that NutriMirror has given me the tools and knowledge to maintain this for the rest of my life. It's easy to use, it's free, and it's changed my life. It's given me such control over what I eat, and since my food intake is so much healthier now, it's lead me to a very good sense of well-being. I've never been happier."

· ·

"Thanks to this site I have completely changed the way I look at food. I have discovered new foods and have found a good balance between what I like to eat and what I should eat. More importantly, my cholesterol went down 33 points, my LDL by 24 points and my triglycerides by 14 points! It was proof that I am healthier and taking charge of my life."

"NutriMirror has helped me to change my relationship with food one bad habit at a time. Through the support and advice I get from fellow members and the feedback I get everyday from my own personal log, I have been able to break some pretty destructive dieting habits. I'm finally at a point where I don't diet and it is the healthiest I have been. I attribute this to the direct feedback I receive from my log and the loving community!"

"I lost 100% of my excess body weight and am keeping it off thanks to the eighteen months I have been using NutriMirror. Truly a miracle tool!"

"As a Physical Therapist I am constantly emphasizing the importance of balance (physical, nutritional, psychosocial, and emotional) to have a healthy life. This site allows folks to see how all these parameters fit together. I've told many of my patients and colleagues about this site and I hope they take advantage of it—they'd be foolish not to! Bravo to you for making this available."

"I've lost forty-two pounds, and gained a world of knowledge of what my eating habits were doing to me, both nutritionally and physically. I would recommend NutriMirror to anyone. It's not just for those who'd like to lose weight. But if you do have some weight you'd like to lose, this is the place to start."

"I have always had great success losing weight with Weight Watchers … and tremendous success at putting that weight right back on again. What's so great this time around is that I am focusing on my whole health. NutriMirror has shown me the obvious. Thank you so, so much!"

"I am a physical therapist and I love this site and that it lets you look at nutrients, not just calories and fat grams. The graphs are so easy to read. Thanks so much!"

"My husband and I have both done Weight Watchers, however I love, love, love NutriMirror better because you are able to see your total nutritional intake, not just how many points you have for the day."

. . . .

"I found this site quite by accident. But now that I have, I plan on staying for a long time. This site makes it all so easy. You have it all in front of you in green and red. Thank you for keeping this site free!"

. . . .

"I started using NutriMirror in July of '09. I started because I was having health issues and hoped that keeping track of my food intake would help me figure it out. Thanks to NutriMirror, the issues (which had sent me to the E.R. four times in the previous twelve months) are completely under control. Also, I've shed thirty pounds. For the first time in my life, I feel in control of food. It doesn't happen overnight, but if you use the tool and turn to the journal room for support, your health will benefit more than you would expect."

. . . .

"I started using NutriMirror just to make myself aware of what I was putting in my mouth. I am short and have struggled with my weight all my life. I always exercise and thought I was eating right. I was convinced all I needed was portion control. Once I started logging my foods it made me aware. I have a tendency towards emotional eating and not paying attention to what goes in my mouth. When you log your foods you include EVERY LITTLE BITE. That was the clue for me. From June to December I went from a size almost 14 to a size 6–8. I even lost a little weight during the holidays. I am confident that I will be able to keep it off because I have to be accountable to myself. The key is to be aware so that you can make good choices."

"This website is amazing! I started using it in January and I have already lost weight and inches and I eat so much better! There is unbelievable support here as well!"

"Since joining, I have lost forty-five pounds (five more to go). What I look forward to most is using the site to help create a healthy lifestyle to maintain. Taking control of your life … that is what this site is all about. Keep up the great work!"

"I just wanted to say I love NutriMirror. It has changed my life in a big way. I couldn't have lost the weight I have lost so far without it. I love how it tells me everything that goes in my body from vitamins to fiber and cholesterol, not only calories. And I love that I can keep track of my exercise and find out how many calories I'm really burning. I really love that the site is this amazing, and it's free!"

"I never knew that being all green could be so exciting! I made it! For the first time I'm all green! I struggled with it every day and today I played around with my menu and I did it! About thirty minutes ago I was under only in fiber by three percent. So, I added twenty peanuts and there I went! ALL GREEN! This site is the best tool I've ever come across. I have faith that I will stay healthy and continue to lose weight with NutriMirror. I love all the people on here too. What a great thing this NutriMirror is!"
"NutriMirror has made becoming a healthier person easier and I plan on making it a part of my every day life forever so that when I do reach my goal I never slip back into bad habits."

"NutriMirror has helped me lose one hundred pounds and to maintain that loss. I really don't believe that would have been possible without this website. Thank you again."

"The people on this site are supportive, engaging, funny, interesting, and quite knowledgeable. I have noticed that no matter what your question, or what you are struggling with, someone else has been there and can help you get through. I have found NutriMirror to be the most helpful weight loss program I've ever tried. In less than five weeks I have lost thirteen pounds, and I feel better than I have ever felt in my life. It's all about health here with weight loss as a great side effect."

"My jeans are too big! I am so happy, today I put on a pair of jeans that were too tight when I bought them and now I have been walking around all morning pulling them up! Also, yesterday someone told me I looked like I had lost weight and asked me what my secret was—NutriMirror!"

"I married my husband in 1995. A year later I noticed that my ring was getting tight. Today for the first time I was able to put my ring on. I couldn't believe it. I kept sliding it on and off. My husband was tickled to death. We laughed and laughed. Just watching the sodium in my diet did the trick. I am soooo excited about the other things I can accomplish with this website as a tool to reach my goals."

"I know it sounds sappy but for the first time in my life I actually feel in charge instead of food being in charge! You guys will never know how much you have done for me!"

"It has been officially thirty days since I started using this site. Here is what has changed about me: I've lost 11 pounds and two inches around my waist/hips; I no longer have food on my mind ALL the time; I don't return to the fridge every time I am bored; I've learned my limits, and when to stop eating; I've learned how to make healthier choices; I haven't had ONE headache since I started (I used to get them every other day); I feel better physically and mentally. Thank you NutriMirror!"

"You will find that NutriMirror is a wonderful family of supportive people. There are people in all different stages of their journey so there is always someone able to guide and help you through their personal experiences. You won't believe all of the inspirational people here. This is a 'no fail' tool IF it is used properly. I say this because I played around for a few months with no success and just recently started really following the site, logging honestly, planning ahead, and fitting exercise in, and I am feeling so much better and am starting to see results. I can't wait to hear of your success too in the future. Welcome!"

"I am new here. I've been following Weight Watchers which became a game to see how much junk I could eat and stay in the 'points.' Cookies, crackers, ice-cream—I was 'allowed' to eat any of it. I just had to keep track of the points. I was eating, sure, but I wasn't eating well. With NutriMirror, I am compelled to watch the 'green.' It has completely changed the way I think. I've been looking at how every food compares nutritionally rather than what I think I can get away with."

"I am so in love with NutriMirror. I have not lost this much weight in over fifteen years. I am so excited. It is so easy to use this site. Thank you so much. I know I will reach my goal. It will take a bit longer than I wanted, but then we all seem to think it will drop off in mass amounts. Now I realize that is not the way to go. This really works and I am never hungry. I got my husband started yesterday and he really likes listing his food and exercise. Having his support is fantastic."

"This site is fantastic! NutriMirror will definitely help you lose weight. You will learn the nutritional value of your foods and the sodium value, too! The NutriMirror site is pretty easy and fun. If you need any help the members here are very helpful and encouraging! Welcome aboard, you'll make some great friends, too!"

"I used to 'cheat.' I would actually call it 'closet binging.' I would eat all kinds of bad things in secret and then eat normally when others were around. Then, when I started NutriMirror, I realized that I was only 'cheating' myself. I was not taking responsibility for what I was putting in my body, but I'm the only one who can be responsible for it. No one forced me to wolf down all those cookies, chocolates, ice cream, etc. Using NutriMirror has made me more accountable to myself and in the end, that's all that really matters."

. . . .

"I have consistently logged my food every day, save a vacation or two I took where it was not feasible. I have consistently worked towards green every day and have had a green homepage for almost a year now. And I have consistently exercised in some fashion nearly every day.

The benefits I have reaped from doing the above: 1. Lost 28 lbs with nary a plateau. 2. Lost virtually all of my cravings for sugar-laden treats. 3. Have no problem skipping the dessert/treat aisle at the store. 4. 'Forget' to eat my 100 cal dark chocolate bar that I bring to the movies. 5. Don't even think about going out to dessert after a wonderful sushi meal. 6. Enjoy the fact that I have lots and lots of fruits and veggies and healthy 'green' snacks in my house. 7. Love my healthy snack choices like they are dessert! 8. Enjoy meals out like I have never had a meal out before. 9. I no longer feel guilt or shame when I go red and eat French-fries and a half a cheeseburger or any other 'bad' food I choose.

Bottom line: I feel so good now I don't ever want to go back and since I have NutriMirror I don't ever have to. What I want you to hear is that if you use this tool consistently, work hard at tweaking your logs to get them green, and then just keep plodding away at it every day, you WILL get to where you want to go. You WILL get to your weight goal and you also WILL make permanent changes to your eating habits. You will have lasting success at being healthy and living a full and energetic life. I have no doubt about that because I am proof positive that NutriMirror works!"

"NutriMirror can be so much more than a food log if you choose it to be. Not only does it keep track of more than just calories, but there is a wonderful community that will support you along the way! Remember, go GREEN!"

"You will find NutriMirror members very supportive. The key is to not to think of this as a 'diet.' NutriMirror is a tool to help you make healthier food choices and to see where the improvements need to be and to reach your goals by staying in the green. I still enjoy my sweets and goodies, even ice cream as long as I log it and I stay in the green. Happy Logging."

"I will be dreaming GREEN tonight! FINALLY, I did it—an ALL GREEN day! I have been totally DANCING around my house tonight after logging in everything! Anyone wanna dance with me? Thanks, NutriMirror. You make this lifestyle change fun!"

"So many diets do not take in the whole picture. I am continually shocked at how many health marketed products are high in fat and sodium … Getting green on my macro and micro nutrients is one of the most fun things I have ever done!"

"I will never take my body or health for granted. Thank you God for blessing me with the ability to do the things I do and thank you NutriMirror for giving me the tools to utilize my body to its fullest potential."

"The cool thing about NutriMirror is that we are always 'rookies' learning new things from each other. I learn something new here daily. It's a fabulous resource!"

"This site is changing the way I look at food. Now I love to log in and I find that I am checking food labels and really enjoying it. In the past I would always check food labels and never had the tools to figure out how to add everything up. It was so difficult to keep a food journal. This site makes eating right so easy."

"I was exercising a lot and could not lose weight. I became so frustrated. Then I found NutriMirror and started 'seeing' what I was actually eating. It is no wonder I wasn't losing. Even though I was exercising I was still eating more than I was burning; what an eye opener. I also struggled with eating the right amount but now I really try to eat the amount set out to meet my weight loss goal. I may not be losing weight as fast as some of my co-workers who aren't using NutriMirror but I feel healthier and think that I am making real lifestyle changes. I have been focused on food and weight since I was fifteen years old and for the first time it is making sense to me!"

"Don't look for shortcuts—look for foods that you love that make your logs green! Once you get your home page green and keep it that way, and eat ALL of your allotted weight loss calories, weight loss happens automatically. I've been here five months and have lost forty-nine pounds, and haven't been hungry or deprived for one minute. NutriMirror is awesome!"

"Today is my four-month anniversary with NutriMirror. I am glad to still be here learning how to eat healthy and stay green! Since it's my four-month mark, I thought I'd give four things I have learned: 1. NutriMirror has a lot of wonderful people who are not only supportive but have lots of helpful suggestions. 2. Sodium is not your friend no matter what shape it comes in! 3. I CAN and have lost weight. So far it's 53 pounds! 4. NutriMirror is for life. Thanks to all of you for your support!

"I CAN eat cheese! This website has taught me many things, but one of the most important things I'm learning is that I don't need to eliminate things from my diet that are 'bad' … like cheese. As long as I'm watching my calories, and eating in moderation, I'm allowed to sprinkle a little cheese on my beans and rice. It's not going to make me gain a bunch of weight. I truly appreciate the accountability this site provides. Knowing how many calories I've eaten and how many are left for the day leads you into making smarter choices and shows you what you can get away with. Thanks, NutriMirror."

"Is it possible? I broke my 5k record today at 22:29. It has to be NutriMirror, because I haven't changed anything else. Thanks, NutriMirror!"

"Wow, I can't believe I've actually stuck with it and logged a food journal for one full month! And as of this morning I've lost eight of the twenty pounds that I set as my goal when I started. WHOOHOO! NutriMirror has been an awesome tool and you guys are great motivators. Thanks to all that share their stories, ideas, recipes, and food journals … Someone asked me tonight what diet I was doing to lose weight! I told her I wasn't dieting, I was doing NutriMirror. I can't wait to weigh myself (never thought I would be saying that) … I am officially obsessed with NutriMirror."

"I woke up this morning and had, for the first time in months, no swelling in my legs. Since my emergency surgery at the end of 2007 on my right thigh I have had swelling/water retention, especially in my right leg where four abscesses were removed. It may not last but even one morning with no swelling is great. I credit NutriMirror. The other thing NutriMirror is doing for me is allowing me to see exactly my intake and somehow that gives me the strength to make better choices or even stop eating for the day. Wow! Cravings have run my life for years and now they are greatly reduced. Thanks again for all your work, advice, and free NutriMirror."

"When I found NutriMirror I was just looking for a place to keep a journal for my dieting. But as you all know, I found much, much more than that! What I found is a powerful tool to help me change the way I eat for a lifetime. And I found an incredible community of fantastic people to help me on my new journey to a healthier and longer life. So a BIG thanks to you all for embracing me in my Battle of the Bulge! I feel empowered, invigorated, motivated, enthusiastic, and (this may sound weird) loved by a bunch of strangers who have taken me under their wings. I can't wait to be here long enough to give something back and to be able to help others in the ways that I have been helped.
I love you guys!"

. . . .

NutriMirror is guiding us to the key for lifetime weight control. It's an
Understanding that in our journey 'after' does not exist. We learn
The truth about balancing calories and nutrition. Finding pleasure
Reflected in choices that move us to balance. A slow approach
In weight loss is better and we are happy without deprivation.
Mindsets that daily help us choose food wisely and frequently leads to an
Improved state of well-being and a winning strategy. Learning that
Realistic physical activity is beneficial to our health and weight control. With
Results that are not perfect but allow us to forgive our lapses. Overcoming
Obstacles knowing that to manage performance, we must measure it. Old ways are
Rejected by the Eight Guiding Truths. Our success lasts a lifetime.

—Thank you from NYLatinJazz

Monica Callan, RD, Reviews *Balanced Days, Balanced Lives* and NutriMirror.com

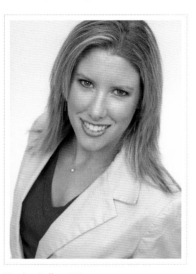

Monica Callan, RD.

Monica Callan is a Registered Dietitian and certified Personal Trainer specializing in weight management, heart health, and behavior change.

My name is Monica Callan, and I am a registered dietitian and personal trainer. I was raised by parents who took to an interest in healthy living in the 1970s. They role modeled good health through gardening, cooking fresh foods at home, daily family dinner, and plenty of fun physical activity. As a result, self-care comes naturally to me. The experiences of my youth, and the value system created by my parents, led me to my career path.

Some of my professional experience includes specializing in weight management, behavior change, and heart health. I have also developed personalized fitness routines, appeared on television as a nutrition expert, and I go into people's homes to declutter their kitchens. I am passionate about guiding people towards living their best life. I understand the process of behavior change well, the challenges that people face, and what gives people their best chance at successfully living a healthy lifestyle.

My connection to this book, its co-creator Jim Ray, and NutriMirror.com has been an interesting journey. Jim hired me to sit down with him and listen to his ideas about an online nutrition and fitness logging system that his son, Michael, was creating to help Jim manage his weight loss and hypertension. He asked that I complete a write-up determining if I thought his ideas were viable and needed for the marketplace. In summary, my bottom line was that there wasn't a need for another online tool of this kind. I thought there were enough already available.

About six months later, he contacted me again, letting me know he had gone ahead with his ideas despite my feedback, and asked me to review the website he and Michael had developed. I was so profoundly impressed with what I saw. I hadn't grasped the scope of what he was trying to describe, and hadn't realized just how unique his program would be. When I expressed how great I thought NutriMirror.com had turned out, he said something that I will never forget. "When I expressed my vision to you, and you said you didn't think it was a good idea, I felt like I had shown you a photo of my grandchild, and you said he was ugly!"

So, I have served as a consultant to Jim throughout the entire process, watching the vision grow, with life-changing results for the many thousands of people who have taken advantage of the NutriMirror.com tool.

This book is an offshoot of that website. However, this book is of standalone benefit even if the reader never visits the website. It is so unique, because the forty-two contributors all draw from real experiences, sharing the choices that have made them successful. They give the reader real-life food options, not some impersonally created generic menus. Individual contributors describe the daily choices that have helped them succeed at mastering the challenges of what to eat and how to exercise when striving for nutritional balance and weight control. Here you find real people, real food, real stories, and real success!

The stories speak to experiences that I've seen throughout years of my practice. The *Eight Guiding Truths* are the behavioral essence of what I as a health professional want people to understand. Unfortunately, I have not seen many who have grasped these concepts and actually put them into practice on a lifelong basis. Most people try to bypass these truths with shortcuts. But always they end up circling back to old behaviors, feelings of failure, and frustration. What is marketed as a shortcut to health is usually a long detour heading back to the wrong direction.

In general, people are so confused and misdirected when it comes to weight control and nutritional balance. This book, and the NutriMirror.com tool, start people at the top of the hierarchy of skill levels—self-management. The goal of every program should be to create independent problem solvers. With these two resources, you have what you need to be your own creative problem solver from the very beginning. You are equipped to go to work on the most important possession you own, your body.

Congratulations for embarking on this journey. You're on your way to living your best life.